# CHIROPRACTIC SPINOGRAPHY

## A Manual of Technology and Interpretation

SECOND EDITION

# CHIROPRACTIC SPINOGRAPHY

## A Manual of Technology and Interpretation

**SECOND EDITION**

**Roy W. Hildebrandt,** D.C., D.A.C.B.R. (Hon.)

*Professor, Division of Clinical Sciences*
*National College of Chiropractic*
*Lombard, Illinois*

*formerly Associate Professor and Chairman*
*Department of Roentgenology*
*Palmer College of Chiropractic*
*Davenport, Iowa.*

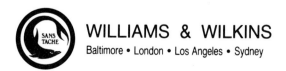

**WILLIAMS & WILKINS**
Baltimore • London • Los Angeles • Sydney

*Editor:* Jonathan W. Pine, Jr.
*Associate Editor:* Carol Eckhart
*Copy Editor:* Caral Shields Nolley
*Design:* Bert Smith
*Illustration Planning:* Joe Cummings
*Production:* Raymond E. Reter

*Printed in the United States of America*

First Edition 1977

**Library of Congress Cataloging in Publication Data**

Hildebrandt, Roy W.
   Chiropractic spinography.

   Includes bibliographies and index.
   1. Radiography in chiropractic. 2. Spine—Radiography.
I. Title. [DNLM: 1. Chiropractic. 2. Spine—radiography.
WE 725 H642c]
RZ251.R33H55 1985        616.7'307572        84-23704
ISBN 0-683-04002-2

Composed and printed at the
Waverly Press, Inc.

85  86  87  88  89
10  9  8  7  6  5  4  3  2  1

"No man of science could subscribe to all of Galileo's beliefs, or to all of Newton's beliefs, or to all of his own beliefs of ten years ago."

W. I. B. BEVERIDGE

# Preface

The primary motivation for writing a book is that a need is perceived to exist for it. In attempting to define the need for this particular book it was pointed out in the Preface to the First Edition that *spinography*, as an innovative new approach to the radiological examination of the spinal column for evidence of biomechanical irregularities, was originated by the chiropractic profession in 1910; that over the intervening years the profession developed a wide array of specialized x-ray equipment and procedures which could be considered worthwhile original contributions to x-ray science and art; that it was taught in some form in every chiropractic college; and that it was being used to some extent as a helpful clinical tool by nearly every doctor of chiropractic (as well as some medical and osteopathic physicians) around the world.

However, it was also pointed out that no organized, relatively comprehensive text on the subject existed, which was considered regrettable for three principal reasons; *first*, it was considered regrettable because original knowledge was in danger of being lost to history; *second*, it was considered regrettable because no standardized teaching and reference text on the subject was available; and *third*, it was considered regrettable because the related knowledge was not compiled in such a form as to allow for its critical review by the scientific community at large.

Consequently, the need for such a book was reasonably well established and the first edition, as a *beginning effort* to found a repository for related knowledge as a whole and to provide a much-needed instructional text of basic concepts and methodologies, was compiled: (*a*) by attempting to gather together some of the more reliable knowledge which had evolved over the years (from both within and outside the chiropractic profession); and (*b*) by putting forth some added innovations developed by the author as a result of more than 30 years of study, research and teaching of the subject. The hope was that this book, in addition to serving its tangible purpose as a basic text and reference manual, would also serve the somewhat intangible purpose of illustrating that chiropractic spinography, rather than being an illegitimate offspring of accepted medical radiology, is a logical, clinically useful, *respectable* roentgenological specialty in its own right. However, as far as the first edition itself was concerned, two points were made which are still applicable to this new volume:

1. The information presented which may be peculiar to basic chiropractic concepts is in no way considered absolute, either as it may concern the ideas of the author or the ideas of others from whom the author may have drawn information; to state or imply otherwise would be presumptuous since, to this time, chiropractic spinography has been somewhat provincial and has not had the benefit of adequate critical review by the scientific community at large
2. Although this compilation purports to be a relatively comprehensive treatise on chiropractic spinography, it is not to be considered the totality of the subject as a whole; it is essentially a *core text* of basic knowledge which must be supplemented by other related writings (including various general radiological texts and proprietary spinographic system manuals) for a more complete understanding

At this time of reflection on that first edition, it is gratifying to be aware that it has reasonably well fulfilled its purpose and objectives; it has been recognized within the chiropractic profession as the primary repository of related knowledge, it has been accepted as a core text on the subject by a number of chiropractic colleges, and it has served as a means of communicating such chiropractic knowledge to the scientific community at large for critical review. Above all, perhaps, it has been accepted by membership of the profession's academic community as a good start toward bringing some degree of order and reason into an otherwise respectable roentgenological procedure which was sinking into a quagmire of individual entrepreneurial systems of application.

The privilege of preparing this second edition is accompanied by the opportunity to supplement, revise, expand and, to some extent, condense the material previously presented. All chapters have undergone re-working, some have undergone major revisions, and new ones have been added. It is hoped that these revisions and additions will be well received.

Chapter 1 has been extensively revised to affect a more informational introduction to the subject of chiropractic spinography as a whole. The major parts of the previous Chapter 1 discussion of spinal biomechanics (including the historical review of basic chiropractic theory) have been moved to those chapters to which they more logically apply. Reference support for Chapter 1 has been extensively augmented. Of particular note in Chapter 1 is the addition of a *statement of purpose and objectives* of chiropractic spinography which attempts to spell out the parameters of this procedure in terms

of general consensus within the chiropractic profession (particularly its academic community); a perogative that has in the past been left to the advocates of various and sundry entrepreneurial systems of spinographic analysis procedure.

Chapter 2 on *X-Ray Physics and Radiological Technology* and Chapter 3 on *Radiation Health Physics and Protection* have been added to this second edition so that the volume can be used more completely as a *primary* core text. However, the material presented should be regarded as the minimal basic knowledge necessary to introduce the student (those in assistantship as well as doctoral programs) to the rudiments of safe and effective x-ray technology procedure. As in the case of most other topics in this book, supplementary reading from other more comprehensive texts on these subjects is recommended; the extent of such supplementary reading being determined by the objectives of the particular academic program in question—technologist, general practice doctoral, or postgraduate specialty.

All other chapters have been significantly upgraded and the volume has been divided into three distinct parts to facilitate its use in related, but perhaps separated, academic courses of study. Additionally, the Appendix has been augmented with a review of the *Systems Internationale* (SI) metric measurement procedures and an updated Glossary.

In conclusion, it is to be emphasized that this book is not now, nor conceivably will it ever be, complete. Criticisms, suggestions and contributions aimed at improvement of future editions are sincerely welcomed.

ROY W. HILDEBRANDT, D.C.

# Acknowledgments

It is with sincere gratitude that I extend recognition to those pioneers in the chiropractic profession—both past and present—who have in some manner contributed to development of the body of knowledge on which this book is heavily based.

Gratitude is also extended to those of the chiropractic academic community who have encouraged and supported my efforts in the field of chiropractic spinography over the past two decades, to the officers and members of the American Chiropractic College of Roentgenology who have honored me for my efforts, and to my students of years gone by who made my efforts worthwhile.

Finally, I extend my appreciation to Williams & Wilkins for their encouragement to complete this new volume, for their interim patience, and for their expert assistance in preparation for publication.

R. W. H.

# Contents

## Part 3
## PRINCIPLES OF SPINOGRAPHIC INTERPRETATION

# CHAPTER 1

# Introduction to Chiropractic Spinography

## PURPOSE AND OBJECTIVES

Chiropractic spinography is a roentgenological diagnosis procedure which utilizes postural (weight-bearing) x-ray views for the principal purpose of examining the spinal column and pelvis for evidence of clinically-significant biomechanical irregularities. Specific consideration is given to the identification and evaluation of *spinal curvatures* (scolioses, kyphoses and lordoses) which may compromise efficient body mechanics as a whole and/or vertebral orthodysarthrias (the biomechanical element of the chiropractic vertebral subluxation syndrome) which may compromise efficient function of individual "vertebral motor units;" i.e. the biomechanical interrelationship of two contiguous vertebrae.

The primary objectives of chiropractic postural spinography interpretation procedure are: (*a*) to confirm preliminary non-roentgenological evaluations (case history, physical examination, etc.) which may have suggested the presence of clinically significant biomechanical irregularities; (*b*) to assess their nature and possible effects on normal body function; and (*c*) to determine the probable cause for their development, and their treatment or referral requirements.

Inherent within these objectives of chiropractic postural spinography interpretation procedure is the understanding that, as in all other diagnostic roentgenology procedures, the ultimate goal is to seek out all possible information that may have value to the accurate diagnosis and effec-

tive treatment of a patient's health problem, including pathologic, morphologic and/or traumatic disorders which may have a contributing effect on the development (or aggravation) of biomechanical irregularities of the spinal column and pelvis, in addition to their possible significance as specific health problems in themselves.

In consideration for the need to hold patient x-ray exposure to a minimum, while obtaining the greatest amount of useful information to assist in the accurate diagnosis and effective treatment of a patient's health problem, the *chiropractic application* of postural spinography procedure (when such procedure is indicated) considers the standard weight-bearing veiws (anteroposterior and lateral full spine, and supplemental postural—standing or sitting—views) to be the *primary* roentgenological procedure. In these cases, all other views (for specific confirmation of pathology, trauma or abnormal development) are then considered the *secondary* roentgenological procedure. In effect, this protocol considers the postural spinographic views to be *diagnostic films* with the *added dimension* of providing information of a biomechanical nature which is not provided by standard diagnostic films, whether taken in the reclining or upright positions.

However, it is to be *emphasized* that under no circumstances do postural x-rays supplant the need for indicated specific views for the diagnosis of pathology, trauma or abnormal development as "primary" views when the need for such is

1

identified at the time of initial examination, or at any later period.

## CLINICAL SIGNIFICANCE OF SPINAL BIOMECHANICAL IRREGULARITIES

Biomechanical irregularities of the spinal column are accepted today as serious health problems which are estimated to afflict a large percentage of the population (1). The following, paraphrased from a presentation on *Body Mechanics* by John G. Kuhns, M.D., provides a good overview (2):

> For good health and efficient function, the body must be used in good balance and alignment with no strain or excessive activity in any part... In dealing with faulty body mechanics, we strive to improve the function of various organs by taking away excessive loads from the various systems of the body. In this way, we can usually avoid irreversible changes in structure and serious faults in function before nature's powers of adaptation have been broken. Correcting bad body mechanics is of great value in improvement or recovery from many chronic diseases...
>
> "It has been found that 80% of the children and young adults in this country have detectable postural deformities and varying degrees of faulty body mechanics... In childhood, faulty mechanics and its accompanying deformities develop insidiously. If these continue throughout the growing years, fixed deformities can result, as well as less efficient function of the body with impaired health in later life. These deformities do not disappear spontaneously, but slowly become worse. Their correction is a serious problem in later life. With age, the milder faults in body mechanics, which were compensated for in youth, cause more serious symptoms and increasing deformities. Osteoarthritis develops about the joints and is often accompanied by muscular spasms and pain caused by irritation of spinal nerve roots.
>
> "A large share of patients with faulty body mechanics will be found constitutionally inadequate in all their tissues... All of the internal organs are attached directly or indirectly to the skeleton and, with displacements of the skeleton, the organs are displaced and their nerve and blood supply become pressed or stretched... In general, the symptoms which arise from faulty body mechanics can be grouped into five headings: (*a*) fatigue, (*b*) sprains, (*c*) deformity, (*d*) traumatic arthritis, and (*e*) visceral disturbances." [From Kuhns JG: Body mechanics. *The Cyclopedia of Medicine, Surgery and the Specialties.* Philadelphia, FA Davis Co., 1974, vol 2, pp 347–358 (2).]

The deleterious effects of poor body mechanics resulting from spinal curvatures, including acute visceral disturbances and chronic degenerative joint disease, (Fig. 1.1, 1.2) are well accepted by the clinical community at large today, and need for early diagnosis and treatment is emphasized (2–7). Additionally, since 1895 the chiropractic profession has postulated a far-reaching theory that minute biomechanical aberrations of the spinal column (interarticular orthodysarthrias) may physically affect closely related nervous tissue (the neurological element of the chiropractic subluxation syndrome) in such a manner as to set up viscerosomatic-somatovisceral reflexes which may result in the development of pathophysiological processes anywhere in the body (Fig. 1.3) (8–11). Although this theory has not as yet been scientifically substantiated, considerable support is given to it today by the scientific community (12–31), and research is presently an ongoing process within and outside the chiropractic profession (Fig. 1.4) (32, 33).

## BASIS OF X-RAY EXAMINATIONS

In view of requirements to properly establish justification for all diagnostic x-ray procedure in accordance with clinical need, it was well established in the preceding discussion that spinal biomechanical irregularities can have serious adverse effects on the human body (even without consideration of the chiropractic subluxation syndrome) and do justify their examination by roentgenological means. However, the decision to x-ray a particular patient is not automatic, but requires careful and detailed evaluation of each individual case; the final decision being made on the basis of *professional judgment* on the part of the attending doctor. Although such judgments are not always a clear-cut decision, the following

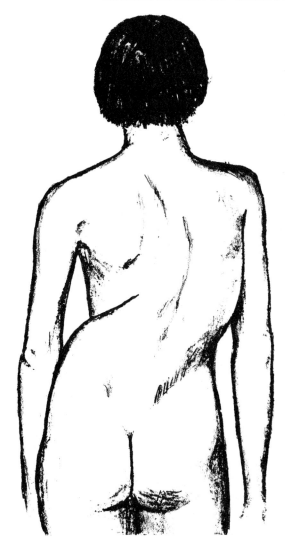
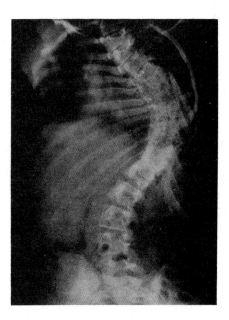

**Figure 1.1.** Idiopathic scoliosis. This severe type of spinal curvature usually begins about the age of 9 to 10 and often progresses insidiously until puberty, at which time it can reach a severe stage which is life threatening to the individual. Extreme thoracic curvature often shortens the torso and raises the diaphragm to the point where cardiorespiratory function is impaired. Surgery may be required at this stage to improve the patients general wellbeing.

ascending steps are generally followed in reaching a considered opinion:

1. The doctor should first determine that a health problem exists (or potentially exists) which requires diagnostic evaluation; such determination being based on a preliminary case history and consultation.
2. The doctor should secondly determine whether or not the health problem evident (or suspected) requires x-ray evaluation; such determination being based on physical examination, orthopedic and neurological examination, palpatory and postural examination, etc.
3. The doctor should thirdly determine that the anticipated radiation dose to the patient (and fetus in the case of pregnancy) from x-ray exposure (if conducted) will not constitute an iatrogenic hazard out of proportion to the anticipated diagnostic benefits to the patient.
4. The doctor should finally determine that the particular type of roentgenological examination selected as the procedure of choice will provide the greatest amount of

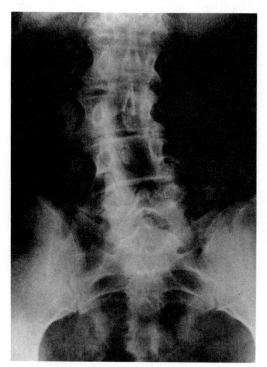

**Figure 1.2.** Chronic spinal degenerative joint disease of the lumbar and sacroiliac articulations. It may be logically hypothesized that such conditions may result after longstanding existence of interarticular microtraumatic orthodysarthrias.

useful information to aid in the accurate diagnosis and effective management of the patient's health problem, with the least amount of radiation exposure required consistent with the desired technical results; i.e. that the diagnostic quality of the films justify their being taken in the first place.

In consideration of the concern for radiation exposure in diagnostic x-ray procedure, it is recognized that all such procedures constitute some degree of risk. However, when properly considered and conducted the risk is minimal, and justifiable in terms of value to the patient.

While it is important that all x-ray exposure to the patient be kept as low as possible consistent with the desired roentgenological objective, caution must also be exercised that one does not overreact to the extent that such procedures are not used when there is a reasonable justification of need. As a matter of perspective in this

issue of radiation exposure in diagnostic roentgenology, the following from *X-Ray Examination—A Guide to Good Practice*, issued by the *American College of Radiology* in cooperation with the *Bureau of Radiological Health* of the *US Department of Health, Education, and Welfare* (USDHEW), (34) is of value:

1. In almost every medical situation, when the physician feels there is a reasonable expectation of obtaining useful information from roentgenological examination that would affect the care of the individual, potential radiation hazard is not the primary consideration.
2. In diagnostic roentgenology, the goal is to obtain the desired information using the smallest amount of radiation that is practical.
3. Emphasis should be given to the technical means (collimators, gonadal shielding, etc.) by which radiation dose can be reduced without impairment of the medical value of the procedure.
4. Each physician should give due consideration to the potential somatic consequences of radiation exposure to the pa-

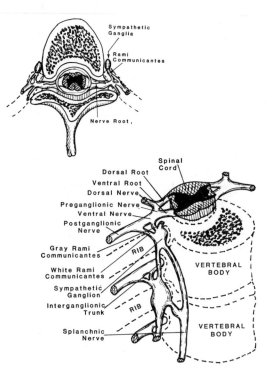

**Figure 1.3.** Neurological elements which may be compromised at the site of a spinal interarticular orthodysarthria.

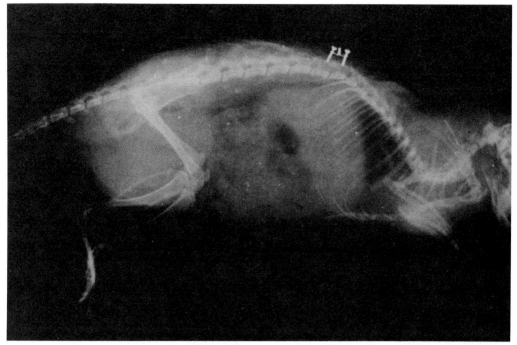

**Figure 1.4.** Experimental induction of vertebral orthodysarthrias in a laboratory animal.

tient, and to the genetic effects upon mankind as part of his or her responsibility to public health.

5. The physician should retain complete freedom of judgment in the selection of roentgenographic procedures, and should conform with good technical practices.

## RATIONALE FOR CHIROPRACTIC POSTURAL ROENTGENOLOGY

It has been confirmed that biomechanical irregularities of the spinal column and pelvis do constitute significant health problems and that roentgenological examination is an important means of evaluating these problems in terms of their diagnosis and treatment. However, the question now arises as to how such roentgenological evaluations are best performed—by using postural (weight-bearing) or reclining techniques, or full spine or sectional exposure procedure. Although there has been some difference of opinion within the chiropractic profession regarding these questions, the predominant opinion is that a single full spine (especially the anteroposterior

view) exposure in the standing, weight-bearing attitude is most desirable (35–39).

The use of such postural full spine roentgenographs for the evaluation of biomechanical disorders has, of course, been utilized to the greatest extent within the chiropractic profession. However, in recent times such procedures have also been recommended by members of the medical profession as the most efficient means of evaluating spinal scolioses. In this regard, the following quotes bring out several significant points (40–42):

"In scoliosis, the axial skeleton (spine and sacrum) is involved in lateral deviation and rotation. Therefore, a film visualizing the entire axial skeleton is necessary. The 36-in anteroposterior (AP) standing film (taken at a distance of 72 in) is an excellent answer to this need. On such an x-ray picture the involved spinal anatomy can be seen as one unit. The AP view is recommended, since it provides the most clinical information relative to lateral deviation and rotation of the vertebrae. The 36-in standing spine film shows all curves and their relationship to one another while the spine is being subjected to the normal gravitational forces. This size roentgenogram also includes the sacrum and shows the iliac apophyses, which is useful in evaluating the completion of spinal growth. [From Hoppenfeld S: *Scoliosis: A Manual of Concepts and Treatment.* Philadelphia, Lippincott, 1967, pp 50–51 (40).]

"Generally, it is wise to obtain a scoliosis series of x-rays on a new patient. This should include erect anteroposterior and lateral views of the spine from the occiput to the sacrum. An AP 14 × 36-in cassette is useful in larger children and adults." [From Keim HA: *Scoliosis: Ciba Clinical Symposia,* Summit, NJ, Ciba Pharmaceutical, 1972, pp 22–44 (47).]

"Ultimately, accurate diagnosis of type, location, extent, apex and exact measurement of the curves requires accurate x-ray evaluation of the erect spine. Routine x-rays on a 14 × 17-in film, which is a standard diagnostic film taken of the prone patient, does not give full evaluation. Nor are these views standardized, so films from various clinics or various countries cannot be compared. Also, failure to include the pelvis in the x-ray does not reveal the level of obliquity of the sacral base or the remaining growth evaluation of the iliac apophyses. Without an upright view, the effect of gravity upon the scoliosis is not observable. It is now standardized internationally that x-rays be taken on a 36-in film with the anode at a distance of 72 in." [From Cailliet R: *Scoliosis: Diagnosis and Management.* Philadelphia, FA Davis Co., 1975, pp 52–54 (42).]

To summarize the basis for the use of postural full spine films in the evaluation of biomechanical irregularities of the spinal column and pelvis, the following points are emphasized:

1. The human body is structurally designed to function most efficiently in the upright—bipedal—postural attitude, and biomechanical disorders within its musculoskeletal system (particularly the spinal column and pelvis) are most significantly illustrated when examined under weight-bearing conditions which take into account the effects of stress on the articulations and the efficiency of neuromuscular control of body posture.
2. The human spinal column (including its pelvic support mechanism) is structurally designed to function as a complete axial organ unit in which biomechanical events in any one area are mechanically and neuromuscularly transmitted throughout the entire structure and, therefore, continuity of biomechanical impressions are only observable when the spinal column and pelvis are x-rayed in their entirety at a given point in time.

Consequently, there is good reason for the justification of postural spinography procedure wherein the spinal column and its pelvic support mechanism are x-rayed (particularly in the sagittal-anteroposterior plane) in their entirety at a given point in time, under weight-bearing conditions, when the objective is to make a biomechanical evaluation. However, in some cases it is understood that sectional views (taken in the standing, sitting, or reclining positions) may be necessary to supplement the full spine views, or replace them when technical conditions disallow them; i.e. in those cases where the patient is excessively obese, unable to stand without support, etc.

## QUALIFICATIONS OF CHIROPRACTIC POSTURAL SPINOGRAPHY

Since its first use in 1933, (43) chiropractic full spine postural roentgenology has evoked cosiderable controversy regarding certain qualifications which some within and outside the chiropractic profession have considered good reason(s) to limit or disallow its use. These qualifications, or criticisms, primarily relate to: (*a*) difficulties in obtaining films of adequate quality to allow for a reasonably complete diagnosis—pathological as well as biomechanical; (*b*) alleged excessive radiation exposure to the patient as compared to what they would receive if the same spine area was x-rayed by three separate sectional exposures; and (*c*) increased radiographic distortion which is thought by some to prevent accurate evaluation (particularly by measurement) of spinal structural configurations.

Because of the potential seriousness of these criticisms, it is important that they be adequately considered in terms of their reality.

### Quality Control Considerations

Postural full spine procedure, admittedly, does present some difficulties in the aspect of radiographic image quality control. These difficulties for the most part relate to (a) the often extreme variations in body thickness and/or density; (b) the mass of the body; and (c) the instability of the standing patient. Each of these are considered as follows:

## VARIATIONS IN BODY THICKNESS AND/OR DENSITY

The often extreme variations in body thickness and/or density can result in unacceptable variations in film exposure if not adequately controlled—the thicker and/or more dense areas of the body can result in excessively light (under exposed) areas on the film, and the thinner and/or less dense areas of the body can result in excessively dark (over exposed) areas on the film. In a small number of cases this problem may not be sufficiently preventable, however, in the majority of cases the exposure can be adequately controlled by the use of available technical means; such as, compensating filters to reduce the amount of exposure to the thinner or less dense areas of the body, high kilovoltage technics to more evenly penetrate the body, etc.

## MASS OF THE BODY

The mass of the complete body torso can result in the production of large amounts of *secondary radiation* emissions, or *scatter* of primary x-rays, which can result in "fogging" of the film to the extent that the image quality is materially reduced. However, as in the case of variations in body thickness and/or density, technical means are available by which this film fogging can be adequately controlled; such as, by the use of primary x-ray beam collimation, radiographic grids, etc.

## INSTABILITY OF THE STANDING PATIENT

The instability of the standing patient (as compared to the stability of a reclining one) can result in excessive *blurring* of the film image due to motion during the expo-

sure, in much the same manner as it occurs in photography. Although such motion is much more difficult to control than with a reclining patient, technical means are available by which such motion blurring of the film image may be adequately controlled; such as, by the use of immobilization equipment, use of very short (high speed) exposures, etc.

Consequently, although it is more difficult than in sectional and/or reclining x-ray procedures, good quality postural full spine films can be produced by diligent attention to all related technical factors (which will be discussed in greater detail in the chapters on radiographic and spinographic technology).

In the case of small- to medium-sized individuals, postural full spine films can be produced with diagnostic quality that is almost indistinguishable from sectional and/or reclining views. In the case of medium- to large-sized individuals, films can be produced that illustrate reasonably good diagnostic quality, although some areas may be marginal in the larger individuals. In the case of large to obese individuals, consideration may need to be given to postural sectional views. In the case of very obese individuals, it may not be possible to take x-rays of some spinal areas with the patient in the standing position. Nevertheless, with proper x-ray equipment and rigid attention to all related technical details, 80–90% of the cases should present no insurmountable problems (Fig. 1.5).

## Radiation Exposure Considerations

The contention that full spine roentgenography exposes the patient to greater amounts of radiation than when the same full spine areas are exposed in sectional procedures is without basis in fact. Actually, when properly produced, full spine roentgenographs expose the patient to less radiation than standard sectional views. This reduction of radiation in full spine procedure is accomplished by three basic factors: (a) the *longer focal-film* distance (FFD) used in full spine procedure (72

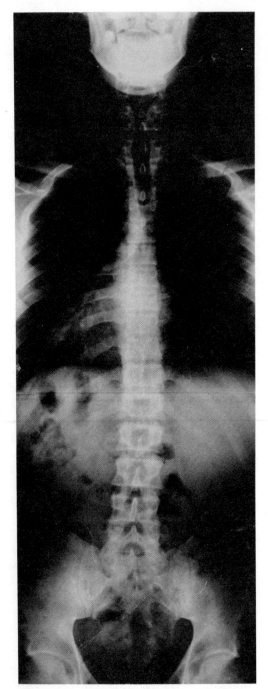

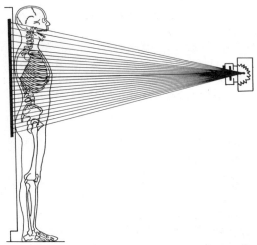

**Figure 1.6.** Schematic diagram of an antero-posterior full spine projection in one exposure at a 72-in focal-film distance.

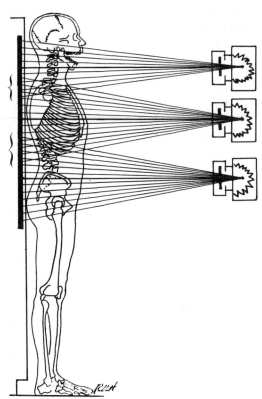

**Figure 1.5.** Anteroposterior full spine film of a medium- to large-sized individual (195-lb male) illustrating reasonably good diagnostic quality. Technical factors were 110 kVp, 100 mAs, 72-in focal-film distance.

**Figure 1.7.** Schematic diagram of an antero-posterior full spine projection in three exposures. Note projectional overlaps.

inches in full spine procedure as opposed to 40 inches in standard sectional procedures); (b) the avoidance of *projectional* overlap that is necessary in sectional procedures to project all spinal structures to the film (Fig. 1.6, 1.7); and (b) the *higher kilovoltage* technics generally used in full spine procedure.

For confirmation of this contention that postural full spine roentgenography actually exposes the patient to less radiation than when the same full spine areas are exposed in sectional procedures, we can refer to a study conducted by the US-DHEW Bureau of Radiological Health (44). In this study, anteroposterior full spine and sectional views were taken of a phantom patient in which radiation dose-measuring devices were attached to (and implanted within) various body areas. (Tables 1.1–1.3).

It was shown that the *skin dose* exposure in the case of an anteroposterior full spine view (taken according to recommended high kilovoltage technics) was 126.8 mR, while sectional views of the same full spine areas (taken according to standard technics) were 844.3, 176.2, and 103.9 mR, respectively. All films were considered to be within an acceptable range of diagnostic quality.

It will be noted that the increased exposure to the lumbar and thoracic areas in the sectional procedures were significant enough in themselves, but when it is considered that the areas of thoracolumbar and thoracocervical overlap received skin dose exposures of 1020.5 and 280.1 mR, respectively, the point that "if the entire full spine is to be x-rayed, less radiation exposure will be received by the patient in a single exposure" seems indisputable.

## Radiographic Distortion Considerations

Radiographic distortion is the process by which component parts of the three-dimensional human body are projected to the flat, two-dimensional film by a *point-source* emission of x-rays from the x-ray tube which results in an increase in size and a change in shape of the film images as compared to the actual size and shape of the body structures themselves (Fig. 1.8). This radiographic distortion phenomenon is an inherent physical characteristic of x-ray projection—although it can be reduced in

magnitude it cannot be eliminated—and it can have a profound effect on spinographic analysis procedures which are based on the measurement of lines drawn on the film images of body structures.

On the surface this criticism of spinographic analysis procedure may seem valid, but when the subject is studied more in-depth it is found that rather than being unmanageable, radiographic distortion itself is measurable insofar as it is affected by known physical principles. Therefore, it is possible to establish distortion correction factors which may validate information gained by measurement of lines drawn on the film. Such correction factors have been established for various medical radiology procedures (Figs. 1.9, 1.10) (45), and there is no reason why similar distortion correction concepts cannot also be applicable to spinographic analysis procedure.

Also, it is possible to establish radiographic projection constants whereby the patient is positioned in a known, stabilized position relative to the x-ray tube and the film to the extent that measurements are reliable within certain ranges of accuracy. Such "positioning constants," as opposed to the use of distortion correction factors, have generally been the "procedure of choice" in chiropractic spinography analysis.

Consequently, this criticism of chiropractic spinography procedure is not necessarily, *in itself*, any more valid than those relating to quality control and radiation exposure. In the final analysis of these criticisms, it appears most likely that they are simply the "reasons" given by critics to justify a more basic argument; the *belief* that spinography procedure is unacceptable *on any terms* insofar as its existence is based on an unproven theory in the first place—the chiropractic subluxation. However, this *belief* is not necessarily valid either.

## FUNDAMENTALS OF SPINOGRAPHIC INTERPRETATION

In relation to the purpose and objectives of this volume, spinographic interpretation

**Table 1.1.**
**AP full spine exposure values measured at selected phantom sites during various diagnostic radiographic technics**

| Technique | Total filtration[a] (mm of Al) | Type of collimator | Screen speed | kVp | mAs | Entrance exposure | Exit exposure | Average thyroid exposure | Average male gonad exposure | Average female gonad exposure | Average eye exposure |
|---|---|---|---|---|---|---|---|---|---|---|---|
| | | | | | | | | All values reported in mR | | | |
| 1. Swinging diaphragm | 3.54[b], 5.15[c], 6.01[e] | | Par[d] | 90 | 100[b], 250[c], 300[e] | 126.6, 292.5, 315.9 | 27.6, 15.4, 15.4 | 126.7 | 269.2 | 70.6 | 126.6 |
| 2. Swinging diaphragm | 4.57[b], 6.18[c], 7.04[e] | | Par[d] | 90 | 100[b], 250[c], 300[b] | 68.2, 189.7, 199.1 | 12.1, 8.4, 8.4 | 69.4 | 181.6 | 45.3 | 64.8 |
| 3. Swinging diaphragm | 4.57[b], 6.18[c], 7.04[e] | | Par[d] | 110 | 10[b], 50[c], 75[e] | 13.9, 63.9, 78.3 | 1.7, 3.3, 5.0 | 16.9 | 85.3 | 26.6 | 8.9 |
| 4. Common[f] (one screen) | 4.52[g], 8.23[k] | Dial-X[h,i] | Hi[j] | 80 | 200 | 240.4 | 9.8 | 133.8 | 67.1 | 23.8 | 84.9 |
| 5. High kVp (one screen) | 4.52[g], 8.23[k] | Dial-X | Hi[j] | 100 | 60 | 108.8 | 4.6 | 69.4 | 47.2 | 15.5 | 43.1 |
| 6. High kVp (one screen) | 4.52 | Dial-X | Hi[j] | 100 | 60 | 129.4 | 3.6 | 70.4 | 104.9 | 30.9 | 45.4 |
| 7. Common[f] (one screen) | 4.52 | Dial-X | Hi[j] | 80 | 200 | 242.7 | 8.4 | 137.2 | 193.8 | 43.6 | 86.0 |
| 8. Common[f] (one screen) | 7.02 | Picker[l] | Hi[j] | 80 | 200 | 216.0 | 7.1 | 126.6 | 16.9 | 36.5 | 8.5 |
| 9. High kVp (one screen) | 7.02 | Picker | Hi[j] | 100 | 60 | 126.8 | 2.6 | 70.0 | 10.6 | 25.3 | 2.3 |
| 10. Common[f] (split screen) | 7.02 | Picker | Combined[m] | 95 | 250 | 480.9 | 20.1 | 281.2 | 41.7 | 104.7 | 21.9 |
| 11. High kVp (split screen) | 7.02 | Picker | Combined[m] | 100 | 75 | 111.3 | 3.6 | 68.8 | 8.3 | 25.3 | 3.4 |
| 12. Common[f] (split screen) | 4.52[g], 8.23[h] | Dial-X[i] | Combined[m] | 95 | 250 | 353.4 | 14.7 | 268.9 | 82.6 | 54.0 | 167.2 |
| 13. High kVp (split screen) | 4.52[g], 8.23[k] | Dial-X[i] | Combined[m] | 100 | 75 | 116.5 | 6.7 | 99.7 | 27.1 | 18.1 | 55.2 |
| 14. High kVp (split screen) | 4.52 | Dial-X[i] | Combined[m] | 100 | 75 | 176.8 | 10.8 | 105.9 | 153.6 | 44.1 | 63.9 |
| 15. Common[f] (split screen) | 4.52 | Dial-X[i] | Combined[m] | 95 | 250 | 484.3 | 26.0 | 299.3 | 440.2 | 115.5 | 176.7 |

[a] Includes 1-mm aluminum equivalent filtration from x-ray tube.
[b] Cervical.
[c] Thoracic.
[d] Par, lower 3/5s of screen.
[e] Lumbar.
[f] Technique used by the majority of chiropractors as determined by Dr. JW Howe.
[g] Upper 1/3 of beam.
[h] Dial-X Collimator Model DM; Dial-X Instruments, Inc., 331 W. Merrick Road, Valley Stream, NY (Serial No. 3133).
[i] 14 × 36-in (36 × 91-cm) field. Field size as listed by manufacturer.
[j] Hi,
[k] Lower 2/3 of beam.
[l] Picker Radiographic Collimator; Delux Model 2089, Picker X-Ray Company, White Plains, NY.
[m] Upper 2/5s of screen.

**Table 1.2.**
**AP regional spine exposure values measured at selected phantom sites during various diagnostic radiographic technics**

| Technique | Total filtration[a] (mm of Al) | Type of collimator | Screen speed | kVp | mAs | Field size[b] | Entrance exposure | Exit exposure | Average thyroid exposure | Average male gonad exposure | Average female gonad exposure | Average age eye exposure |
|---|---|---|---|---|---|---|---|---|---|---|---|---|
| | | | | | | *in* | | | All values reported in mR | | | |
| 16. Common[c] lumbar | 4.52 | Dial-X[d] | Par | 85 | 100 | 14 × 17 | 745.7 | 21.5 | 9.2 | 36.8 | 133.8 | 5.7 |
| 17. High kVp lumbar | 4.52 | Dial-X | Par | 110 | 10 | 14 × 17 | 132.2 | 6.7 | 2.0 | 9.5 | 32.2 | 1.4 |
| 18. High kVp lumbar | 7.02 | Picker[e] | Par | 110 | 10 | 14 × 17 | 166.1 | 4.4 | 0.8 | 3.5 | 30.3 | 0.6 |
| 19. Common[c] lumbar | 7.02 | Picker | Par | 85 | 100 | 11 × 17 | 844.3 | 16.0 | 2.3 | 6.4 | 104.6 | 0.5 |
| 20. Common[c] thoracic | 4.52 | Dial-X | Par | 75 | 50 | 14 × 17 | 176.2 | 4.5 | 26.7 | 1.8 | 5.4 | 2.7 |
| 21. DuPont thoracic (12) | 4.52 | Dial-X | Par | 90 | 100 | 14 × 17 | 837.9 | 32.7 | 137.0 | 11.5 | 33.9 | 11.9 |
| 22. High kVp thoracic | 4.52 | Dial-X | Par | 100 | 15 | 14 × 17 | 171.6 | —[f] | 30.5 | 2.0 | 7.8 | 2.3 |
| 23. High kVp thoracic | 7.02 | Picker | Par | 100 | 15 | 8 × 17 field (14 × 17 film) | 184.5 | 4.1 | 3.4 | ND[g] | 2.5 | ND[g] |
| 24. DuPont thoracic (12) | 7.02 | Picker | Par | 90 | 100 | 8 × 17 field (14 × 17 film) | 882.7 | 21.5 | 19.9 | 3.9 | 12.4 | 4.0 |
| 25. Common[c] thoracic | 7.02 | Picker | Par | 75 | 50 | 8 × 17 field (14 × 17 film) | 201.3 | 4.5 | 4.5 | 1.7 | 3.3 | 1.7 |

[a] Includes 1-mm aluminum equivalent filtration from x-ray tube.
[b] 14 × 17 in = 36 × 43 cm; 11 × 14 in = 28 × 36 cm; 8 × 17 in = 20 × 43 cm. Field size as listed by manufacturer.
[c] Technic used by the majority of chiropractors as determined by Dr. JW Howe.
[d] Dial-X Collimator Model DM; Dial-X Instruments, Inc., 331 W. Merrick Road, Valley Stream, NY (Serial No. 3133).
[e] Picker Radiographic Collimator; Delux Model 2089, Picker X-Ray Company, White Plains, NY
[f] Measurement unavailable—capsule came open and powder lost during study.
[g] ND, nondetectable.

**Table 1.3.**
**AP cervical spine exposure values measured at selected phantom sites during various diagnostic radiographic technics**

| Technique | Total filtration[a] (mm of Al) | Type of collimator | Screen speed | kVp | mAs | Field size[b] in | Entrance exposure | Exit exposure | All values reported in mR | | | |
|---|---|---|---|---|---|---|---|---|---|---|---|---|
| | | | | | | | | | Average thyroid exposure | Average male gonad exposure | Average female gonad exposure | Average eye exposure |
| 26. High kVp cervical | 7.02 | Picker | Par | 84 | 10 | 8 × 10 | 57.3 | 4.5 | 45.7 | ND[c] | ND[c] | 4.2 |
| 27. DuPont cervical (12) | 7.02 | Picker | Par | 70 | 40 | 8 × 10 | 137.6 | 7.7 | 102.5 | 0.5 | ND[c] | 8.2 |
| 28. Common[d] cervical | 7.02 | Picker | Par | 60 | 50 | 8 × 10 | 103.9 | 4.3 | 74.4 | ND[c] | 0.3 | 5.7 |
| 29. High kVp cervical | 4.52 | Dial-X | Par | 84 | 10 | 8 × 10 | 58.3 | 4.2 | 45.9 | ND[c] | 0.7 | 47.5[e] |
| 30. DuPont cervical (12) | 4.52 | Dial-X | Par | 70 | 40 | 8 × 10 | 139.8 | 6.8 | 103.2 | ND[c] | 0.4 | 119.5[e] |
| 31. Common[d] cervical | 4.52 | Dial-X | Par | 60 | 50 | 8 × 10 | 100.0 | 5.5 | 71.5 | 0.4 | 0.2 | 85.3[e] |

[a] Includes 1-mm aluminum equivalent filtration from x-ray tube.
[b] 8 × 10 in = 20 × 25 cm. Field size as listed by manufacturer.
[c] ND, nondetectable.
[d] Technique used by the majority of chiropractors as determined by Dr. JW Howe.
[e] These high readings of average exposure to lens of eye must be due to the oversized field of the Dial-X collimator. Entrance beam was aligned at same place on the phantom for each collimator. Evidently, the Picker collimator is much more exact in defining field size.

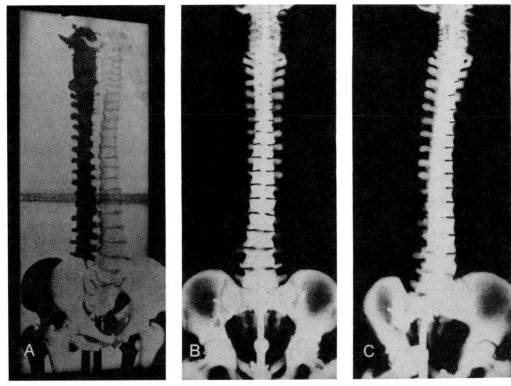

**Figure 1.8.** Demonstration of spinographic distortion. *A*, three-dimensional model positioned as for a standard AP full spine view. *B*, radiograph of model which was positioned without any rotation relative to the film. *C*, radiograph of model as it is distortionally projected when rotated 6° anterior (away from the film) on the left side. Note change in size and contour of the pelvis, and appearance of a spinal curvature which did not actually exist but appeared so due to projection of AP spinal curves to the film as the model was rotated.

(as opposed to spinographic analysis) is the process of evaluating postural full spine radiographs for evidence of biomechanical irregularities which may have clinical significance. The first step in that process is the visual examination of the films to ascertain the general configuration of the patient's pelvis and spinal column, comparing them to what would ordinarily be considered *normal* or *correct* in essentially the same manner as one makes a diagnosis of pathology by comparing the particular impressions on the film with what might be considered normal tissue density, shape, size, etc.

In the event that the patient's pelvis and spinal column does not ascribe to what would ordinarily be considered normal con-

figuration, further evaluation is made to determine the presence, nature and magnitude of specific biomechanical irregularities which may be directly or indirectly responsible. Included in this visual examination is the observation of any pathology, trauma or abnormal development which may be a contributing (or aggravating) factor to the biomechanical irregularities, or which may constitute specific disease conditions subject to referral consideration.

Visual spinographic examination of the pelvis and spinal column for biomechanical irregularities requires a good comprehension of two specialized elements of interpretive knowledge, in addition to the basic knowledge required for general radiographic interpretation: (*a*) normal pelvic

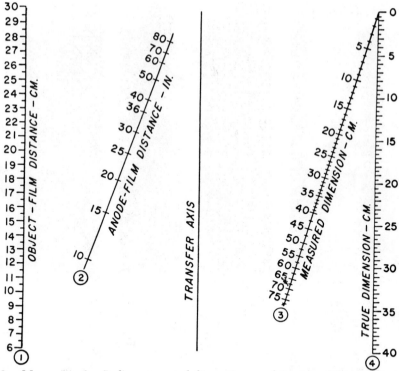

**Figure 1.9.** Monogram for finding corrected dimensions and for converting a given target-film distance to another target-film distance. To use, draw a straight line from (*a*) the object-film distance through (*b*) the anode-film distance to (*c*) the transfer axis; draw a second line from the transfer axis point through (*d*) the measured dimension to (*e*) the true dimension. [Adapted from Lusted and Keats (51)].

and spinal biomechanics, and (*b*) the physics of radiographic projection. It is by the visualization of the film images, through a mental picture of these two considerations, that one is able to make an accurate biomechanical diagnosis.

To assist in the complete spinographic interpretation process, various angles may be measured on the film to equate specific relationships of contiguous pelvic or spinal structures. Such measurements may or may not be made in all cases, depending to some extent on the following objectives:

1. To arrive at a judgment of possible biomechanical irregularity in borderline cases where visual impressions are inconclusive,
2. To arrive at a decision as to corrective procedure to be employed,
3. To make comparative evaluations of subsequent studies for an estimate of corrective progress following a course of treatments, and/or
4. To collect data on normal and/or abnormal

biomechanical values for clinical research purposes.

In conclusion, it should be emphasized that impressions of biomechanical irregularities as portrayed on the spinographs are in themselves only *suggestive* of clinical significance; the final decision being based on a correlation of all x-ray findings (pathological as well as biomechanical) with the patient's case history; physical examination; orthopedic, neurologic and postural examination, etc. However, it should also be emphasized that the absence of a positive correlation at a given point in time does not necessarily rule out the possibility of biomechanical instabilities which may have potential clinical significance at a later time; it has previously been pointed out that spinal biomechanical irregularities which originate in childhood or early adulthood may not reach a point of clinical significance as a manifest health problem until many years later.

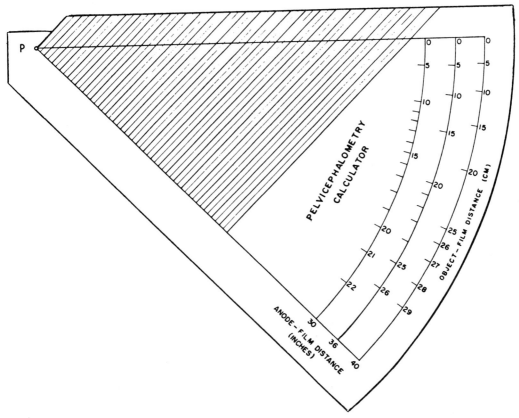

**Figure 1.10.** Pelvicephalometry calculator for estimating radiographic distortion rate between fetal head and maternal pelvic outlet. Standard size approximately 10 in long and 8 in wide at base. [Adapted from Lusted and Keats (51)].

## References

1. Kelsey JI, White AA, Patides H, Bisbee GE: The impact of musculoskeletal disorders in the United States. *J Bone Joint Surg* 61A:959–964, 1979.
2. Kuhns JG: Body mechanics. *The Cyclopedia of Medicine, Surgery and the Specialties.* Philadelphia, FA Davis, 1974, vol 2, pp 347–358.
3. Belstead JS, Edgar Ma: Early detection of scoliosis. *Br J Med* 2:937–938, 1978.
4. Hugo AK: Scoliosis. *Ciba Clin Symp* 30:1–30, 1978.
5. Kane WJ, Brown JC, Hensinger RN, Keller RB: Scoliosis and school screening for spinal deformity. *Am Fam Physician* 17:123–128, 1978.
6. Rogala EJ, Drummond DS, Gurr J: Scoliosis: incidence and natural history. *J Bone Joint Surg* 60A:173–176, 1978.
7. Haldeman S: The pathophysiology of the spinal subluxation. In Goldstein S (ed): *The Research Status of Spinal Manipulative Therapy.* NINCDS monograph no. 15, 1976, pp 217–226.
8. Hildebrandt RW: The scope of chiropractic as a clinical science and art: an introductory review of concepts. *J Manipulative Physiol Ther* 1:7–17, 1978.
9. Irving RE: Pain and the protective reflex generators: relevance to the chiropractic concept of spinal subluxation. *J Manipulative Physiol Ther* 4:69–71, 1981.
10. Janse J: History of the development of chiropractic concepts: terminology. In Goldstein S (ed): *The Research Status of Spinal Manipulative Therapy.* NINCDS monograph no. 15, 1975, pp 25–42.
11. Drum DC: The vertebral motor unit and intervertebral foramen. In Goldstein S (ed): NINCDS monograph no. 15 1975, pp 63–75.
12. Korr IM: The spinal cord as an organizer of disease processes: some preliminary perspectives. *J Am Osteopath Assoc* 76:89–99, 1976.
13. Korr IM: The spinal cord as organizer of disease processes. II. The peripheral autonomic nervous system. *J Am Osteopath Assoc* 79:82–90, 1979.
14. Korr IM: The spinal cord as organizer of disease processes. III. Hyperactivity of sympathetic innervation as a common factor in disease. *J Am Osteopath Assoc* 79:232–237, 1979.
15. Korr IM: The spinal cord as organizer of disease processes: axonal transport and neurotrophic function in relation to somatic dysfunction. *J Am Osteopath Assoc* 80: 451–459, 1980.
16. Miller WD: Treatment of visceral disorders by

manipulative therapy. In Goldstein S (ed): *The Research Status of Spinal Manipulative Therapy* NINCDS monograph no. 15, 1975, pp 163–172.

17. Sato A: The somatosympathetic reflexes: their physiological and clinical significance. In Goldstein S (ed): *The Research Status of Spinal Manipulative Therapy.* NINCDS monograph no. 15, 1975, pp 163–172.

18. Sharpless SK: Susceptibility of spinal roots to compression block. In Goldstein S (ed): *The Research Status of Spinal Manipulative Therapy.* NINCDS monograph no. 15, 1975, pp 155–161.

19. Schaumburg HH: Pathology of spinal root compression. In Goldstein S (ed): *The Research Status of Spinal Manipulative Therapy.* NINCDS monograph no. 15, 1975, pp 141–147.

20. Sunderland S: Anatomical perivertebral influences on the intervertebral foramen. In Goldstein S (ed): NINCDS monograph no. 15, 1975, pp 129–140.

21. Upton ARM: Differentiation between lesions in the primary and secondary divisions of the nerve roots. In Buerger AA, Tobis JS, (eds): *Approaches to the Validation of Manipulative Therapy.* Springfield, Ill, Charles C Thomas, 1977, pp 72–138.

22. Feinstein BF: Referred pain from paravertebral structures. In Buerger AA, Tobis JS (eds): *Approaches to the Validation of Manipulative Therapy.* Springfield, Ill, Charles C Thomas, 1977, pp 139–174.

23. Coote JH: Somatic sources of afferent input as factors in aberrant autonomic, sensory and motor function. In Korr IM (ed): *The Neurobiologic Mechanisms in Manipulative Therapy.* New York, Plenum Press, 1978, pp 91–127.

24. Sunderland S: Traumatized nerves, roots and ganglia: musculoskeletal factors and neurobiologic consequences. In Korr IM (ed): *The Neurobiologic Mechanisms in Manipulative Therapy.* New York, Plenum Press, 1978, pp 137–166.

25. Ochs S, Chan SY, Worth R: Calcium and the mechanism of axoplasmic transport. In Korr IM (ed): *The Neurobiologic Mechanisms in Manipulative Therapy.* New York, Plenum Press, 1978, pp 359–367.

26. Nigro MA: Trophic changes in afflictions of the motor unit. In Korr IM (ed): *The Neurobiologic Mechanisms in Manipulative Therapy.* New York, Plenum Press, 1978, pp 375–391.

27. Sunderland S: The anatomy of the intervertebral foramen and mechanisms of compression and stretch of nerve roots. In Haldeman S (ed): *Modern Developments in the Practice of Chiropractic.* New York, Appleton-Century-Crofts, 1980, pp 45–64.

28. Luttges MW, Gerren GA: Compression physiology: nerves and roots. In Haldeman S (ed): *Modern Developments in the Principles and Practice of Chiropractic.* New York, Appleton-Century-Crofts, 1980, pp 65–92.

29. Sato A: Physiological studies of the somatosympathetic reflexes. In Haldeman S (ed): *Modern Developments in the Principles and Practice of Chiropractic.* New York, Appleton-Century-Crofts, 1980, pp 93–105.

30. Haldeman S: The neurophysiology of spinal pain syndromes. In Haldeman S (ed): *Modern Developments in the Principles and Practice of Chiropractic.* New York, Appleton-Century-Crofts, 1980, pp 119–141.

31. Suh CH: Computer-aided spinal biomechanics. In Haldeman S (ed): *Modern Developments in the Principles and Practice of Chiropractic.* New York, Appleton-Century-Crofts, 1980, pp 143–170.

32. Lin H, Fujii A, Rebechini-Zasadny H, Hart DL: Experimental induction of vertebral subluxation in laboratory animals. *J Manipulative Physiol Ther* 1:63–66, 1978.

33. Rebechini-Zasadny H, Tasharski CC, Heinze WJ: Electromyographic analysis following chiropractic manipulation of the cervical spine: a model to study manipulation-induced peripheral muscle changes. *J Manipulative Physiol Ther* 4:61–63, 1981.

34. X-ray Examinations—*A Guide to Good Practice.* Washington DC, US Department of Health, Education and Welfare, Public Health Science, 1971.

35. Coelho LR: If spinography is dead, so is chiropractic. *ICA Rev Chiropractic* Nov.:8–10, 1977.

36. Field TH, Buehler MT: Improvements in chiropractic full spine radiography. *J Manipulative Physiol Ther* 4:20–25, 1981.

37. Howe JW: The role of x-ray findings in structural diagnosis. In: Goldstein S (ed): *The Research Status of Spinal Manipulative Therapy.* NINCDS Monograph No. 15. 1975, pp 239–247.

38. Winterstein JF, Leverone RA: Full spine radiography: its methods and value. *Dig Chiropractic Econ* 17:26–30, 1974.

39. Vampa AJ: Recognition of the full spine radiograph. *Dig Chiropractic Econ* May/June:31–34, 1980.

40. Hoppenfeld S: *Scoliosis: A Manual of Concepts and Treatment.* Philadelphia, Lippincott 1967, pp 50–51.

41. Keim HA: Scoliosis. *Ciba Clinical Symposia.* Summit, NJ, Ciba, pp 22–44, 1972.

42. Cailliet R: *Scoliosis: Diagnosis and Management.* Philadelphia; FA Davis 1975, pp 52–54.

43. Sausser WI: Entire body x-ray technique perfected. *Natl Chiropractic J* 17–18, 1935.

44. Levine JI, Howe, JW, Rolofson JW: *Radiation Exposure to a Phantom Patient During Simulated Chiropractic Spinal Radiography.* Washington DC, Department of Health, Education and Welfare, US Bureau of Radiological Health, Radiation Health Data and Reports 1971; 212–245.

45. Lusted LB, Keats TE: Atlas of roentgenographic measurements, 4th edition. Chicago, Year Book Medical Publishers 1978, pp 2–3.

# PART 1

# FUNDAMENTALS OF SPINOGRAPHIC X-RAY PROCEDURE

# CHAPTER 2

# X-Ray Physics and Radiologic Technology

## RADIATION AND THE NATURE OF X-RAYS

In the context of this discussion, radiation can be defined as "the propogation of energy through space or matter." This definition excludes such manifestations as sound because sound cannot travel through a vacuum (1).

All radiations can be classified into one of two categories; corpuscular and electromagnetic.

### Corpuscular Radiations

Corpuscular radiations generally consist of accelerated (moving) submolecular (atomic) particles, with or without an electrical charge (i.e. negative, positive or neutral). Typical corpuscular radiations are: α-rays, which consist of accelerated helium nuclei; β-rays, which consist of accelerated electrons; and protons, which are accelerated helium nuclei.

Corpuscular radiations move at a relatively high rate of speed (but less than the speed of light) and their kinetic (movement-induced) energy interacts with matter depending upon three factors; (a) size of the particles, (b) velocity of the particles, and (c) electrical charge of the particles.

### Electromagnetic Radiations

Electromagnetic radiations are a distinct, inherent form of energy generally produced by the action of accelerated electrons. Typical forms of electromagnetic radiations are: 60-cycle alternating current (AC) radiations; radio and television waves; infrared, visible light and ultraviolet rays; and x-rays and γ-rays. Electromagnetic radiations are described in terms of their *nature* and *physical properties*.

## NATURE OF ELECTROMAGNETIC RADIATIONS

Electromagnetic radiations as a combination of an electric and magnetic field; possess no mass, weight or electrical charge; and exhibit a dual *particle* and *wave* nature (1, 2).

### Particle Nature of Electromagnetic Radiations

The particle nature of electromagnetic radiations is generally considered an "assumed" characteristic since the particles exist not as particles of mass or matter (as in the case of corpuscular radiations), but rather as discrete "bundles" of energy called *photons*.

The electromagnetic radiation photons travel at the speed of light (186,000 miles/s) and the energy carried by each represents the minimum *unit* of energy or *quantum* (plural, quanta) carried by the radiation. The energy inherent within the photon is measured in terms of the *electron volt* (i.e. one million electron volt γ-radiation means that each photon carries the energy of 1 MeV.) and the total energy carried by the radiation is expressed in multiples of the energy of each photon.

## Wave Nature of Electromagnetic Radiations

The wave nature of electromagnetic radiation resides in the concept of it being a continuously oscillating electric and magnetic field moving through space (Fig. 2.1). The distance between each successive oscillation or wave—wavelength—is a measure of intensity of a particular form of electromagnetic radiation; the shorter the wavelength of a particular form of electromagnetic radiation, the greater its intensity.

Although all forms of electromagnetic radiations are essentially the same, varying only in terms of their photon energy and wavelength intensity. By virtue of these variations, each type is somewhat arbitrarily (there is some degree of overlapping) assigned a position on a scale referred to as the *electromagnetic spectrum* (Fig. 2.2).

## PHYSICAL PROPERTIES OF ELECTROMAGNETIC RADIATIONS

All electromagnetic radiations share the following physical properties in common (1):

1. They travel in a vacuum at the speed of light;
2. They travel in straight lines; they can be deflected from their original paths, but the new direction is linear also;
3. When interacting with matter, they are either absorbed (release their energy to the matter) or are scattered;
4. Their interaction with matter may result in their reflection, refraction or diffusion;
5. They are unaffected by either magnetic or electric fields;
6. They can be polarized; and
7. They produce interferences.

In addition to these properties, electromagnetic radiations exhibit a large number of different physical properties that depend upon the energy of the photons and may not be shared by radiations of different energies.

## SPECIFIC PHYSICAL PROPERTIES OF X-RAYS

X-rays are a form of electromagnetic radiation which is differentiated from all

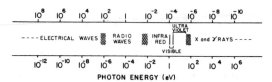

**Figure 2.2.** The electromagnetic spectrum.

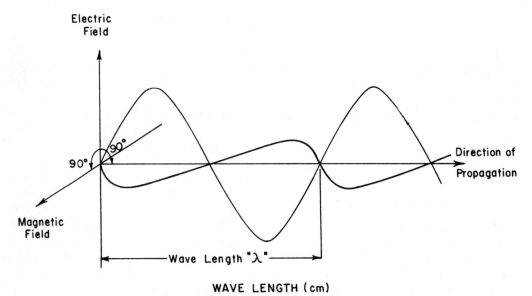

**WAVE LENGTH (cm)**

**Figure 2.1.** The wave nature of x-rays.

other forms only by virtue of its photon energy and wavelength intensity. However, in addition to the physical properties previously cited for electromagnetic radiations in general, x-rays also exhibit the following properties:

1. Their extremely short wavelength enables them to penetrate materials that absorb or reflect visible light;
2. They cause certain substances to fluoresce, i.e. to emit radiation in the longer wavelengths; e.g. visible light and ultraviolet radiations;
3. They affect photographic film, producing a record that can be made visible by chemical development processing; and
4. They cause biological damage (somatic and genetic) by their ability to *ionize* tissue atoms.

## IONIZING ELECTROMAGNETIC RADIATIONS

When electromagnetic radiations interact with the atoms of matter, the energy of the photon may be released to one or more electrons. With this excessive energy, an electron may eject itself from the atom's orbit, thus forming an *ion pair* composed of the ejected, *free*, negatively charged electron (negative ion) and the now positively unbalanced nucleus (positive ion).

The greater the energy and intensity of a particular form of electromagnetic radiation, the greater the extent of ionization that may occur when it interacts with matter. This ionization process is the mechanism by which injury occurs to human tissue, and also the mechanism by which radiation energy and intensity may be measured; e.g. by determining the number of ion pairs formed in a given amount of matter.

## X-RAY PRODUCTION AND CONTROL

In radiographic procedure, x-rays are produced by an *x-ray generator unit* which, in principle, is a relatively simple electronic device composed of: (*a*) an x-ray tube, (*b*) a low voltage (filament) transformer, (*c*) a high voltage transformer, and (*d*) a control panel (Fig. 2.3). The x-ray tube is the pri-

mary component of the x-ray generator in the production of x-rays; all other components, generally speaking, being for the purpose of assisting the x-ray tube in its function.

A typical x-ray tube is composed of an air-evacuated glass enclosure in which two electrodes are mounted in opposing directions to each other: (*a*) a *cathode* (the negative electrode) in which a *filament* (very similar to that of an ordinary light bulb) is mounted in an electron *focusing cup*, and (*b*) an *anode* (the positive electrode) on which a tungsten *target* is imbedded on its inner, bevelled, end (Fig. 2.4).

### Production of X-Rays

The method of producing x-rays within an x-ray tube is basically a two-stage process (Fig. 2.5). *First,* the x-ray tube filament is heated to a state of incandescence by a low voltage electrical current (in milliamperes) from the filament transformer to release free electrons by the process of *thermionic emission. Second,* a high voltage electrical current (in kilovolts) from the high voltage transformer is passed through the filament to propel the free electrons against the anode target with intense force, thus producing x-rays by: (*a*) releasing the kinetic energy of the suddenly stopped electrons (bremsstrahlung or *braking* radiation), and (*b*) releasing the *binding energy* of the ionized target atoms (characteristic radiation). The area of actual electron bombardment on the anode target surface is called the *focal spot*, and from this point the x-rays produced pass outward, in straight lines, in all directions.

### Control of X-Ray Production

The controls which are basic to most all radiographic x-ray generator units are: (*a*) a main panel switch, (*b*) a line voltage compensator (may be automatic), (*c*) a milliamperage (mA) control and meter, (*d*) an exposure timer, (*e*) major and minor kilovoltage (kVp) controls and meter, and (*f*) an exposure switch (Fig. 2.6). The usual

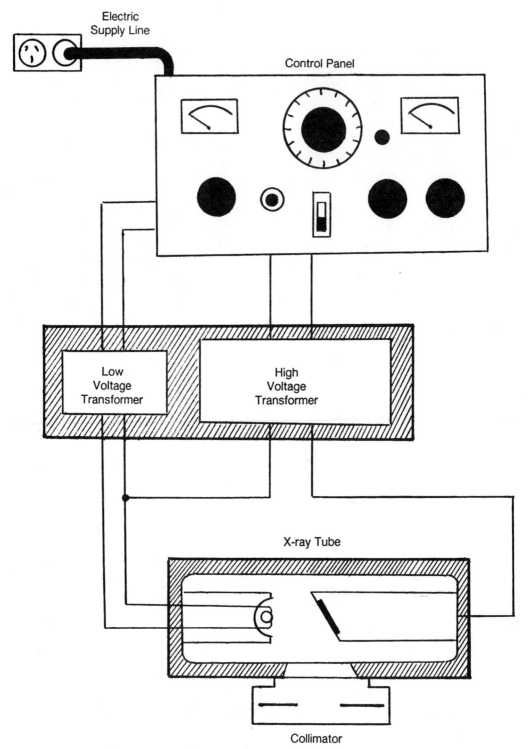

**Figure 2.3.**    Schematic diagram of an x-ray generator unit.

procedure for using these controls to set up for and to make an exposure are as follows:

1. *Turn on the main panel switch*

The main panel switch is an "on/off" *circuit breaker* switch which turns off automatically in the event of an electrical overload in the x-ray generator circuits.

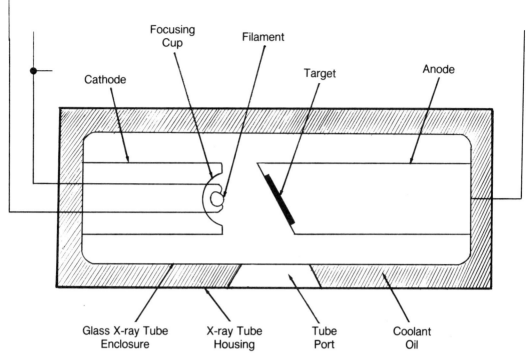

**Figure 2.4.**   Schematic diagram of an x-ray tube.

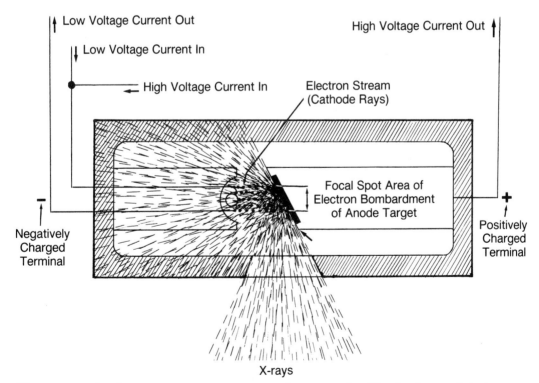

**Figure 2.5.**   Production of x-rays in the x-ray tube as a result of bombardment of electrons on the target, propelled at intense speed from the filament by a high voltage electrical current.

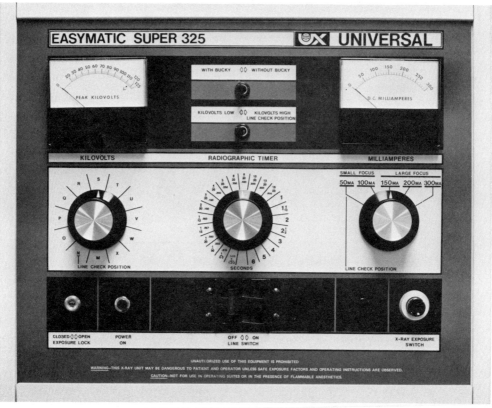

**Figure 2.6.** Control panel of a typical 300 mA/125 kVp x-ray generator unit. (Courtesy of Universal X-Ray, Inc.)

2. *Survey the panel for correct operation*
   When the main panel switch is turned on, the kVp meter should indicate whatever settings are on the major and minor kVp controls. The mA meter should not show any reading, since this meter is only activated when x-rays are being produced.

3. *Check and adjust line voltage control*
   The line voltage control (if present on a particular unit) "preadjusts" the x-ray generator to any fluctuations (higher or lower than optimum) in the incoming line voltage.

4. *Set milliamperage (mA) and timer (s) controls*
   The mA control "preadjusts" the x-ray generator for the amount (quantity) of mA that will be required for an exposure—50, 100, 150, 200, etc. The timer "preadjusts" the x-ray generator for the length of time, in seconds or fractions thereof, that the x-rays will be produced when the exposure is made. The combinations of mA and exposure time in seconds (mAs) preset on these two controls will determine the total quantity and intensity of the x-rays that will be produced. The desired amount of mAs (or

quantity and intensity of the x-rays) can be achieved by various combinations of the two controls, for example:
   50 mA for 2 s = 100 mAs,
   100 mA for 1 s = 100 mAs,
   200 mA for ½ s = 100 mAs.

5. *Set the major and minor kilovoltage (kVp) controls*
   The major kVp control usually adjusts the kVp indicated on the kVp meter in increments of 10s; the minor in increments of 2s. The amount of kVp then selected and shown on the kVp meter will determine the amount of force or *penetrability* of the x-rays that will be produced.

6. *Miscellaneous preparatory procedures*
   If an actual radiograph were to be taken, at this point the patient would be positioned, the film (in its lightproof cassette) would be put in place, and the collimator (x-ray beam-confining device) would be adjusted to the area of radiographic interest.

7. *Make exposure*
   The exposure is made by pressing the remote exposure switch (or panel button) and holding it down until the exposure is

automatically terminated by the exposure timer. During the exposure, the mA meter should indicate a reading consistent with the preset mA, and then should return to zero at the end of the exposure.

Although the foregoing listed controls and procedures are common to most x-ray generators, some variations may be found—mA and kVp pushbuttons instead of knobs; combined mA and timer (mAs) controls, etc.

## X-RAY GENERATOR ELECTRONICS

The x-ray generator unit is basically a simple electronic device to operate. However, to operate it most effectively and safely, one should have some knowledge of certain electronic principles of the particular unit being operated. These electronic principles relate primarily to the method of alternating current *rectification* and type of *x-ray tube* used in a particular generator unit.

### X-Ray Generator Unit Rectification

The main line electrical supply to an x-ray generator unit in the United States (may vary in some other countries) is 110–120 or 220–240 V; 30–100 (or more) A; 1, 2 or 3 phase; 60 cycles per second (cps); alternating current (AC). While the voltage, amperage and phase of the electrical supply to a particular x-ray generator unit may vary, the 60 cps/AC factor is a constant which is of present concern to this discussion of x-ray generator unit rectification.

In the standard electrical supply in the United States, the current (flow of electrons through the conducting wires) changes direction (alternates from positive to negative and negative to positive) 60 times/s (Figs. 2.7, 2.8). While some components of the x-ray generator (for example, transformers) require this alternation of current flow to function, the x-ray tube will only produce x-rays when the high voltage current is flowing through it in a negative (−) to positive (+) direction; e.g. from cathode to anode. This fact is the basis for the two types of x-ray generators that

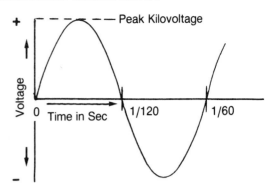

Figure 2.7. Single phase, 60 cycle/s (cps) alternating current (AC) wave form.

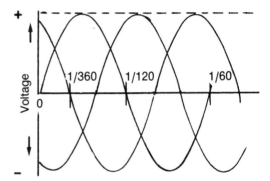

Figure 2.8. Three phase, 60 cycles/s (cps) alternating current (AC) wave form.

are commonly encountered; e.g. *self-rectified* and *full wave rectified.*

## SELF-RECTIFIED X-RAY GENERATOR UNITS

In the self-rectified x-ray generator, x-rays are produced during each 1/60th of a second that the current is flowing from negative to positive (cathode to anode) through the x-ray tube. During the next 1/60th of a second, when the current reverses direction and attempts to flow from positive to negative (anode to cathode) through the x-ray tube, no x-rays are ordinarily produced because usually there are few "free electrons" available at the anode to carry the current across to the cathode filament. Thus, the "inverse" current of the alternating current cycle is "self-rectified" within the x-ray tube by dissipating itself as heat within the anode (Figs. 2.9, 2.10).

26 CHIROPRACTIC SPINOGRAPHY

Aside from this being a relatively inefficient way to produce x-rays, self-rectification also can be very destructive to the x-ray tube because of the intense heat that may be developed in the anode, during both the x-ray production and rectification phases. During the x-ray production phase, only about 1% of the electrons bombarding the anode target produce x-rays; the remainder are dissipated in the anode as heat. Add to this the heat produced through the self-rectification process, and the total amount can be very intense and damaging to the x-ray tube. Therefore, this system of rectification can only be used with smaller x-ray generator units.

## FULL WAVE X-RAY GENERATOR UNITS

The previously described self-rectification process is also referred to as "half-wave" rectification, since only half of the

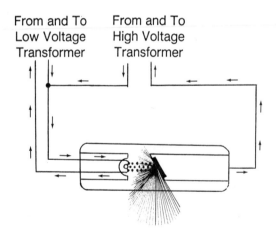

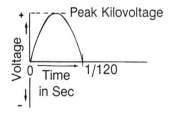

**Figure 2.9.** Self-rectified x-ray generator. Production of x-rays during positive phase of AC cycle. Time of x-ray production is one-half of the 60 cps, or for a period of 1/120th of a second.

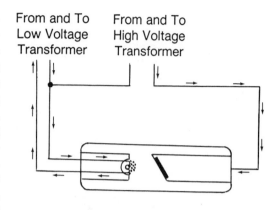

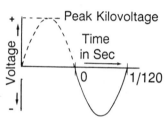

**Figure 2.10.** Self-rectified x-ray generator. Dissipation of negative (inverse) phase of the AC cycle in the anode as heat. Time of heat production is one-half the 60 cps, or 1/120th of a second.

alternating current cycle is used to produce x-rays. In larger x-ray generator units, in order to use both halves of the cycle to produce x-rays, and, at the same time, prevent the high voltage inverse current from being routed to the x-ray tube anode, a system of *four* rectifiers (electronic one-way valves) are inserted between the high voltage transformer and the x-ray tube. By the use of such a system of "full wave" rectification, the high voltage inverse current is reversed so that it also passes through the x-ray tube from cathode to anode (Figs. 2.11, 2.12). In this manner the efficiency of the x-ray tube is increased by producing x-rays during both halves of the alternating current cycle, and preventing the high voltage inverse current from dissipating itself as heat within the anode.

## X-Ray Tubes

Depending upon the maximum operating range of a particular x-ray generator unit

From and To   From and To
Low Voltage   High Voltage
Transformer   Transformer

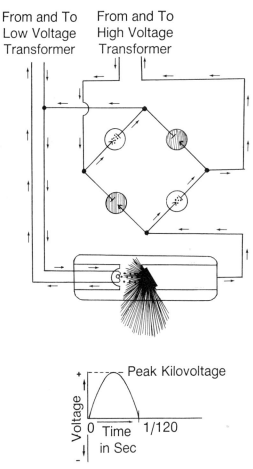

Figure 2.11. Full wave rectified x-ray generator. Production of x-rays during positive phase of AC cycle. Current is routed through x-ray tube from cathode to anode by rectifier component.

(in mAs/kVp values) x-ray tube design takes into consideration two basic factors: (*a*) heat tolerance, and (*b*) focal spot size; i.e. the width of the electron bombardment area in millimeters. In respect to these two factors, a *paradox* exists in that "the larger the focal spot the greater the heat tolerance, but the smaller the focal spot the better will be the quality of the x-ray image produced on the film."

## STATIONARY ANODE X-RAY TUBES

The stationary anode x-ray tube is the simple type which was used in our explanation of how x-rays are produced—an an-ode is composed of a length of copper rod (copper is used for its heat dissipating quality) on which a tungsten target is imbedded on its inner beveled surface, and a cathode with a filament is mounted in an electron focusing cup (Fig. 2.13). In some cases, stationary anode x-ray tubes may be found with two filaments and two corresponding focal spots (usually superimposed) on the tungsten target; the larger focal spot (up to 5 mm in width) being used for relatively heavy exposure loads, and the smaller focal spot (2–2.5 mm in width) being used for

From and To   From and To
Low Voltage   High Voltage
Transformer   Transformer

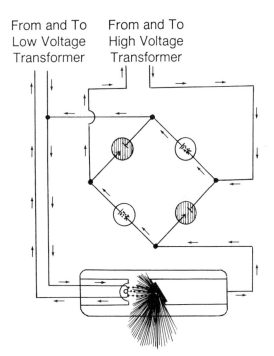

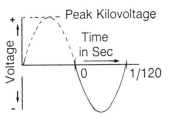

Figure 2.12. Full wave rectified x-ray generator. Production of x-rays during the negative (inverse) phase of the AC cycle. Although line current was reversed in polarity (direction of travel through circuit) the rectifer component rerouted it through the x-ray tube from cathode to anode to produce x-rays during the inverse phase.

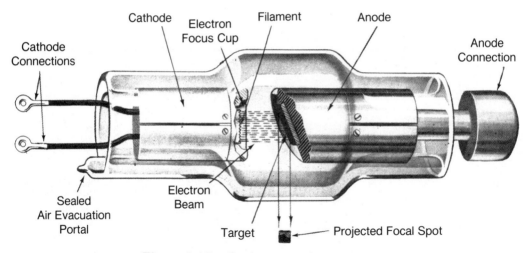

**Figure 2.13.**   Stationary anode x-ray tube.

relatively light loads. Selection of large or small focal spots may be either manual (according to manufacturers instructions) or automatic when exposure values (mAs/kVp) are selected which allow for the smaller, or require the larger, focal spot.

## ROTATING ANODE X-RAY TUBES

The ultimate in x-ray tube design is the rotating anode type which allows for much greater heat loads on smaller focal spots by bombarding the electrons on a rotating anode disk, rather than on a stationary target, thus distributing the heat load over a surface from 100–200 times greater than that of the stationary target. Most rotating anode x-ray tubes are of the *double focus* type which provide focal spots of about 1 and 2 mm in width. Consequently, rotating anode x-ray tubes are most desirable because they provide smaller focal spots for better film quality, while at the same time allowing for heavier heat loads (Fig. 2.14).

## X-RAY TUBE COLLIMATORS

A *collimator* is a device which is mounted on the x-ray tube housing (tubehead) to: (a) restrict unnecessary exposure to the patient by confining the x-rays to the specific field of radiographic interest, (b) improve film image quality by minimizing the production of scattered (secondary) radia-

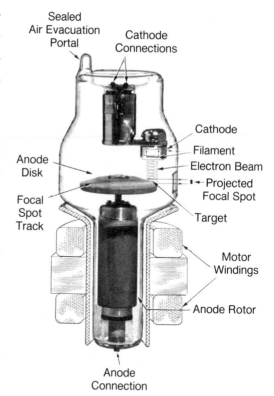

**Figure 2.14.**   Rotating anode x-ray tube.

tion, and (c) allow for precision placement of the x-ray tube for a particular procedure by use of its x-ray representative light beam (Fig. 2.15).

A collimator is composed of a case which contains two sets of x-ray opaque (x-ray

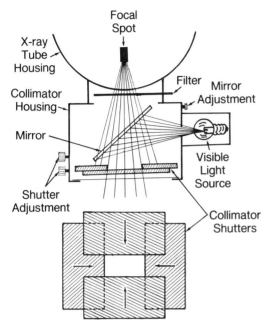

**Figure 2.15.** X-ray tube collimator. When mirror is properly adjusted, the visible light and x-ray beams are projected to the same radiographic field on the patient and film.

resistant) shutters to restrict the primary x-ray beam to a desired lateral and horizontal field on the patient and film. The collimator incorporates a visible light source which is projected by a mirror through the shutters to the exact same area where the x-rays will be projected (assuming that the unit is properly adjusted), thus it can be used to preposition the x-ray tube to the patient and film prior to taking a radiograph (Fig. 2.16).

In selecting a collimator to be used in chiropractic spinography procedure, care should be taken to ensure that the shutters of the particular collimator selected will open to a minimum of 14 × 36 inch at a 72-inch focal-film distance.

## X-RAY TUBE LOAD RATING CHARTS

Ordinarily, the x-ray tube installed in a particular x-ray generator should be of sufficient capacity to withstand the reasonable loads (combinations of mAs and kVp) which may be required in standard roent-

genographic procedures, and in relation to the loads the particular unit is designed to deliver. However, it cannot be assumed that such is the case with a particular exposure, therefore, a *tube load rating chart* for the unit in question should be consulted for any individual exposure which may exceed the x-ray tube limit.

To read a tube load rating chart (Fig. 2.17), refer to the mA and kVp to be used for a particular exposure using a specific size focal spot, and at the intersection of these lines follow upward to the maximum exposure time (in seconds or fractions thereof) which would be allowed at those mAs/kVp settings. The exact arrangement of tube load rating charts for different x-ray tubes may vary, but the basic principles

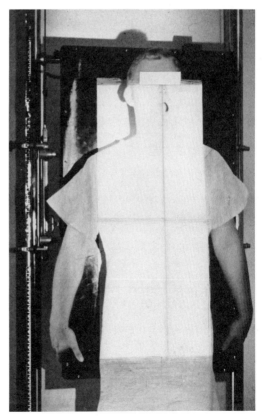

**Figure 2.16.** Collimator light adjustment prior to taking an anteroposterior full spine postural radiograph. Note projected position cross-lines, and restriction of eyes from primary x-ray beam.

2.4 mm  Stationary Anode Tube

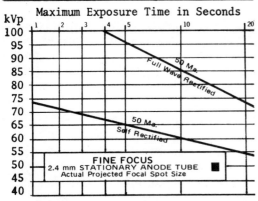

5.2 mm  Stationary Anode Tube

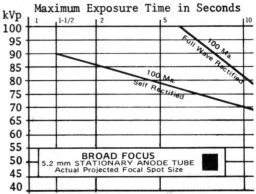

0.8 mm  Rotating Anode Tube

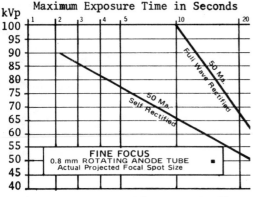

1.8 mm  Rotating Anode Tube

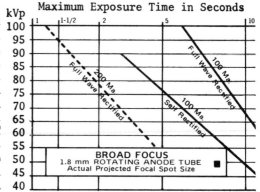

**Figure 2.17.**  X-ray tube load rating charts.

are the same. The charts illustrated here are for explanatory purposes only; the chart for the particular x-ray tube under consideration should be consulted in actual practice.

## X-RAY IMAGE FORMATION AND RECORDING

An *x-ray image* is effected when a composite beam of x-rays (comprised of photons of varying wavelengths) passes through a body of varying densities and thicknesses. The exact mechanism of this *selective absorption process* (interaction of radiation with matter) will be further discussed in Chapter 3 on *Radiation Health Physics and Protection*; however, suffice it to say at this point that the selectively absorbed x-rays emitting from the body constitutes the *actual* x-ray image. This x-

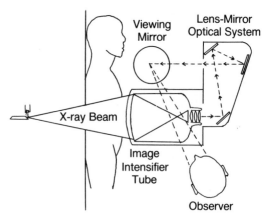

**Figure 2.18.**  Conversion of invisible x-ray image into a visible image by the use of an electronically intensified fluoroscopic unit. (Viewing through lens-optical system, rather than by direct viewing of the intensifier tube output lenses, allows for observer to see image without being in the direct line of the primary x-ray beam.)

ray image (pattern of selectively absorbed x-ray photons emitted from the body) is initially invisible to the naked eye, but may

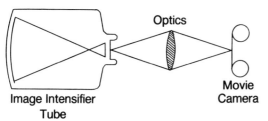

**Figure 2.19.** Cinefluorography (cineroentgenography) unit.

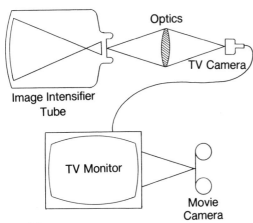

**Figure 2.20.** Kinefluorography.

be made visible by various methods; such as in *fluoroscopy/fluorography* (Figs. 2.18–2.20). However, of particular interest to this present discussion is the discussion of *radiography/spinography* which is the process of recording x-ray images on x-ray film (Fig. 2.21) (3).

### X-Ray Film

X-ray film generally used in radiographic procedure is composed of a blue-tinted plastic base, coated on both sides (duplitized) with an emulsion of light-sensitive silver bromide crystals (x-ray film used for duplicating purposes has emulsion on one side only). The silver bromide crystals are then *overcoated* with a layer of protective gelatin which dissolves during chemical development processing to allow the silver bromide crystals to be darkened in accordance with the x-ray image pattern exposed within their structure.

X-ray film is available in various speeds (sensitivity to x-rays and visible light) and various sizes. X-ray film speed varies from slow to fast, the slower speeds providing greater image detail and the faster speeds allowing for less amount of x-rays for the

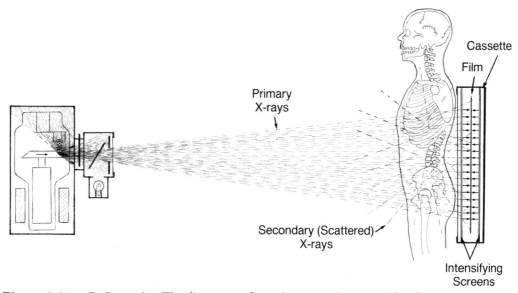

**Figure 2.21.** Radiography. The direct recording of an x-ray image on film. Primary x-rays are *selectively absorbed* by the adjacent density differences of the various body tissues and the resulting image pattern is recorded on the film as a *latent image* after being brightened (intensified) by the intensifying screens which are mounted on the inside of the front panel and back cover of the cassette.

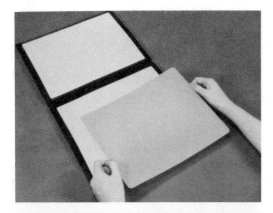

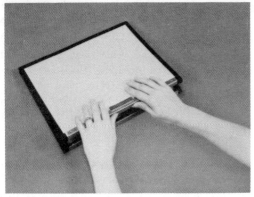

**Figure 2.22.** Loading of film into cassette. (Courtesy of the Eastman Kodak Co.)

same amount of exposure. The sizes generally used in chiropractic spinography procedure are: 8 × 10 in (20.3 × 25.4 cm), 10 × 12 in (25.4 × 30.5 cm), 14 × 17 in (35.6 × 43.2 cm) and 14 × 36 in (35.6 × 91.4 cm).

## Cassettes and Intensifying Screens

Cassettes are lightproof cases in which the x-ray film is *loaded* (under photographic darkroom conditions) for handling during the radiographic procedure and for assisting in the exposure process by the fluorescent action of their inner-mounted intensifying screens. A cassette is constructed of a strong metal framework; a light proof, radiolucent (aluminum or Bakelite) front; and a hinged back cover with an inner layer of lead foil to prevent backside scattered x-rays from fogging the film. With the film placed in the cassette, the back cover is secured in place with a series of spring clamps or other locking devices (Figs. 2.22, 2.23).

Intensifying screens, which are cardboard-like sheets coated on one side with a phosphor (visible light-emitting) substance, such as calcium tungstate or barium

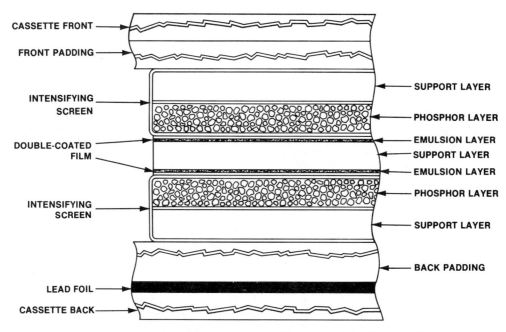

**Figure 2.23.** Cross-section of loaded cassette. (Courtesy of the Eastman Kodak Co.)

lead sulfate, are an integral part of the cassette. One screen is attached (with double-sided tape) to the inside front cassette panel and another to the inside of the back cover so that when the film is loaded into the cassette it will be tightly "sandwiched" between the screens. Although the illustration in Figure 2.21 shows a separation of the film and screens (to demonstrate screen fluorescence exposure of the film), they are actually in close contact with each other.

The purpose of the intensifying screens is to utilize the visible light of the phosphor coating, when energized by x-rays, to assist in exposing the films, thus requiring less actual x-rays to produce a radiograph. As in the case of x-ray film, intensifying screens are available in various speeds;

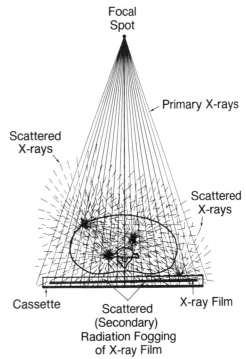

**Figure 2.25.** Production of scattered radiation within the body and its superimposition as secondary radiation fog over the latent image.

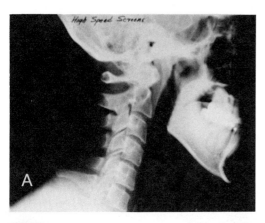

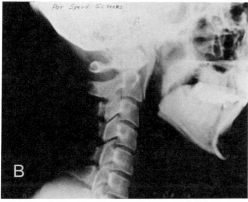

**Figure 2.24.** Comparative 72-inch focal-film distance exposures of the lateral cervical spine showing effect of screen speed on film definition. *A*, high-speed screens. *B*, par speed screens. Loss of image sharpness is nearly indistinguishable.

again, the slowest producing the best film detail and the fastest requiring the least amount of radiation to produce the same amount of film exposure. The various speed screens available, from slowest to fastest, are: (*a*) detail, (*b*) par, (*c*) high, and (*d*) high-plus. As in the case of film speed, high speed (particularly the type referred to as "rare earth") intensifying screens are recommended for chiropractic spinography procedure to reduce patient radiation exposure. Although this may result in some slight loss of image detail, this effect is adequately offset by the longer focal-film distances used in spinography as compared to general radiography (Fig. 2.24).

## CONTROL OF SCATTERED RADIATION FILM FOG

When the *primary* x-rays pass through the body, some photons collide with the inherent atomic structures resulting in the generation of scattered (or secondary) radiation (Fig. 2.25). This scattered radiation will result in a fogging of the film image unless some means are employed to minimize its effect. The standard methods of control incorporate the use of *collimation* and *radiographic grids.*

## Collimation

The smaller the area of the body exposed during the radiography procedure, the less scattered radiation that will be generated by the body (and surrounding equipment) to fog the film. Consequently, "tight" collimation of the primary x-ray beam to the specific area of radiographic interest is an important consideration in holding scattered radiation film fog to a minimum (Fig. 2.26).

## Radiographic Grids

A radiographic grid is a device composed of vertically aligned thin lead strips interspaced with more or less equally thin radiolucent-material spacers. The grid is placed in front of the cassette for the purpose of

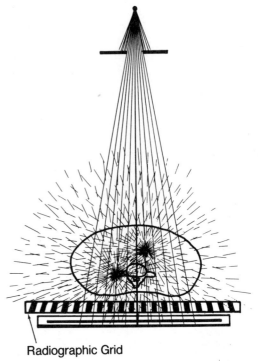

Radiographic Grid

**Figure 2.27.** The effects of radiographic grids on the minimization of secondary radiation fog.

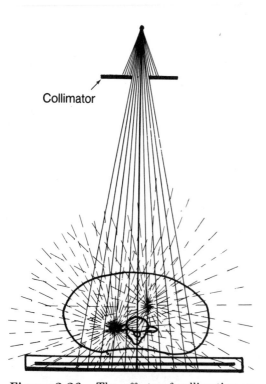

Collimator

**Figure 2.26.** The effects of collimation on the minimization of secondary radiation fog.

minimizing the amount of scattered radiation that will reach the film. The mechanism of the grid's effect is to allow the majority of the primary x-rays (which comprise the selectively absorbed x-ray image) to pass through the radiolucent spacer material to carry the x-ray image of the body to the film, but the scattered radiation emitting from the patient's body (and surrounding equipment) is, to a large extent, restricted by the lead strips (Fig. 2.27).

In selection of a grid, various factors, such as: (*a*) grid ratio, (*b*) lines per inch, (*c*) grid focus, and (*d*) grid cut-off are important considerations.

## GRID RATIO

The primary factor in the effectiveness of a grid to *clean up* scattered radiation is the grid ratio, which is determined by the depth of the lead strips as compared to the width of the space between them—the greater the ratio of a grid, the more effective its action in cleaning up scattered radiation

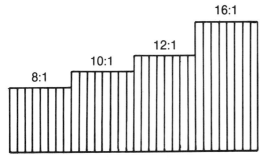

**Figure 2.28.** Schematic of generally available grid ratios. The greater the grid ratio, the better the clean up of secondary radiation.

(Fig. 2.28). However, as the grid ratio is increased, more and more primary x-rays are absorbed along with the scattered radiation, therefore, it is necessary to increase kilovoltage proportionally to achieve the same amount of film exposure as compared to what may have been required for a grid of lower ratio. Consequently, grids are usually "matched" to the highest kVp that might be used with a particular radiographic unit installation. The following are recommended matches of kVp to grid ratio:

| Highest kVp | Recommended Grid Ratio |
|---|---|
| 80 | 8:1 |
| 100 | 10:1 |
| 110 | 12:1 |
| 120 | 16:1 |

## GRID FOCUS

The lead strips and spacers in most grids are angled to conform to the divergence of the primary x-rays from the x-ray tube. Because the focal-film distances used in various radiographic procedures vary, grids are made to be used at specific ranges of focal-film distance, thus, a characteristic of a particular grid is its focus. A discussion of the various ranges of grid focus is not germane to this presentation, since in chiropractic spinography the principal grid will be a 14 × 36-in size which is designed to be used at a general range of 60 in.

## GRID CUT-OFF

Grid *cut-off* is the amount of lateral x-ray tube shift or angulation which will be allowed by a particular grid before the primary x-rays are completely restricted from reaching the film (Fig. 2.29). Grid cut-off becomes more acute—positioning of the central ray 90° to the center of the grid becomes more critical—as grid ratio increases (Fig. 2.30). Grid cut-off may also occur as the result of using focal-film distances that are too short or too long with respect to the grid focus.

## LINES PER INCH

Lines per inch refers to the number of lead strips per inch in a particular grid and is of primary importance in relation to the

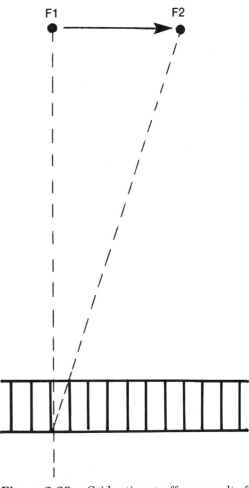

**Figure 2.29.** Grid ratio cut-off as a result of lateral shifting of the x-ray tube (*F1* to *F2*). X-ray tubes must be aligned as close as possible to a 90° relationship to the center of the film.

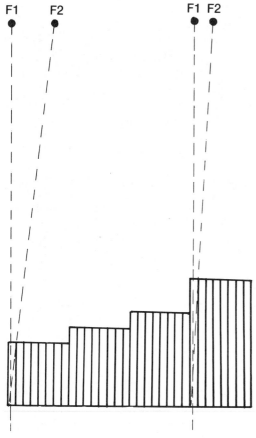

**Figure 2.30.** Increase of grid cut-off with increase of grid ratio.

manner by which the grid is to be used: in a *stationary grid holder* or a *Potter-Bucky unit.* When a grid is to be used in a stationary grid holder, a fine line type (110–120 lines/in) is recommended in order that the lead strip line exposed on the film is not excessively visible. When a grid is to be used in a Potter-Bucky unit (a device in which the grid is shifted laterally during the exposure to "blur out" the lead strip line), a coarser, less expensive grid of 60–80 lines/in may be used. Potter-Bucky grid units (commonly referred to as a "Bucky") are available in two basic types: (*a*) single stroke, and (*b*) reciprocating.

1. *Single stroke Bucky*
   The single stroke Bucky is one in which the grid makes one single lateral pass in front of the cassette during the exposure.

Its travel is by spring action, triggered automatically when the exposure switch is pressed. The grid's travel time during the pass is coordinated with the x-ray exposure time by setting a timer (connected to a hydraulic speed control) on the Bucky cabinet. The single stroke Bucky must be readied by "cocking" before each exposure.

2. *Reciprocating Bucky*
   The reciprocating Bucky is one in which the grid movement is by a built-in motor which moves the grid continuously during the exposure.

### Grid Unit Selection

Stationary grids and Buckys are usually incorporated into some form of radiographic unit, such as a stationary or motorized reclining-upright table (Fig. 2.31), spinographic postural radiography unit, etc. These units provide for the insertion of various size cassettes into a *self-centering cassette tray* (automatically centers the cassette to the center of the unit and central ray) which may then be slid under (or behind) the grid, and moved caudally or cephalically relative to the patient. (Note: spinographic postural radiography units will be discussed in Chapter 4).

Whether to use a stationary grid or movable Bucky in a radiographic unit has been a matter of some debate for many years. In the early days, when only 50–60 line grids were available, the use of a Bucky was mandatory. However, with the advent of the modern fine-line grids of up 120 lines/in, there is a question of the need or desirability of Bucky units. Ter-Pogossian (4) discusses the disadvantages of the Bucky and advantages of the stationary grid as follows:

"The most serious drawback to the use of moving grids are the disadvantages associated when a Bucky, which are costly and subject to failures, does not perform well for very short exposures, and may introduce undesirable motion of the film. For these reasons, and because of the availability of grids with large numbers of strips per inch which render grid strip shadows almost unnoticeable, there is a tendency to abandon moving grids in favor of stationary grids."

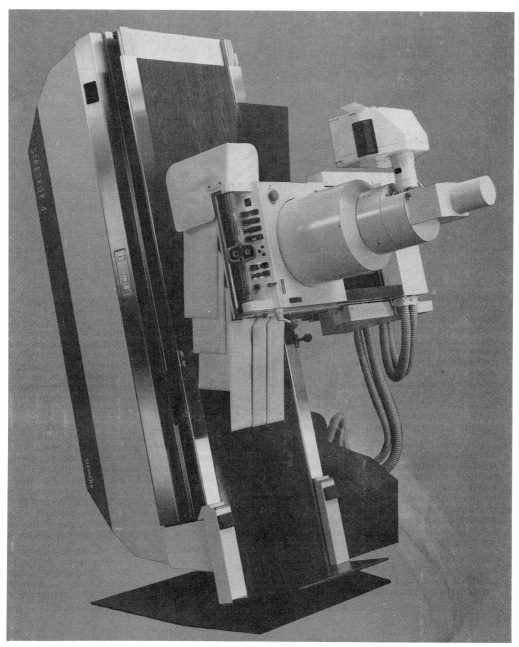

**Figure 2.31.** General radiography unit equipped with image intensification fluoroscopy. Table tilts from horizontal to vertical for reclining or upright procedures. (Courtesy of Siemans X-Ray Co.)

## RADIOGRAPHIC TECHNIC AND QUALITY CONTROL

A radiographic image and its photographic implantation on the x-ray film (as previously discussed) is the result of a proc-

ess of *selective absorption* of a composite beam of x-rays (composed of photons of varying wavelengths; penetrabilities) passing through a body of varying densities and thicknesses. Such selectively absorbed x-rays affect a corresponding *selective expo-*

*sure* on the film emulsion, which is called a *latent image* (invisible) before, and a *manifest image* (visible) after, chemical development processing. This process of selective absorption and selective film exposure is dependent upon the following factors (3–6).

### Inherent Factors

Inherent factors are those characteristics of the body (or part thereof) which are responsible for the selective absorption process, without which an x-ray image would not occur. These inherent factors may be referred to as subject density and subject contrast.

## SUBJECT DENSITY

Subject density is the overall compactness and/or thickness of a body part, and the *quantity* of x-rays which are allowed to pass through to expose the film is *indirectly proportional* to such part-density; i.e. at given x-ray machine settings of mAs and kVp the quantity of x-rays passing through the part increases as part-density decreases, and decreases as part-density increases.

## SUBJECT CONTRAST

Subject contrast is the adjacent density differences of the body part, and the *quality* of x-rays which are allowed to pass through to expose the film is *directly proportional* to such contrast; i.e. at given x-ray machine settings of mAs and kVp, the quality of the x-rays passing through the part increases as part-contrast increases, and decreases as part-contrast decreases. (Note: subject contrast is the primary factor in x-ray image formation because without sufficient adjacent density differences selective absorption, and therefore selective film exposure, would not occur).

### Film Exposure Factors

Film exposure factors are those individual characteristics of a radiograph which collectively determine the quality (detail) of the photographically recorded manifest image. These film exposure factors are density, contrast and definition.

## FILM DENSITY

Film density is the overall darkness or lightness of the film in general; such density being referred to as a *photographic effect*. The ideal film is considered one in which the density is held to a minimum consistent with adequate exposure to visualize the images. Film density should be such that all images throughout the radiographic field are clearly visible with normal illumination.

## FILM CONTRAST

Film contrast is the range of exposure difference within the image; such contrast being considered a *photographic effect*. The ideal film is considered one in which contrast is held to a relatively *long scale* (gradual grayish tones rather than extreme black and white) in which penetration of all parts within the radiographic field are sufficient to illustrate the inherent subject contrast of all body parts.

## FILM DEFINITION

Film definition is the sharpness of the image, such sharpness being considered a *geometric effect* having to do with physical factors not directly associated with the foregoing photographic effects of film density and contrast. The ideal film is one in which the definition of all structures (down to the trabecular structure of bone) is as sharp and clear as possible.

### Radiographic Control Factors

The objective of radiographic technic is to produce consistently acceptable radiographs capable of the most complete interpretation with the least amount of exposure to the patient. This objective cannot be reached unless one is sufficiently knowledgeable of all technical factors and is rig-

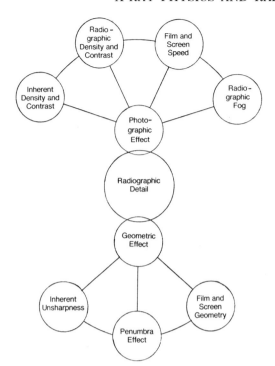

**Figure 2.32.** Factors of radiographic quality control.

idly attentive to all related details. Without such knowledge and attention to details, *consistency* in producing good quality radiographs is not possible.

The radiographic control factors are those x-ray generator and accessory unit calibrations and procedures which affect the three considerations of film density, film contrast and film definition. As previously noted, the first two of these are *photographic factors*, while the third is an independent *geometric factor* (Fig. 2.32).

## CONTROL OF PHOTOGRAPHIC FACTORS

Control of the photographic factors of film exposure is by the correlated adjustment of: (*a*) the milliampere-seconds/focal-film distance (mAs/FFD), and (*b*) the kilovoltage (kVp).

1. *Photographic effects of mAs/FFD*
   Combined, the mAs/FFD have a single effect on film density; i.e. the overall darkness or lightness of the film in general. Individually, the mAs and FFD contribute to film density as follows:

   a. *Effect of mAs on film density*
      The mAs determines the quantity of radiation produced by the x-ray tube, and film density is *directly proportional* to the mAs selected; i.e. if mAs is doubled, film density will be doubled; if mAs is reduced by half, film density will be reduced by half. Generally, the amount of increase or decrease in mAs to affect a visible change in film density is about 20–30%.

   b. *Effect of FFD on film density*
      The FFD determines the quantity of radiation that reaches the film (as compared to the quantity produced by the x-ray tube) and film density is *inversely proportional* to the square of the FFD; i.e. if the FFD is doubled, film density will be reduced to one-fourth its original amount; if FFD is reduced by half, film density will be increased by 4 times its original value, these changes assuming that mAs is left constant.

   (Note: in a particular radiographic procedure, the FFD is usually held to a constant relative to a particular radiographic procedure and mAs is varied to control film density. However, if FFD is changed for that particular procedure, mAs must be accordingly varied to maintain the original film density.)

2. *Photographic effects of kVp*
   The kVp determines the quality and penetrability of the radiation produced by the x-ray tube, and has a dual effect of controlling: (*a*) film density and (*b*) film contrast.

   a. *Effect of kVp on film density*
      Although kVp does not have a direct effect on the "quantity" of radiation produced (a primary function of mAs), by virtue of its control of radiation "quality" it does

have a primary effect on how much radiation penetrates the body part to expose the film; thus kVp is also a factor of film density control. However, unlike mAs, kVp control of film density is nonlinear and more critical in that approximately a 16% increase or decrease in kVp is equivalent to a 100% increase or a 50% decrease in mAs; whereas it requires a 20–30% change in mAs to affect a visible change in film density, only a 3–5% change of kVp is required to affect the same amount of visible change.

b. *Effect of kVp on film contrast*
Because the kVp determines the penetrability of the radiation produced by the x-ray tube, it controls the range of exposure differences within the film image; e.g. contrast. As kVp is increased (with an ap-

propriate decrease in mAs to maintain normal film density), the body part is penetrated more evenly and film contrast becomes more *long scale*; i.e. grayish. As kVp is decreased (with an appropriate increase in mAs to maintain normal film density), the body part is less evenly penetrated and film contrast becomes more *short scale*; i.e. more black and white (Fig. 2.33). (Note: Short scale—relatively low kVp and high mAs—contrast radiographic technics are generally used in regional diagnostic x-ray procedures where accentuation of images of a confined body area may be desirable. However, in chiropractic spinography procedures, long scale—relatively high kVp, low mAs—technics are recommended to reduce radiation exposure to the patient, and improve over-

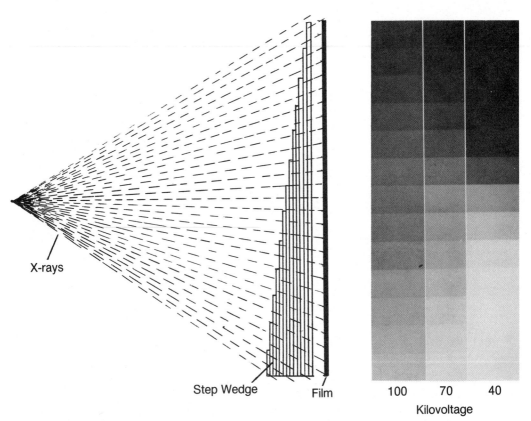

X-rays

Step Wedge          Film          100          70          40

Kilovoltage

**Figure 2.33.** The use of an aluminum step-wedge penetrometer to illustrate change in contrast scale with change in kilovoltage.

all film image quality by more even penetration of the wide range of body densities and contrasts involved).

## CONTROL OF GEOMETRIC FACTORS

The geometric factors of radiographic quality control, as previously discussed, has to do with *definition*—sharpness—of the film image. This geometric sharpness of the film image is related to an inherent physical characteristic of x-ray image formation referred to as *penumbra effect* (Fig. 2.34). Penumbra effect is related to two considerations; penumbra of *projection* and penumbra of *diffusion*.

1. *Penumbra of projection*

   Penumbra of projection is that inherent unsharpness of the x-ray film image caused by individual photons of radiation arising from different locations on the focal spot of the x-ray tube target, which projects specific areas of the object to the film from slightly different angles, thus resulting in an unsharpness of the image. Penumbra of projection is influenced by the following individual considerations (Fig. 2.35):

   a. *Focal spot size*

      Smaller focal spots project less degree of angulation of radiation from the focal spot, to the object, to the film—thus resulting in less penumbra and sharper film images.

   b. *Focal-film distance*

      Longer focal-film distances project less degree of angulation of radiation from the focal spot, to the object, to the film—thus resulting in less penumbra and sharper film images.

   c. *Object-film distance*

      Closer object-film distance projects less degree of angulation of radiation from the focal spot, to the object, to the film—thus resulting in less penumbra and sharper film images.

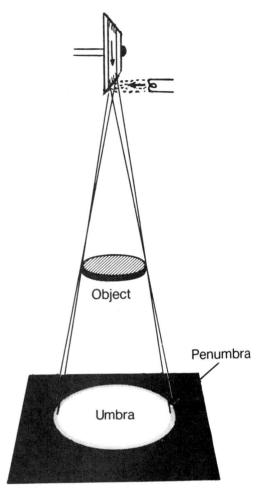

**Figure 2.34.** Production of penumbra of projection as an effect of x-rays arising from different points on the anode target, projecting at different angles to subject and film.

   d. *Motion*

      Motion of the object, film or x-ray tube during an exposure causes a *waving* of the penumbra of projection *back and forth* across the film while the image is being photographically recorded, thus increasing the penumbra from all causes, and resulting in a severe loss of image sharpness.

   e. *Rotating anode imbalance*

      In cases where a rotating anode x-ray tube has been subjected to excessive heat overloads, the anode disk may become unbalanced and

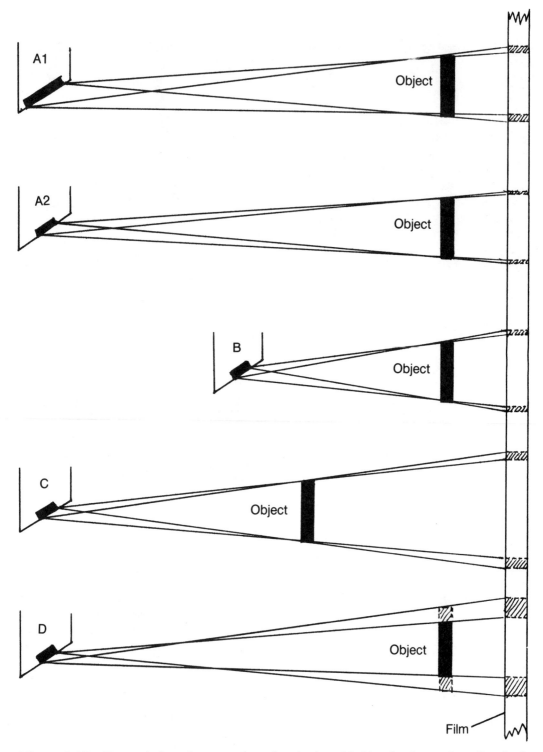

**Figure 2.35.**   Factors influencing penumbra of projection: *A1–A2* = focal spot sizes, *B* = focal-film distance, *C* = object-film distance, and *D* = object motion.

result in a wavering during operation which will cause excessive increase in penumbra and severe loss of image sharpness.

2. *Penumbra of diffusion*

Penumbra of diffusion is primarily that inherent characteristic of the intensifying screens which results in the fluorescent image occurring from the selectively absorbed x-rays *blurring* outward to expose the film with a degree of image unsharpness. Two factors of intensifying screen penumbra of diffusion are of consideration; screen speed and screen contact:

a. *Intensifying screens*

Due to the smaller size fluorescent crystals used in the construction of slower speed screens, the penumbra of diffusion is less (as compared to faster speed screens), thus resulting in sharper film images. However, in chiropractic spinography the loss of sharpness due to the use of recommended high speed screens is generally offset by the longer focal-film distances used; e.g. 60–70 in. in spinography as compared to 40 inch in general radiography.

b. *Intensifying screen contact*

When a cassette does not efficiently "sandwich" the film tightly between the front and back intensifying screens, due to the cassette being warped or having loose hinges or clamps, the diffusion of the visible fluorescent light between the film and screens results in a severe loss of image sharpness. If the fault cannot be adequately corrected by straightening the cassette and/or tightening the hinges and clamps, it is necessary that it be replaced.

3. *Inverse square law*

All factors of penumbra are increased in inverse proportions to the square of the distance (inverse square law). For example, if the focal-film distance is

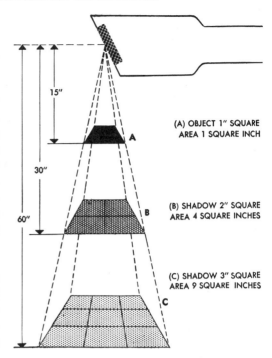

**Figure 2.36.** Inverse square law affect on radiation intensity and projectional geometry.

(A) OBJECT 1" SQUARE
AREA 1 SQUARE INCH

(B) SHADOW 2" SQUARE
AREA 4 SQUARE INCHES

(C) SHADOW 3" SQUARE
AREA 9 SQUARE INCHES

doubled, the size of the x-ray image (and its penumbra) is decreased 4 times; if the focal-film distance is decreased by half, the size of the image (and its penumbra) will be increased 4 times. The inverse square law, as previously discussed, also applies to the effect of FFD on film distance (Fig. 2.36).

## Radiographic Technic Calibration

The radiographic technics (mAs, kVp and FFD factors) used for various procedures (body part, view, etc.) in a particular x-ray laboratory are established in accordance with the characteristics of a particular x-ray generator, film and screen speed, etc. Because of the inherent variabilities of a particular installation, no common radiographic technic is practical, although *technic charts* are available which give approximate values which can be adapted to a particular installation by trial and error. Also, technic calculators are available by

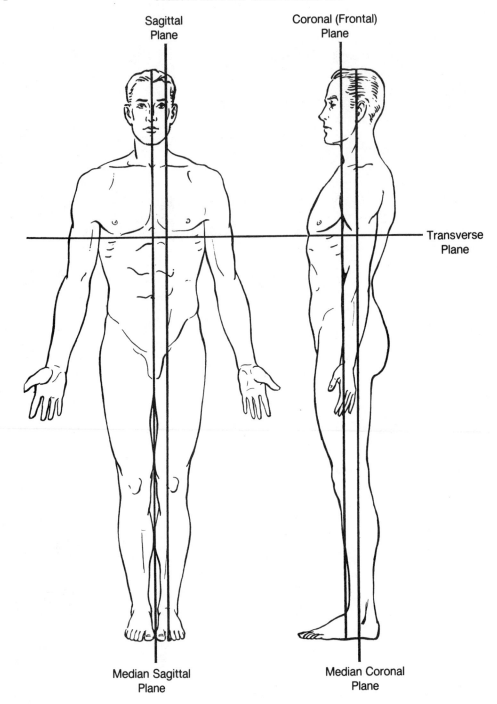

**Figure 2.37.** Body planes.

which the various factors may be estimated.

In either case, radiographic technics generally incorporate a system whereby all factors (mAs, kVp and FFD) are held to a constant (in accordance with film and screen speed) except one which is used as the variable to control film exposure. The two basic methods generally used are the *optimum kVp* and the *optimum mAs* technics.

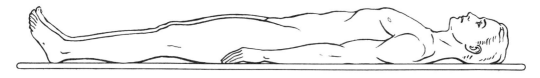

SUPINE

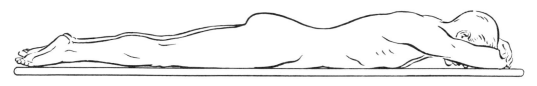

PRONE

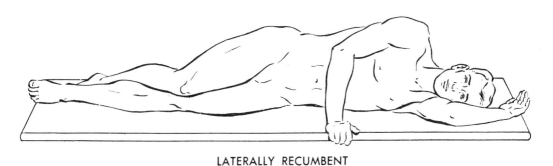

LATERALLY RECUMBENT

**Figure 2.38.** Body positions.

## OPTIMUM MAS TECHNIC

Optimum mAs technic is that in which the mAs that is determined appropriate for a particular radiograph (part, view, position, etc.) is held to a constant and the kVp is varied by a ±5–10% (2–4 kVp/cm of part thickness to control film density. This type of technic is most often used in general radiography, but is considered by some to be least desirable in spinography procedure because when the kVp is varied to control film density, film contrast is also changed. For example, as the kVp is lowered for smaller individuals, contrast scale may become excessively short; as it is raised for larger individuals, contrast scale may become excessively long. Also, because kVp is a critical control factor (requires only about a 5% variation to affect a visible change in film density), the lattitude for technic error is minimal.

## OPTIMUM KVP TECHNIC

Optimum kVp technic is that in which the kVp that is determined appropriate for a particular radiograph (part, view, position, etc.) is held to a constant and the mAs is varied by a ±25–30%/cm of part thickness to control film density. This type of technic is considered by some to be most desirable in spinography procedure because, with the kVp held to a constant (and high enough to thoroughly penetrate a particular part on almost all individuals, regardless of thickness of part), the contrast scale remains essentially the same on all exposures. Also, because mAs is not a critical control factor (requires at least a plus

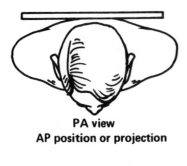

**PA view**
**AP position or projection**

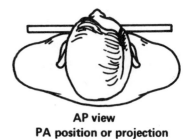

**AP view**
**PA position or projection**

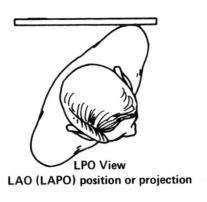

**LPO View**
**LAO (LAPO) position or projection**

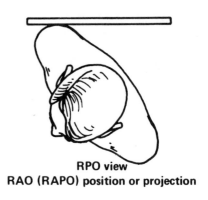

**RPO view**
**RAO (RAPO) position or projection**

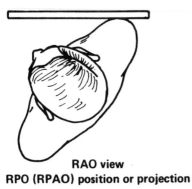

**RAO view**
**RPO (RPAO) position or projection**

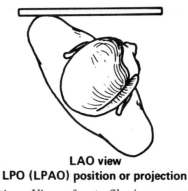

**LAO view**
**LPO (LPAO) position or projection**

**Figure 2.39.** Radiographic views, positions and projections. View refers to film image, position refers to patient placement and projection refers to direction of x-ray transmission through the body.

or minus change of 25% to affect a visible change in film density), the lattitude for technic error is considerably greater than with the optimum mAs system.

## RADIOGRAPHIC POSITIONING

In radiographic procedure certain standardized terminology is used to denote orientation of body planes (Fig. 2.37); patient attitudes (Fig. 2.38) and views-positions-projections (Fig. 2.39). Films are identified (for convenience as well as for legal identification purposes) in accordance with the following requirements:

1. Patient's name, or case number which is identified in a log;
2. Date of procedure;
3. Name of laboratory, or doctors office, where the procedure was conducted;

4. Left or right side and/or left or right extremity of patient; and
5. Position of patient; erect or reclining.

Identification of films is usually by the use of lead letters and numerals which are placed in an aluminum holder and taped to the front of the Bucky, grid or cassette. Flasher marker systems are also used wherein the information is typed on a file card and exposed on the film in the darkroom before it is developed.

## FILM PROCESSING

At the time of the exposure of the film to x-rays, a *photochemical* reaction takes place in the silver halide or silver bromide crystals which constitutes a *latent* (invisible) *image*. Film processing, then, is a chemical process whereby the exposed crystals are developed (darkened) to affect the *manifest* (visible) *image*; such processing being done under strict photographic dark-

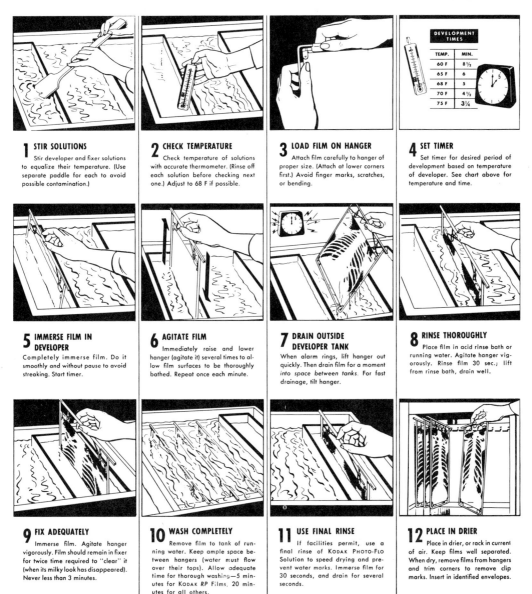

**1 STIR SOLUTIONS**
Stir developer and fixer solutions to equalize their temperature. (Use separate paddle for each to avoid possible contamination.)

**2 CHECK TEMPERATURE**
Check temperature of solutions with accurate thermometer. (Rinse off each solution before checking next one.) Adjust to 68 F if possible.

**3 LOAD FILM ON HANGER**
Attach film carefully to hanger of proper size. (Attach at lower corners first.) Avoid finger marks, scratches, or bending.

**4 SET TIMER**
Set timer for desired period of development based on temperature of developer. See chart above for temperature and time.

**5 IMMERSE FILM IN DEVELOPER**
Completely immerse film. Do it smoothly and without pause to avoid streaking. Start timer.

**6 AGITATE FILM**
Immediately raise and lower hanger (agitate it) several times to allow film surfaces to be thoroughly bathed. Repeat once each minute.

**7 DRAIN OUTSIDE DEVELOPER TANK**
When alarm rings, lift hanger out quickly. Then drain film for a moment *into space between tanks*. For fast drainage, tilt hanger.

**8 RINSE THOROUGHLY**
Place film in acid rinse bath or running water. Agitate hanger vigorously. Rinse film 30 sec.; lift from rinse bath, drain well.

**9 FIX ADEQUATELY**
Immerse film. Agitate hanger vigorously. Film should remain in fixer for twice time required to "clear" it (when its milky look has disappeared). Never less than 3 minutes.

**10 WASH COMPLETELY**
Remove film to tank of running water. Keep ample space between hangers (water must flow over their tops). Allow adequate time for thorough washing—5 minutes for KODAK RP Films, 20 minutes for all others.

**11 USE FINAL RINSE**
If facilities permit, use a final rinse of KODAK PHOTO-FLO Solution to speed drying and prevent water marks. Immerse film for 30 seconds, and drain for several seconds.

**12 PLACE IN DRIER**
Place in drier, or rack in current of air. Keep films well separated. When dry, remove films from hangers and trim corners to remove clip marks. Insert in identified envelopes.

**Figure 2.40.** Basic steps in manual processing of x-ray film in darkroom. (Courtesy of the Eastman Kodak Co.)

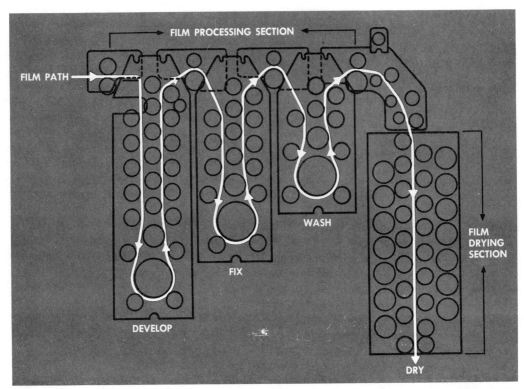

**Figure 2.41.** Illustration of an automatic processor unit. Any length film up to 14-inch wide may be processed through the roller system in 1–3 min depending upon the type of processor, solution temperature, film exposure factors, etc. (Courtesy of the Eastman Kodak Co.)

room conditions. After the film has been initially processed in the *developer* solution for a specified period of time at a specified solution temperature (time-temperature development), it is briefly rinsed in clear running water; placed into the *fixer* solution (to stop the development process) for approximately twice the development time; and washed thoroughly in clear running water to remove all residual chemicals before being dried. Film processing may be accomplished *manually* in the darkroom or by the use of an *automatic* processor (Figs. 2.40, 2.41) (6).

1. *Manual processing*
   In manual processing the first requisite is that the darkroom is in fact dark to the extent that there are no cracks or pin holes of light showing around the door or partition joints. The darkroom should be equipped with an adequate size stainless steel processing tank; fitted with a tight, lightproof cover; and with an adequate wa-

ter supply maintained at a temperature of 68°. Other equipment includes a sufficient number of film hangers for each size film that will be used, a visible light and x-ray-proof film storage case, and a safelight which corresponds to film manufacturer's recommendations.

2. *Automatic processing*
   Automatic processors are self-contained units which develop, rinse, fix, wash, and dry in as little as 90 s—from dry to dry. Since the processing of exposed film is a very critical step in radiographic procedure which should be stabilized to a constant, the automatic processor is to be highly recommended.

### References

1. Ter-Pogossian MM: *The Physical Aspects of Diagnostic Radiology.* New York, Harper Row, 1967, 7–25.
2. Howe JW, Stowe RS: *Basic X-Ray Physics and Principles of X-Ray Protection.* Lombard, Ill, National College of Chiropractic, 1977, 8–47.

3. Fuchs AW: *Principles of Radiographic Exposure and Processing*, ed 2. Springfield, Ill, Charles C Thomas, 1973, 3–8.

4. Ter-Pogossian MM: *The Physical Aspects of Diagnostic Radiology.* New York, Harper Row 1967, 278.

5. Jacobi CA, Paris DQ. *Textbook of Radiologic Technology.* St. Louis, Mosby, 1972.

6. *The Fundamentals of Radiography.* Rochester, NY, Eastman Kodak, 1980.

# CHAPTER 3

# Radiation Health Physics and Protection

## INTERACTION OF RADIATION WITH MATTER

Of particular concern to this discussion are the interactions of those ionizing radiations which occupy the x- and γ-ray range of the electromagnetic spectrum. The three basic mechanisms of absorptive interaction of x- and γ-radiation with matter are: the *photoelectric effect*, the *Compton effect*, and *pair production*. (1, 2).

### Photoelectric Effect

The photoelectric effect is the basic process of radiation absorption in matter, the mechanism being an ionization of atoms by a relatively low energy photon which dissipates *all* of its energy to an orbital electron. The electron, then having an excess of energy, ejects itself from its orbit around the nucleus. The ejected, negatively charged electron (now called a negative ion) and the remaining, positively charged nucleus (now called a positive ion) are collectively referred to as an *ion pair*. (Fig. 3.1). The end effect of this ionization process in human tissue is a destruction of its molecular components due to the resultant electrochemical change in its atomic structure. The extent of the destruction (injury) is in direct proportion to the quantity of ion pairs that are formed, which are, in turn, dependent upon the intensity of the radiation.

### Compton Effect

The *Compton effect* is the secondary process of radiation absorption in matter,

whereby a medium energy photon gives up *part* of its energy to an electron which then ejects itself from its orbit around the nucleus in an ionizing photoelectric effect. The remaining photon energy which was not absorbed by the electron travels on, somewhat weakened and in a changed direction, but still capable of further ionization until completely dissipating itself in a final photoelectric effect (Fig. 3.2). The Compton effect is the basic mechanism of scattered or secondary radiation production, generated by the body and surrounding equipment during radiographic procedures.

### Pair Production

*Pair production* is a process of radiation absorption in matter, whereby a high energy photon (in the γ-ray range) gives up most or all of its energy to the nucleus of an atom. This action results in the formation of two new particles of matter called a *negatron* and a *positron*. Pair production (which is not to be confused with photoelectric production of ion pairs) is a unique process which exemplifies the Law of Conservation of Matter and Energy insofar as the formation of the negatron and the positron represents the conversion of energy into matter (Fig. 3.3).

## MEASUREMENT OF RADIATION

Radiation, like electricity, cannot be measured directly, but only indirectly by the effects it produces. In this case, the effects of radiation are ionization; hence,

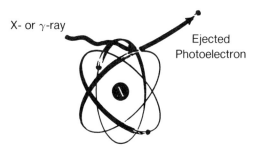

## Photoelectric Effect
### (Primarily Low Energy Photon)

**Figure 3.1.** Photoelectric effect.

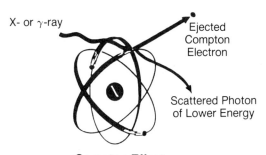

## Compton Effect
### (Primarily Medium Energy Photon)

**Figure 3.2.** Compton effect.

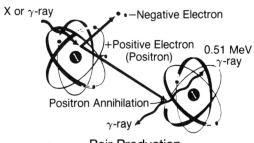

## Pair Production
### (High Energy Photon, >1.02 MeV)

**Figure 3.3.** Pair production.

the term ionizing radiations. Two aspects of radiation measurement are of interest; units of radiation measurement and methods of radiation measurement.

### Units of Radiation Measurement

With the advent of the movement of the scientific community toward conversion of measurements from the English to the metric system, traditional units of radiation measurement—*roentgen, rad* and *rem*—are undergoing a change to metric units; many scientific journals are already requiring their use. However, in consideration of the transitional stage of their current clinical use, both systems will be discussed (3, 4).

## TRADITIONAL UNITS OF RADIATION MEASUREMENT

1. *Roentgen*
   The roentgen is regarded as the standard base unit of *radiation intensity* and one roentgen (1 R) is equivalent to the amount of energy required to produce a total of two billion ion pairs (one electrostatic unit) in 1 cm$^3$ of dry air under controlled conditions.
2. *Rad*
   The rad (roentgen absorbed dose) is the standard unit of radiation *exposure dose* which is assumed to be completely absorbed by the matter irradiated. Under controlled exposure conditions, 1 R of exposure dose is equivalent to 1 rad of absorbed dose.
3. *Rem*
   The rem (rad-equivalent man) is the absorption dose in rads multiplied by the biological effectiveness of the type of radiation used. X- and γ-rays are said to have a "relative biological effectiveness (RBE)" of one; therefore, for each rad of exposure dose, 1 rem of absorption effect may be expected.

## METRIC UNITS OF RADIATION MEASUREMENT

In radiology and allied fields, the *joule per kilogram* (J/kg) replaces the rad and rem; the *reciprocal second* replaces the curie; and the *coulomb per kilogram* (C/kg) replaces the roentgen (5, 6). However, in 1975 the international governmental *Conference* Generale *des Poids et Measures* (CGPM) adopted at the request of the *International Commission on Radiation Units and Measurements* (ICRU), the *gray* (symbol Gy) as a special name for the joule per kilogram for measurement of absorbed dose. It added a note to the effect that the gray could also be used for other physical quantities in the field of ionizing radiations that are expressed in joules per kilogram.

This means that absorbed dose index, *kerma* and specific energy imparted are also expressed in terms of the gray. Also in 1975, the CGPM adopted the *becquerel* (Bq) as a special name for the reciprocal second for measurement of radioactivity. No special name was adopted for the coulomb per kilogram.

Following these CGPM decisions, ICRU recommended that the units curie, rad and roentgen be abandoned and replaced by the SI (System Internationale) units over a period of not less than 10 yr (i.e. the old units should not be completely abandoned before 1985). At the same time it requested all international and national organizations to assist in implementing the change. The present situation is summarized in Table 3.1. It is recommended that, as an interim measure, numerical values should, for most purposes, be quoted in the literature as in the right-hand column of Table 3.1. Attention is drawn to the recommendation that, in order to avoid confusion, dose equivalent (for which the old unit was the rem) should be expressed in *joule per kilogram*, and not the gray.

### Methods of Radiation Measurement

As previously stated, radiation is measured by virtue of its ionizing activity. The following are some of the various methods or types of instruments commonly used to measure ionizing radiations (7).

## RADIATION RATE METERS

Radiation rate meters (Geiger counter, scintillation counter) are meters in which radiation causes a certain amount of ionization in a known volume of air (known number of molecules) in a sealed container. The number of ion pairs thus formed in the air when exposed to radiation is electronically measured and indicated on a meter in terms of roentgens or milliroentgens. Ratemeters measure the *rate* at which radiation is being received (R or mR per second), the total dose being determined by the time element of the exposure.

## RADIATION DOSE METERS

Radiation dose meters (pencil dosimeter and film badge) also determined the amount of radiation by ionization effects, but unlike rate meters, measure total dose received in a given period of time rather than the rate at which it is being received. The pencil dosimeter measures ionization by means of an electroscope and the film badge measures ionization by the amount of film exposure.

## BIOLOGICAL EFFECTS OF RADIATION

The biological effects of radiation are divided into *somatic* (i.e. those which affect individuals directly) and *genetic* (i.e. those which indirectly affect future generations).

**Table 3.1.**
**Radiation quantities and units**

| Quantity | SI unit | Old unit | Example |
|---|---|---|---|
| Absorbed dose: Absorbed dose index; kerma; specific energy imparted) | gray | rad | 15 μGy (1, 5 mrad) |
| Absorbed dose rate | grey per second | rad per second | 15 μGy/s (1.5 mrads/s) |
| Dose equivalent | joule per kilogram | rem | 10 mJ/kg (1 rem) |
| Activity | becquerel | curie | 37 mBq |
| Exposure | coulomb per kilogram | roentgen | 0,258 μC/kg (1 mR) |
| Exposure rate | coulomb per kilogram second (or ampere per kilogram) | roentgen per second | 0,258 μC/(kg·s) (1 mR/s) |

## Somatic Effects

Somatic effects of radiation are the result of direct damage to tissue by the ionization process. In such cases, it is important to understand that the body does not *store* radiation (except to the extent that it may store radioactive particles that continuously emit radiation), but rather it tends to *accumulate* the damage to tissue caused by the ionizing process, which, to some extent, is reparable by normal healing as with any other type of tissue injury. Somatic effects are further subdivided into acute and chronic.

## ACUTE SOMATIC EFFECTS

Acute somatic effects are those which are generally received in a single, large exposure to the whole body, or part thereof. Such large doses are ordinarily possible only with radiation therapy or nuclear industry accidents; highly unlikely in radiography. Table 3.2 presents the expected biological effects of such acute whole body exposure (8).

## CHRONIC SOMATIC EFFECTS

Chronic somatic effects are those which occur from relatively small, repeated exposures (as in radiography) to sensitive tissues or organs, such as the lense of the eye, thyroid, blood-forming organs, etc. This is a hazard of all radiography procedure which is difficult to assess directly, but is assumed to cause some degree of long-term injury in most cases. Consequently, the need to properly consider and conduct all radiographic procedures in terms of need and benefit to the individual.

## Genetic Effects

X-rays have the ability to produce gene mutations and chromosome aberrations. These effects are proportional to the radiation dose absorbed by the cells, and it is presumed that there is no threshhold dose below which these effects are absent. If such effects occur in reproductive cells, undesirable mutations may be passed to sub-

**Table 3.2.**

**Representative dose-effect relationship in man for whole body irradiation.**[a,b]

| Nature of effect | Absorbed dose: x- or γ- (rads) |
|---|---|
| Minimal dose detectable by chromosome analysis or other specialized analyses; not hemogram | 5–25 |
| Minimal acute dose readily detectable in a specific individual (e.g. presented as a possible exposure case) | 50–75 |
| Minimal acute dose likely to produce vomiting in about 10% of people exposed | 75–125 |
| Acute dose likely to produce transient disability and clear hematological changes in the majority of people exposed | 150–200 |
| Median lethal dose (MLD 50/30); fatal in 30 days to 50% of people exposed | 300–400 |

[a] The dose entries in this table should be taken as representative compromises only of a surprisingly variable range of values that would be offered by well qualified observers asked to complete the right-hand column. This comes about, in part, because whole body irradiation is not a uniquely definable entity. Midline absorbed doses are used; the data are a mixed derivative of experience from radiation therapy and a few nuclear industry accident cases (often with more up-to-date dosimetry). Also, the interpretations of such qualitative terms as "readily detectable" is a function of the conservatism of the reporter.

[b] For comparison, an average AP lumbar radiograph exposure will deliver approximately 250 mR, or one-fourth of 1 rad.

sequent generations. These considerations have led to general agreement that unnecessary exposure to the gonads should be avoided.

The significance of gonadal exposure can be appreciated by considering that:

1. The genetic risks to future populations are based on the cumulative radiation doses received by the genetic pool of the total population, and
2. These genetic effects will be randomly dis-

tributed since humans are an outbreeding population.

Consequently, no individual's progeny can be protected by preventing exposure to himself if all others in the population are exposed. On the contrary, protection of one's own progeny is intimately linked to the exposure to others in the population. Therefore, the physician who protects his patients may, in fact, be protecting his own progeny (9).

### Radiation Dose Limits

Although the application of radiation dose limits for minimizing chronic somatic and genetic effects is substantially conditioned by many qualifications, a summary of recommended dose limits is provided in Table 3.3 (8). In order to maintain dose limits to at least (or below) these recommendations, the strict adherence to certain good practices are considered mandatory. These practices (particularly in regard to the diagnostic x-ray laboratory) apply to both employees and patients.

### EMPLOYEES

Although the prospective annual limit for employees working in or near a diagnostic x-ray laboratory is 5 R, actual exposure should be kept as far below that as possible considering that an employee is also a potential patient and candidate for x-ray evaluation (Fig. 3.4). Procedures to be observed are:

**Table 3.3.**
**Dose limiting recommendations**

| Limiting factor | Quantity |
|---|---|
| *Maximum permissible dose equivalent for occupational exposure* | |
| Combined whole body exposure: | |
|    Prospective annual limit | 5 R in any 1 yr |
|    Retrospective annual limit | 10–15 R in any 1 yr |
|    Long-term exposure to age $N$ yr | $(N–18) \times 5$ r |
| Skin | 15 R in any 1 yr |
| Hands | 75 R in any 1 yr (25/qtr) |
| Forearms | 30 R in any 1 yr (10/qtr) |
| Other organs, systems, tissues | 15 R in any 1 yr (5/qtr) |
| Fertile female (respect to fetus) | 0.5 R in gestation period |
| *Dose limits for public, or occasionally exposed individuals* | |
| Individuals or occasional | 0.5 R in any 1 yr |
| Students | 0.1 R in any 1 yr |
| *Population dose limits* | |
| Genetic | 0.17 R average per yr |
| Somatic | 0.17 R average per yr |
| *Emergency dose limits—life saving* | |
| Individuals (over 45 if possible) | 100 R |
| Hands and forearms | 200 R additional (300 total) |
| *Emergency dose limits—less urgent* | |
| Individual | 25 R |
| Hands and forearms | 100 R, total |
| *Family of radioactive patients* | |
| Individual (under age 45) | 0.5 R in any 1 yr |
| Individual (over age 45) | 5 R in any 1 yr |

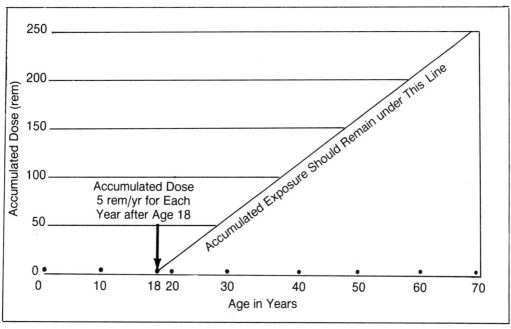

**Figure 3.4.** Maximum allowable occupational x-ray exposure dose.

1. Always utilize proper protective means (stand behind adequate shielding (Fig. 3.5) when making an exposure, etc) to hold dose as low as possible. Using assistants to hold a patient during an exposure should be avoided. When it is absolutely necessary for someone to hold a patient during an exposure, they should be adequately protected by a leaded apron and gloves, and should be cautioned to stand clear of the primary beam.
2. Always wear a film badge (and require all employees to do the same) to monitor any inadvertent excessive exposure. (Note: film badges are subscribed to as a service of commercial film badge laboratories; they are usually returned to the laboratory on a monthly basis for analysis, and reports are issued on a monthly, quarterly and annual basis for each employee).

## PATIENTS

In the case of patients, no specific limits can be set since the need for radiographic diagnostic procedure determines the application. However, every possible means should be exercised to insure that the procedure is justified; that it be conducted with the least amount of exposure consistent with technical need; and that, in the case of radiography, the quality of the films be adequate to provide the information needed to make an accurate diagnosis. Some specific considerations for minimizing exposure dose to the patient are as follows:

1. An efficient, approved type of collimator equipped with a minimum of 2.0 mm of *added* filtration (preferably as much a 5 mm in spinography) is mandatory to minimize exposure of the patient to useless, long wavelength radiation.
2. Collimate closely to the specific area of radiographic interest.
3. Exclude the eyes, thyroid and gonads from the primary beam to the extent possible. Gonadal shielding is particularly important for all persons having reproductive potential.
4. Consider possible pregnancy in the case of all females in the reproductive age group. All such female patients should be routinely asked whether pregnancy may be possible. To the extent possible, exposure to such female patients should be confined to a time span of 10 days following the onset of a menstrual period.
5. Use the highest possible kVp, lowest possible mAs, and longest possible ffd.
6. Keep adequate records of all exposures, including an estimate of dose (Fig. 3.6).
7. Be sure that the x-ray equipment being used meets approved standards and is in proper working order.

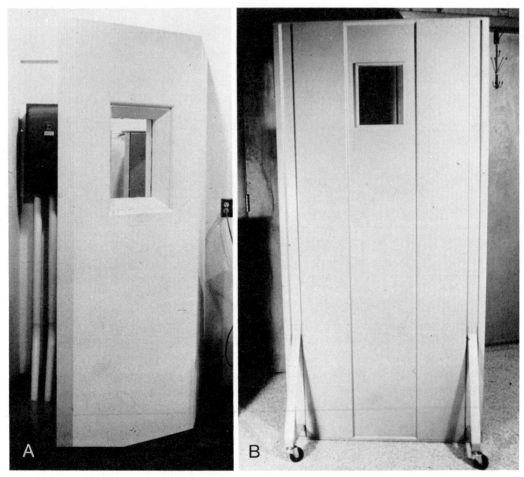

**Figure 3.5.** Employee protection shielding. *A*, permanent; *B*, portable.

## DIAGNOSTIC X-RAY EQUIPMENT STANDARDS

On August 1, 1974, the Federal diagnostic x-ray equipment standard became effective. The following describes some of the major provisions of the standard, practitioner responsibilities, and upgrading of used equipment (10).

### Introduction

The Federal diagnostic x-ray equipment standard is aimed at reducing patient exposure during x-ray examinations. Its significance lies in the fact that 90% of the United States population's exposure from man-made radiation sources is attributed to the diagnostic use of x-rays. More than 130 million people are estimated to receive some kind of x-ray examination each year in this country.

The x-ray equipment standard was issued by the Food and Drug Administration (FDA) under the authority of the Radiation Control for Health and Safety Act (Public Law 90-602). The act requires the Secretary of Health, Education, and Welfare to conduct a radiation control program to include the development and administration of standards to reduce human exposure to electronic product radiation. This responsibility has been delegated to FDA's Bureau of Radiological Health.

Although the standard is patient-protection oriented, it offers many advantages to practitioners and others using diagnostic x-

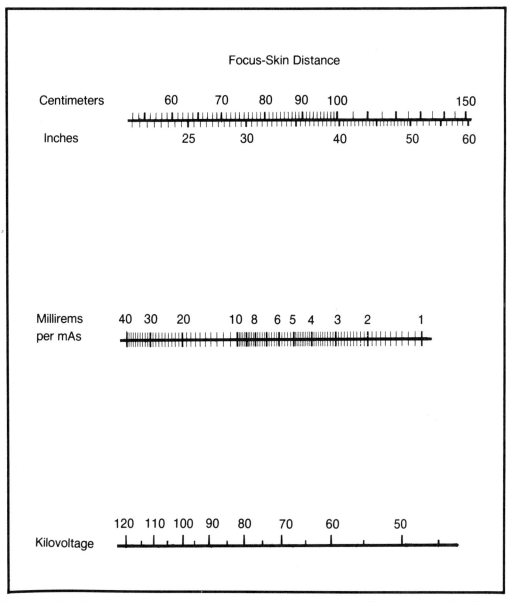

**Figure 3.6.** Nomogram for estimating x-ray exposure to a patient (for use only with full-wave rectified generators fitted with a minimum of 2-mm added filtration; values are estimates and will vary with different x-ray machine installations). To use: connect the *focus-skin distance* (not the focal-film distance) to the *kVp* used in a particular exposure with a ruler and multiply *millirems* (found where ruler crosses the mR per mAs line) by the *milliampere-seconds used in the exposure.* For a diagnostic series determine the mR values for each exposure and multiply. (Adapted from Clark's *Positioning Manual*, edited by L. Kreel and A. Paris. London, Heinemann Medical Books, 1977.)

ray equipment. In essence, the standard calls for equipment capable of providing more reliable diagnostic information with an increased level of radiation protection.

**Major Provision of the Standard**

Two general points should be made about the standard at the outset. First, it is an equipment performance standard. It cannot require equipment design features. A certain type of beam-limiting device, for example, cannot be stipulated. It is up to the manufacturer to determine how to achieve levels of equipment performance mandated by the standard. The other point is that the standard does not regulate diagnostic equipment users. It neither requires health professionals to practice radiology in certain ways or prohibit them from using x-ray equipment for a desired purpose.

The standard applies to major components, as well as complete systems, manufactured after August 1, 1974. With respect to systems in use prior to the effective date, it in no way requires or implies that these units *must* be modified, upgraded or discarded.

Components covered by the standard are tube-housing assemblies, x-ray controls, x-ray high voltage generators, fluoroscopic imaging assemblies, tables, cradles, film changers, cassette holders, and beam-limiting devices. All components made after the August 1, 1974 effective date of the standard must be certified by the manufacturer for compliance with its provisions. Such components must bear permanent certification labels, which are readily visible after component assembly.

## Beam Limitation

One of the most important provisions of the standard is aimed at a major cause of unnecessary exposure—the practice of using an x-ray beam larger than needed to produce diagnostically acceptable radiographs. The standard requires all diagnostic x-ray equipment to be able to limit the beam to the image receptor. However, the requirements for stationary general-purpose radiographic equipment are different from those specified for special-purpose radiographic equipment.

Stationary general-purpose radiographic equipment is defined in the standard as any system that is installed in a fixed location and is not limited by design to examination of specific anatomical regions. It is required

to provide positive beam limitation. This may be achieved by automatic beam-limiting devices or by manually operated collimators. If a manual collimator is used, the system must be equipped with some means, such as electrical interlocks, for preventing the production of x-rays until the collimator is properly adjusted to the receptor size.

Special-purpose radiographic equipment is considered to include, e.g. in dental systems: equipment designed for visualization of specific areas such as chest or skull; and photofluorographic equipment. Beam-limiting requirements for such equipment may be satisfied by fixed apertures or manually adjustable collimators capable of restricting the x-ray field to the image receptor for the various examination procedures for which the equipment is designed.

## Reproducibility and Linearity

Also of major importance are provisions of the standard that require x-ray systems to provide improved exposure reproducibility and linearity. Reproducibility means that the machine must be able to duplicate certain radiation exposures for given voltage, current, and time settings. Linearity means that x-ray output must vary in direct proportion to changes in current settings.

## Beam Quality

The standard prescribes certain acceptable levels of beam quality, which can be achieved through appropriate filtration. Systems that have removable filtration, such as general purpose systems used in mammography, must be provided with a positive means of assuring the presence of at least the added filtration needed to achieve the minimum beam quality required. In those units where the amount of filtration varies depending on examination, positive filtration may be afforded by a filter system interlocked with the voltage selector so that x-rays may not be produced until the required filter is in position. In most cases, however, the filter may be permanently installed.

## Fluoroscopic Exposure Limits

The standard establishes maximum exposure rates for fluoroscopic equipment. This rate varies according to the type of controls provided by the manufacturer, so that it does not interfere with the clinical application.

Patient-entrance exposure rate is limited to 10 R/min for equipment with automatic exposure or brightness control unless an optional high level control is provided. When the optional high level control is present, the exposure limit is 5 R/m for normal operation and is unlimited in the high level position. Fluoroscopic equipment without automatic brightness control also is limited to 5 R/min unless the optional high-level control is present. Warning signals must be sounded automatically when high level fluoroscopic controls are actuated to avoid their accidental use.

## Beam-Limiting Devices for Spot Films

The standard requires beam-limiting devices for spot films to be located between the x-ray source and the patient. This will reduce patient exposure, since, in many cases, the practice has been to use shielding directly in front of the film to confine exposure to the desired portion of the film, instead of obtaining the same result by limiting the beam before it enters the patient.

## Automatic Exposure Control Devices

Another provision requires back-up timers for automatic exposure control devices to insure that the equipment cuts off at a maximum exposure time even if the automatic timer fails.

## Beam-On Indicators

All radiographic systems are required to give visible warnings when x-rays are being generated and audible signals when the exposure has terminated.

## Assembling the System

The interconnection of major components to form a diagnostic x-ray system and the adjustment and testing of the system are the final steps in the x-ray equipment manufacturing process. The standard takes cognizance of this fact by defining the installer or assembler as a manufacturer. An assembler who installs one or more certified components must meet requirements of the standard applicable to such installation. This is true whether he installs an entire system or adds or replaces a single major certified component in an existing system. The provision applies also to a physician who installs a certified component into a system used in his practice.

## Practitioner Responsibilities

Although the standard is directed primarily at the x-ray equipment manufacturer to produce systems and components that perform in a prescribed way, it also places some responsibilities on the owner of the system. These responsibilities cover three areas: maintenance, for the most part; assembly; and variances from the standard.

### EQUIPMENT MAINTENANCE

Equipment manufacturers are required by the standard to furnish purchasers with a schedule of maintenance necessary to keep the system in compliance, as well as instructions with respect to procedures and precautions to be followed because of unique features of the equipment. It is the owner's responsibility, however, to have his x-ray equipment maintained according to the schedule furnished by the manufacturer to insure compliance with the standard for the life of the equipment.

Failure to follow the manufacturer's maintenance instructions could relieve the manufacturer of responsibility for continued compliance. Manufacturers must either repair, replace or refund the cost of certified components that fail, through no fault of the user, to comply with the standard.

In the case where equipment maintenance is performed under a service contract, it is important the contract include a provision to keep the unit in compliance with the standard by strict adherence to the maintenance schedule.

## ASSEMBLY

It should be reemphasized that everyone who assembles a diagnostic x-ray system using certified components becomes a manufacturer under the standard and is subject to procedures required of manufacturer-assemblers. The stipulation applies irrespective of who assembles the unit—company representative or a physician, dentist, other practitioner, or their employees in a private office, clinic, or hospital.

When the practitioner installs certified components into a system containing only compatible components, he must:

1. Install components that are compatible with each other and with components already in the system.
2. Install components called for by the standard.
3. Follow instructions of component manufacturers.
4. Complete a "Report of Assembly of a Diagnostic X-ray System" (Form FD 2579) certifying that all requirements of the standard that are applicable to the installation have been met. Such report forms should accompany component assembly instructions provided by the manufacturer.

A practitioner sometimes may find it necessary to install a certified component into a system that contains components with which it is not compatible. This is allowed only when:

1. No compatible component of a similar design is offered for commercial sale in the United States. An assembler has met his obligation in determining commercial availability of a component if he contacts the manufacturer of the noncompatible component in the existing system to verify that a compatible part is not available.
2. The noncompatible component of the existing system either has not been certified because it was made before the effective date of the standard or has not been listed

as subject to the standard and was purchased as new before August 1, 1974.

Assemblers installing certified noncompatible components also must report such installation on Form FD 2579.

In addition to reporting certified component installations, the assembler of an x-ray system must notify the Bureau of Radiological Health (BRH) of evidence of noncompliance found in the system or its components. He also must report any known or suspected radiation accident arising from operation of a defective system or component.

## VARIANCES FROM THE STANDARD

At times, practitioners may identify a need for specialized equipment that does not meet all conditions of the standard. Radiation Control Act regulations permit the Bureau of Radiological Health, upon application of a manufacturer or assembler, to grant a variance to one or more provisions of the diagnostic x-ray or other electronic equipment performance standards when it is determined that:

1. The variance has limited applicability so as not to justify an amendment to the standard or [granting of a variance] is needed before an amendment can be processed.
2. The issuance of a variance is in keeping with purposes of the Act.
3. The variance either uses alternate means to provide a level of radiation safety at least equal to that provided by equipment meeting all requirements of the standard or provides for a necessary clinical application that cannot be accomplished by— or is inappropriate to—requirements of the standard.

A practitioner requiring equipment that deviates from a particular provision of the standard should request the manufacturer or assembler to obtain a variance from the Bureau of Radiological Health. Of course, if a practitioner is assembling the system, he may submit a variance request directly.

Bureau-approved variances must be published in the *Federal Register* for comment. A period of 45–90 days must be expected from the time the variance application is submitted to the date it becomes effective. Additional information on applying for a variance may be obtained from the bureau.

## Upgrading Used Equipment

The question of upgrading equipment not made under the standard has concerned the Food and Drug Administration, as well as the Congress where legislation has been introduced to require improved radiation protection capability in used x-ray machines. In 1973, FDA proposed an interpretation of the intent of the Radiation Control for Health and Safety Act regulations as requiring used x-ray equipment refurbished, rebuilt or reassembled after August 1, 1974 to comply with the standard for new equipment. The proposal was later modified, however, because of the possibility that it might cause shortages of acceptable used equipment and thus adversely affect health care.

In the end, the regulations were amended to effect a more gradual upgrading of equipment by:

1. Requiring that an x-ray system made before August 1, 1974 that is altered by installation of a certified component will thereafter have to use only certified replacement components. This provision was needed to prevent the degradation of certified systems by the installation of noncertified components.
2. Prohibiting the assembly of uncertified components into systems reassembled and sold after August 1, 1979—5 yr after the standard's effective date. Components not certified under the standard will have to be replaced in such systems.

The 5-yr grace period for application of the standard to reassembled equipment al-lows time for adequate inventories of certified components to be purchased. Furthermore, the period conforms with estimates of the approximate time it will take certified equipment to move into the used x-ray market from hospital radiology departments and other high work load facilities.

In conclusion to this presentation of Federal diagnostic x-ray equipment standards, it should be emphasized that in addition to these requirements, most all state radiation control departments have separate requirements relating to the installation and maintenance of x-ray equipment. These requirements are to be considered in *addition to* the foregoing Federal requirements and must also be taken into consideration.

## References

1. Howe JW, Stowe RS: *Basic X-Ray Physics and Principles of X-Ray Protection.* Lombard, Ill, National College of Chiropractic, 1977, pp 64–95.
2. Ter-pogassian MM: *The Physical Aspects of Diagnostic Radiology.* New York, Harper & Row, 1967, pp 64–95.
3. Schulz RJ: *A Primer of Radiation Protection.* New York, General Analine and Film Corporation, 1962, pp 2–9.
4. Hildebrandt RW: Applications of the international system of units (SI) in the health professions. *J Manipulative Physiol Ther* 2:114–119, 1979.
5. Wyckoff HO: Report of the International Commission on Radiation Units and Measurements. *Radiology* 127:549–552, 1978.
6. *The SI for the Health Professions*: Geneva; World Health Organization, 1975.
7. Jacobi CA, Paris DQ: *Textbook of Radiologic Technology.* St. Louis, Mosby, 1972. pp 62–68.
8. *Basic Radiation Protection Criteria*, NCRP Report No. 39. Washington, DC, National Council on Radiation Protection, 1974.
9. *Gonadal Shielding in Diagnostic Radiology.* DHEW Publication (FDA) 74-8028. Washington, DC, Bureau of Radiological Health, June, 1974.
10. *A Practitioner's Guide to the Diagnostic X-Ray Equipment Standard.* HEW Publication (FDA) 78-8050. Washington, DC, Bureau of Radiological Health, February, 1978.

# CHAPTER 4

# Spinographic Technology and Positioning

## SPINOGRAPHIC X-RAY SYSTEMS

A spinographic x-ray system basically consists of a standard x-ray generator and an upright full spine Bucky-grid component. In some cases, a sitting component may be included for specific radiography of the cervico-occipital complex, and a radiographic table for general diagnostic procedures. In order to insure the best possible technical results, each of these components must meet certain specific, rigid specifications of design, construction and installation.

### X-Ray Generator Unit

Full spine x-ray procedure is unquestionably the most difficult of all skeletal radiography procedures and, accordingly, requires an x-ray generator of sufficient capacity to do the job properly. A 300-mA, 125-kVp generator, equipped with a rotating anode x-ray tube, is the minimum recommended capacity. Additionally, the x-ray generator component of the spinographic x-ray system should incorporate certain requirements of design and installation, and include certain accessory equipment.

### X-RAY TUBESTAND

The x-ray tube should be mounted on a well designed and constructed *floor-to-ceiling* tubestand which allows for accurate alignment of the tube to the Bucky-grid component(s) and is capable of maintaining such alignment through the full range of vertical and horizontal travel (Fig. 4.1). The need and desire for such specificity of alignment should be impressed on the supplier at the time of purchase and, again, on the installer at the time of delivery.

### COLLIMATOR

The x-ray tube must be equipped with a good quality collimator, which meets approved x-ray equipment standards, and which projects a manually adjustable rectangular light beam to a 14 × 36-in (35.6 × 91.4-cm) radiographic field at a 72-in (1.8 m) focal-film distance (FFD). The collimator must be equipped with a minimum of 2-mm filtration (preferably 4–5-mm filtration in chiropractic full spine procedure). The collimator mirror must be adjusted to ensure accurate light/x-ray field congruance.

### COMPENSATING FILTERS

The use of compensating filters for attachment to the collimator in full spine radiography procedure is an absolute requisite for proper quality control and for reducing x-ray exposure to the patient. Five types of compensating filter systems are considered: the *Sportelli wedge*, the *Nolan multiple x-ray filter system*, *Siemans compensating mask*, *Gilardoni* total body radiography (GTBR) *homograph* and the *Victoreen-Nuclear Clear-Pb*® *filter*.

#### Sportelli Wedge System

The *Sportelli Wedge* compensating system is composed of a clear plastic backplate

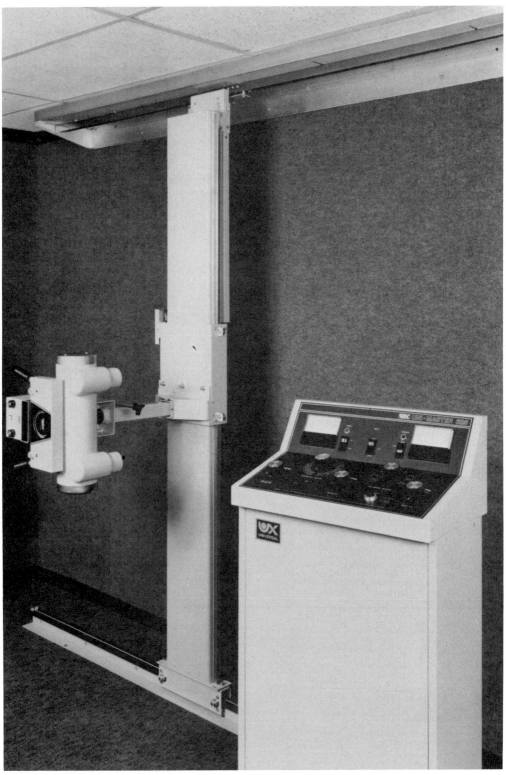

**Figure 4.1.**   Standard floor-to-ceiling tubestand which allows for precisely aligned movement of the x-ray tube, vertically and horizontally, relative to the center of the Bucky-grid unit. (Courtesy of the Universal X-Ray Company.)

(for permanent mounting on the collima-tor) into which one of two filters compo-nents may be inserted—the *anteroposterior* (AP) and *lateral* (1). The anteroposterior component is comprised of a clear plastic holder with a permanently attached alu-minum *base* filter and two wedge-shaped add-on filters. The lateral filter is composed of a clear plastic holder with a permanently attached bracket for insertion of up to five stainless steel add-on filters (Figs. 4.2–4.5).

Both filters are equipped with *shadow-type* gonadal shields (as opposed to more commonly used body contact shields). The anteroposterior component has two shadow gonadal shields, a small for males and a larger for females, which are selected by reversing the direction of insertion of the component into the backplate. The lateral filter component has one large shadow go-nadal shield for use on both males and females.

The anteroposterior filter component is designed for use at a 72–84-in focal-film distance and the lateral filter component is designed for use at a 40–60-in focal-film distance. When inserted into the backplate, the filter components and gonadal shields may be adjusted to a particular individual by raising or lower them in the backplate

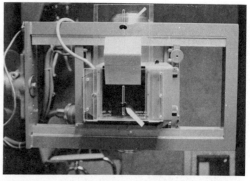

**Figure 4.3.** Collimator-mounted Sportelli wedge system set up for an AP full spine expo-sure. *Arrow* indicates gonad shield. (Courtesy of Dr. L. Sportelli.)

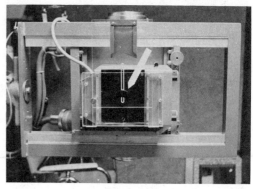

**Figure 4.4.** Collimator-mounted Sportelli wedge system set up for a lateral lumbopelvic exposure. *Arrow* indicates gonad shield. (Cour-tesy of Dr. L. Sportelli.)

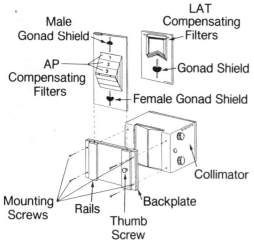

**Figure 4.2.** Schematic view of the Sportelli wedge compensating filter/gonadal shield unit for full spine and regional x-ray procedures. (Courtesy of Dr. L. Sportelli.)

as required while the collimator light is used as a positioning guide (Fig. 4.5).

According to reported phantom dosime-try studies (2), the *Sportelli wedge* system is said to be approximately equivalent to shaped body-contact gonadal shields in ef-fectiveness of radiation dose reduction (Ta-bles 4.1, 4.2). Gonadal shield transmission and undershield scatter was 15% for the AP view and 9% for the lateral view (Table 4.3) which, when adjusted for technical fac-tors, is approximately equivalent to the 92% reduction of gonadal (testes) dose cited by other studies using body-contact go-nadal shields (3, 4).

While Sportelli (and others) may rec-ommend an 84-in focal-film distance for the AP full spine projection, the generally

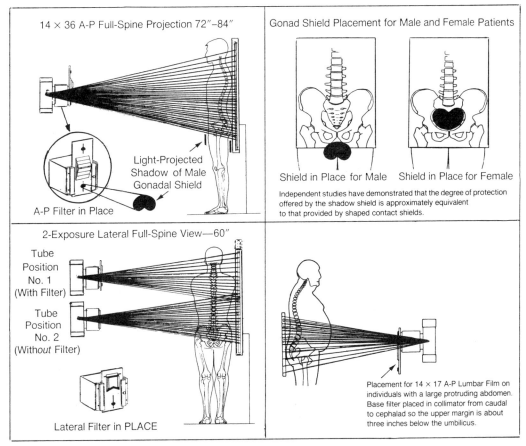

**Figure 4.5.** Application of the Sportelli wedge full spine compensating filter/gonadal shield system.

**Table 4.1.**
**ΛP full spine exposure (Sportelli wedge)**[a]

| Point | Entrance exposure | Entrance exposure with compensator | $\dfrac{\text{Compensate}}{\text{Noncompensated}} \times 100\%$ |
|---|---|---|---|
| 84 kVp, 160 mAs, 84-in SID[b] (patient thickness = 20 cm) | | | |
| Thyroid | 170 mR | 34 mR | 20% |
| Xiphoid | 196 mR | 163 mR | 83% |
| Ovaries | 200 mR | 175 mR | 88% |
| Testes | 20 mR | 17 mR | 85% |
| 92kVp, 250 mAs, 84-in SID (patient thickness = 25 cm) | | | |
| Thyroid | 362 mR | 56 mR | 15% |
| Ovaries | 420 mR | 374 mR | 89% |
| 94 kVp, 400 mAs, 84-in SID (patient thickness = 25 cm) | | | |
| Thyroid | 606 mR | 102 mR | 17% |

[a] Film size/collimator setting = 14 × 36 in (all measurements).
[b] SID, focal-film distance.

**Table 4.2.**
**Lateral full spine exposure (Sportelli wedge)[a]**

| Point | Entrance exposure | Entrance exposure with compensator | $\dfrac{\text{Compensated}}{\text{Noncompensated}} \times 100\%$ |
|---|---|---|---|
| | mR | mR | |
| 96 kVp, 160 mAs, 84-in SID[b] (patient thickness = 30 cm) | | | |
| Thyroid | 252 | 10 | 4% |
| Xiphoid | 277 | 18 | 6% |
| Ovaries | 293 | 245 | 84% |
| Testes | 25 | 15 | 60% |

[a] Film size/collimator setting = 14 × 36 in (all measurements).
[b] SID, focal-film distance.

**Table 4.3.**
**Gonadal shadow transmission (Sportelli wedge)**

| Compensator type | Exposure without shield[a] | Exposure with shield[a] | Transmission[b] |
|---|---|---|---|
| | mR | mR | |
| AP | 561 | 85 | 15% |
| Lateral | 561 | 51 | 9% |

[a] Technic: 94 kVp, 400 mAs, 84-in SID[c] (measurement at central ray)

[b] $\text{Transmission} = \dfrac{\text{Exposure with shield}}{\text{Exposure without shield}} \times 100\%$

[c] SID, focal-film distance.

accepted chiropractic and medical standard is given as 72-in (5–8).

## Nolan Multiple Filter System

The *Nolan multiple filter* compensating system consists of a number of specially designed filters made of aluminum, copper and lead, mounted on plastic slide holders, that insert into a four-groove bracket which is permanently attached to the front of the collimator. By inserting the various filters into the holder, singularly or in series, compensating filter systems may be *constructed* which are in essence *tailored* to each particular patient (Fig. 4.6). The complete system includes a special *Accu-Rad* caliper for measuring the patient and computing the appropriate high kilovoltage (90–100 kV) radiographic technic using the "Siemans-type" point system (9).

The *Nolan multiple filter* compensating system was tested under controlled conditions at the *National Radiation Laboratory* of New Zealand and, although it was found that it took some time to learn the best arrangement of filters to use in a particular case, the full spine films were determined to be of good quality and the skin dose exposures were reduced by 95% over non-compensated technics—gonadal dose was comparable to that of shaped body-contact shields (Table 4.4) (10).

## Siemans Compensating Mask

The *Siemans compensating mask* system is comprised of two collimator-mounted, motor-driven plastic disks which are rotated during exposure so as to gradually introduce an ever-widening band of lead filtering into the primary x-ray beam in such a manner as to reduce exposure to the cervicothoracic area of the spine (Figs. 4.7, 4.8). Separate disks are used for the AP and lateral views. To allow for various patient heights, the rotating mask is arranged at the correct distance from the x-ray tube focal spot with the aid of the collimator light.

The *Siemans compensating mask* system is designed to be used with a heavy-duty, *three-phase* x-ray generator and an elaborate standing Bucky grid unit (discussed later) which permits taking AP and lateral full spine views in single exposures at 8 ft 2-in to 13 ft 2-in (2.5–4-m) focal-film distance (Fig. 4.9). Although the complete Sie-

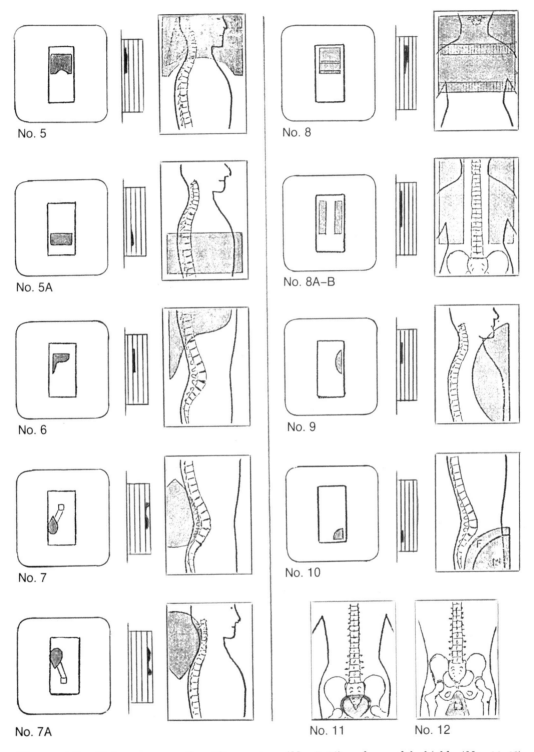

**Figure 4.6.** Nolan compensating filter system (*No. 5–10*) and gonadal shields (*No. 11–12*). Additional compensating filters (*No. 1–4*) are used for variations in average body build. (Courtesy of Dr. J. R. Nolan.)

**Table 4.4.**
**Dose reduction with the Nolan multiple filters system**

| Technic | Filter combination number used | SID[b] | Dose for filtered technic as %-age of dose for unfiltered technic at same setting[a] | | | |
|---|---|---|---|---|---|---|
| | | | Bone marrow | Skin | Ovaries | Testes |
| | | (m) | | | | |
| AP full spine | 3, 8, 8B Female gonad shield | 2 | 55 | 15 | 40 | — |
| AP full spine | 3, 8, 8B Male gonad shield | 2 | 65 | 15 | — | 15 |
| AP cervical thoracic | 3, 8, 8B | 2 | 25 | 15 | — | — |
| Lateral cervical thoracic | 2, 3, 5, 5A, 9 | 2 | 35 | 5 | — | — |

[a] Values have been rounded to next 5% level.
[b] SID focal-film distance.

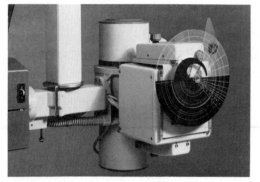

**Figure 4.7.** Siemans compensating mask system. (Courtesy of the Siemans X-ray Co.)

mans system obviously produces full spine films of excellent quality, no information was provided regarding radiation exposure doses—it may, however, be conjectured that they are quite low in consideration of (a) the compensating mask system, (b) the long focal-film distances used, (c) high kVp technics possible with the three-phase x-ray generator, and (d) special radiation barrier shields mounted on the Bucky-grid unit.

## Gilardoni Total Body Radiography (GTBR) System

The *Gilardoni total body radiography* (GTBR) system is comprised of an AP or lateral "homograph" which is inserted into

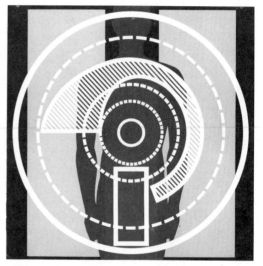

**Figure 4.8.** Schematic view of the Siemans compensating mask system. (Courtesy of the Siemans X-ray Co.)

a holder mounted on a slider guide that allows for distance adjustments relative to the collimator and to the focal-spot/central ray and, thus, allows for adjustment of the *homograph* to a specific focal-film distance and patient height (Fig. 4.10). Gonadal shielding may be incorporated and additional aluminum filters may be added where unusual body-build conditions require—such as in cases of extreme differences in body thickness and/or density.

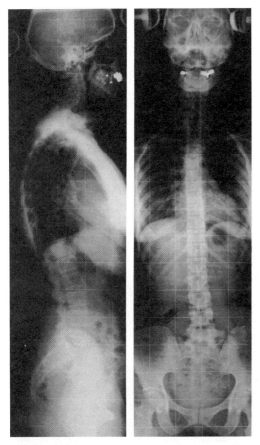

**Figure 4.9.** Lateral and AP full spine views, each taken in a single exposure at a very long focal-film distance using the Siemans compensating mask and Bucky-grid system.

The uniqueness of the GTBR system lies particularly in the design of the *homographs* that are 80 × 200 × 35-mm blocks which incorporate AP or lateral x-ray-absorptive "phantoms" that duplicate (in reduced size) the different parts of the body that may require more or less exposure to produce a "homogenized" film image (Fig. 4.11).

Exposure with the GTBR system on a "normotype" patient is about 50 mAs/100 kVp at an 80-in (2-m) focal-film distance. Exposure skin doses in such a case have been given as 250 mR to the pelvis, 150 mR to the skull and 15 mR to the lungs (Table 4.5).

### Victoreen-Nuclear Clear-Pb® Filter

The *Clear Pb®* compensating system is comprised of a 6½-in (16-cm) wide by 5½-in (14-cm) long by ¼-in (0.635-cm) thick clear plastic *filter holder* attached to a 12 × 12 × ¹⁄₁₆-in (30.5 × 30.5 × 0.16-cm) *mounting plate* (which may be cut to fit collimator accessory trays) on which the *filters, gonad shield* and *breast/lung/paraspinal shields* are attached to two steel rails on the holder with magnetic mounting strips. The filters (72-in AP/PA wedge, 40-in AP/PA wedge, lateral cervical and thoracic) are made of Clear-Pb® lead plastic (30% lead by weight) with 1-in (2.54-cm) wide magnetic mount-

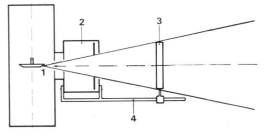

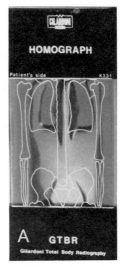
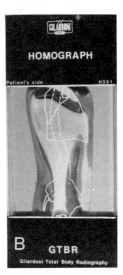

**Figure 4.10.** Gilardoni total body radiography (GTBR) compensating system; *1*, tube focal spot, *2*, collimator, *3*, homograph, *4*, homograph slider guide. *A*, anteroposterior GTBR homograph. *B*, lateral GTBR homograph. (Courtesy of Gilardoni Raggi X, Nucleari-Electromedicali.)

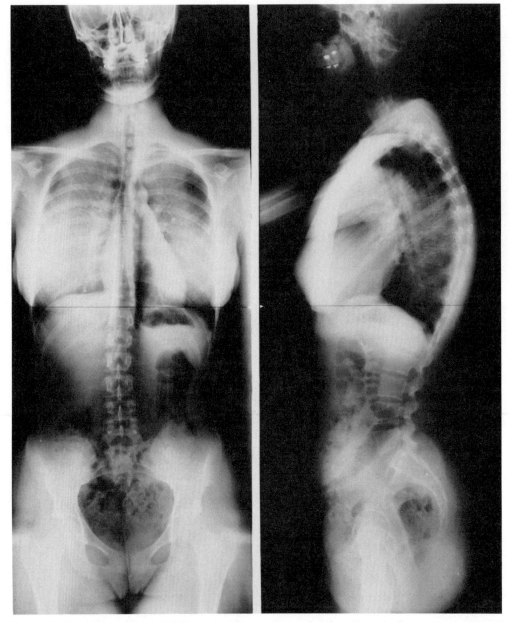

**Figure 4.11.** AP and lateral full spine radiographs, each taken in a single exposure, using the Gilardoni total body radiography (GTBR) system. (Courtesy of Gilardoni Raggi X, Nucleari-Electromedicali.)

ing strips on both sides of each end. The gonad shield is a shamrock-shaped lead insert cemented to a 6½-in long by 1-in high (16.5 × 2.54-cm) clear plastic strip with 1-in (2.54-cm) wide magnetic mounting strips on each end. The two steel breast/lung/paraspinal shields are 2-in (5.1-cm) wide and 3-in (7.6-cm) long (Fig. 4.12).

The Clear-Pb® system, because the various filters and shields are magnetically mounted on a clear plastic holder, is easily

**Table 4.5.**
**Skin and volume dose with standard radiographic unit and Gilardoni total body radiography (GTBR) system (indicative values).**[a,b]

| Technic | Part | Thickness | Grid | FFD | Exposure (rare earth screens) | | HVL Al | Skin dose R[c] | Vol l[d] | Vol dose R-l[e] | THVL |
|---------|------|-----------|------|-----|------|------|--------|-----------|--------|--------|------|
| | | cm | | cm | kVp | mAs | mm | | | | cm |
| Standard | Pelvis (35 × 35 cm) | 20 | Yes | 100 | 70 | 50 | 2 | 0.6 | 24 | 5 | 4.0 (Large field) |
| GTBR | Trunk (35 × 86 cm) | 20 | Yes | 200 | 100 | 50 | 3 | 0.12 Medium | 50 | 2 | 4.5 (Large field) |

[a] GTBR exposure on normotype patient is about 50 mAs with 100 kV and skin dose in correspondence with pelvis about 250 mR, skull 150 mR, lungs 15 mR (medium ~0.12 R).

[b] The abbreviations used are: FFD, focal-film distance; HVL, half-value layer; Al, aluminum; R, roentgen; THVL, total HVL; R-l, roentgen per liter.

[c] GTBR reduces skin dose about 5 times and volume dose about 2.5 times compared with those of standard radiograph through areas and volumes of homogenized total body are about 2 times greater; this is due to the selective prefiltration of different parts (homogenization).

[d] Individual volume dose delivered by natural radioactive background in Mandello Lario, Italy (location of test) is about 35 R-l/yr (60 $\mu$R/h).

[e] Volume dose in R per liter = skin dose (R)x-irradiated part volume (dm$^3$).

adjustable to desired AP/PA and lateral configurations using the collimator light as a guide. According to studies conducted with such lead acrylic type filters (11, 12), the Clear-Pb® system is an effective means of full spine radiographic quality and x-ray exposure control (Tables 4.6–4.8).

(Note: Except for the Siemans compensating mask system on which no data was provided, all of the compensating systems described appear more or less equally effective in reducing radiation exposure to patients in full spine radiography. Depending upon technic factors and care in use, each are also capable of producing good quality, full spine radiographs. The major deciding factors in selection, then, appear mainly related to (a) suitability to a particular x-ray unit and technic procedures, (b) ease of use, and (c) cost.)

### Bucky-Grid Units

The upright, full spine Bucky-grid component of the spinographic x-ray system should be designed to accommodate 14 × 36-in (35.6 × 91.4-cm) and smaller size cassettes; fitted with at least a 10:1 ratio grid (preferably fine-line, stationary) with an approximate focal range of 40–72 in (102–183 cm) and fitted with suitable immobilization devices (Fig. 4.13).

The most elaborate such Bucky-grid unit presently available is the *Siemans*: designed to accept 12 × 36-in (30.5 × 91.4-cm) cassettes; equipped with both immobilization clamps and abdominal compression band; utilizes two primary-ray barrier shields; and is capable of producing excellent anteroposterior and lateral standing full spine radiographs in a single exposure each (Figs. 4.14, 4.15). However, because of the long focal-film distance used, a three-phase x-ray generator is required, thus the complete Siemans system may be cost prohibitive ($125,000-plus) except for large clinic or hospital installations.

Installation of the full spine Bucky-grid unit should give due consideration to two important requisites—it should be positionally oriented to the x-ray tube so as to take proper advantage of the *anode heel effect*, and it should be mounted on a level floor or platform in strict alignment with the central x-ray beam to affect necessary *gravitational-projectional constants*.

The positional orientation of the full spine Bucky grid to the x-ray tube to take advantage of the anode heel effect is a radiographic quality control consideration

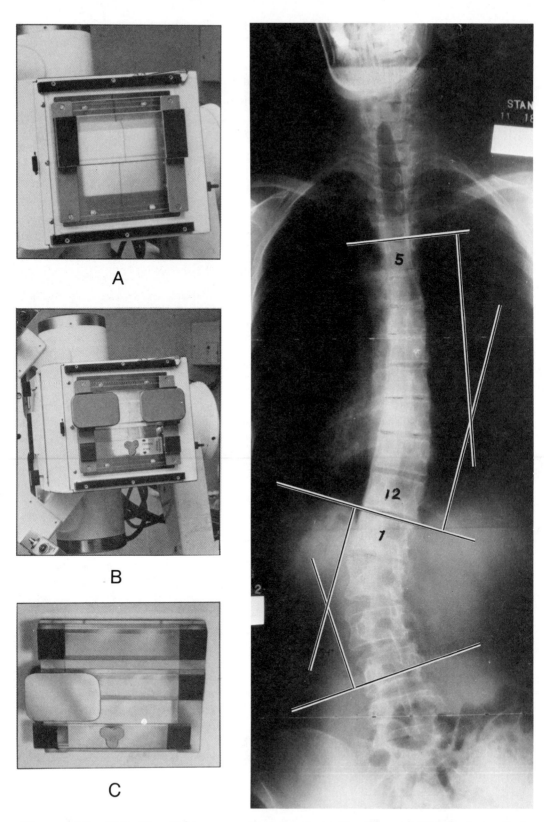

**Figure 4.12.** *Right*, Clear Pb® transparent x-ray compensating filter and AP full spine scoliosis screening film. *Left*, clear Pb units; *A*, illustrating magnetic filter mounting system; *B*, set up for an AP full spine with lung/gonad shields in place; and *C*, set for a lateral full spine view. (Courtesy of Nuclear Associates, Divison of Victoreen, Inc.)

wherein, when these two components are installed so that the anode is in a cephalic position to the standing patient, there will be more uniform exposure of the film from top to bottom. This is due to the fact that the x-rays emitting from the focal spot of the tube are less intense toward the anode heel and more intense away from it, and if directed, accordingly, to the less dense thoracocervical spine area and more dense thoracolumbar spine area, improved image quality will result (Fig. 4.16).

The installation of the full spine Bucky-grid component on a level floor or platform in strict alignment with the central x-ray beam to affect gravitational-projectional constants may be further explains as follows (Fig. 4.17).

1. Because the primary objective of spinography is to evaluate the biomechanical configuration of a patient's pelvis and spinal column as the patient *naturally* assumes a certain *normal attitude* (as dictated by ves-

**Table 4.6.**
**Potential breast exposure reduction (AP projection)**

| Method | Exposure reduction |
|---|---|
| | times |
| Rare earth film/screen | 2–6 |
| Compensating filter | 2–5 |
| Breast shield (or PA | 3–10 |
| projection) | 3–12 |
| Total | ~10–35 |

**Table 4.7.**
**Compensating filter tests[a]**

| | | Patient Measurements | | | |
|---|---|---|---|---|---|
| View | Location | No filter—mean skin exposure | Number of patients | Filter—mean skin exposure | Number of patients |
| | | mR | | mR | |
| AP | Xiphoid | 126 | 3 | 22 | 7 |
| | Umbilicus | 141 | 1 | 108 | 7 |
| Lateral | Xiphoid level | 240 | 3 | 46 | 7 |

[a] Kodak RP/X-REG (14 × 17 inch), 12:1 grid, 102 kVp

**Table 4.8.**
**Exposure with compensating filter and gradient screens[a]**

| Film/screen 14 × 17 in | Compensating filter Technic (AP): single speed rare earth screens | Gradient screens Technic (AP): no filter, gradient rare earth screens |
|---|---|---|
| Grid | 12:1 | 12:1 |
| kVp | 90 | 90 |
| mAS | 50 | 64 |
| Entrance skin exposures: | | |
| Sternoclavical notch | 9 mR | 210 mR |
| Breast region | 30 mR | 210 mR |
| Xiphoid region | 40 mR | 210 mR |

[a] Measurements made using an anatomical phantom.

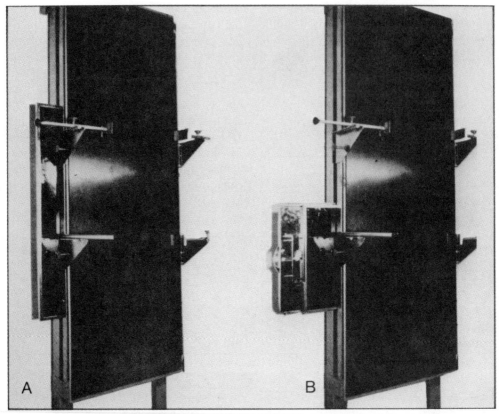

**Figure 4.13.** Standard full spine Bucky-grid unit with attached immobilization clamps. *A,* full spine cassette partially inserted in slot behind inner radiographic grid. *B,* 14 × 17-in (35.6 × 43.2-cm) cassette placed in partially inserted self-centering tray.

tibular and proprioceptive posture control mechanisms) relative to the forces of gravity being exerted on the body, it is necessary that the surface on which the patient is standing in front of the Bucky-grid unit be *level* to rule out biomechanical deviations which are normal compensations to standing on an unlevel surface. Further, the Bucky-grid unit itself must be installed on a level floor or platform in *vertical plumb* with gravity so that the film may be used as a true vertical and horizontal reference to which the inherent biomechanical configuration of the patient's pelvis and spinal column may be equated.

2. Because the patient's pelvis and spinal column are three-dimensional structures which project to the flat, two-dimensional film surface via a divergent beam of x-rays, the resultant radiographic image is magnified and distorted. Since these patterns of magnification and distortion may simulate biomechanical irregularities of the pelvis and spinal column, it is necessary

that they be ruled out in advance by proper equipment alignment.

## Cassettes, Intensifying Screens and Film

The importance of the x-ray film holder cassettes, intensifying screens and film cannot be overestimated. Without proper consideration given to these essential components, good quality full spine radiographs at minimal exposure levels to the patient *are not attainable*, regardless of the sophistication of all other components and technical efforts.

All cassettes should be in the best possible condition (not bent or dented, and without loose hinges or clamps) and should be fitted with high speed (preferably rare earth type) screens. The use of graded/gradient or split-speed screens to control film expo-

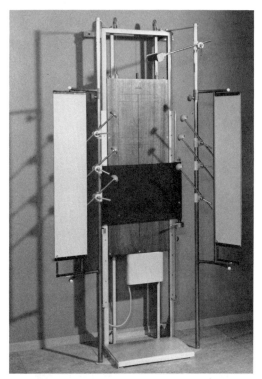

**Figure 4.14.** Siemans full spine Bucky-grid unit with immobilization clamps, compression band and primary ray barrier shields. (Courtesy of the Siemans X-Ray Co.)

sure, as has been promoted in some chiropractic and medical circles (13, 14), are to be considered unacceptable. Also, the use of *grid-lined* intensifying screens for visually equating spatial relationships or structural alignments are to be discouraged insofar as they may obscure important pathological or traumatic details (Fig. 4.9).

The film used in full spine radiographic procedures should be high speed and of proper size for the particular cassette. The use of smaller size films in full spine cassettes is to be discouraged because of the difficulties encountered in aligning each film in the cassette, the problem of taping the films together after processing, inherent viewing distractions, and possible extra cost. The practice of using smaller size films in a full spine cassette (for example: one 14 × 17 in lengthwise, one 11 × 14 in horizontally and one 8 × 10 in horizontally, or two 14 × 17 in vertically) to consolidate

required film stock, to facilitate storage, or to disguise the fact that the films were actually taken under full-spine conditions are insufficient justifications for not using the proper size films.

## INTERPRETIVE CONSIDERATIONS OF SPINOGRAPHIC POSITIONING

Previous discussion of equipment installation elaborated on the need to affect *gravitational* and *projectional constants*, the purpose being to establish bases from which the *unknown* biomechanical configuration of the patient's pelvis and spinal column may be ascertained for comparison to that which may be considered *normally correct*. Without such constants, the configurations seen on the film are ambiguous since there is no way to be certain whether deviations seen on the film are actual biomechanical irregularities or simulations of such due to improper equipment alignment and/or the effect of the patient standing on an unlevel surface.

The question now arises as to how the patient should be positioned relative to the Bucky-grid unit and x-ray tube: (*a*) in a *standardized* attitude of erect posture to

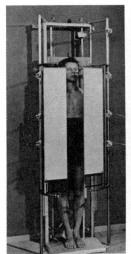
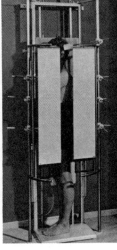

**Figure 4.15.** Positioning of patient in the Siemans full spine Bucky-grid unit for an AP and lateral view. (Courtesy of the Siemans X-Ray Co.)

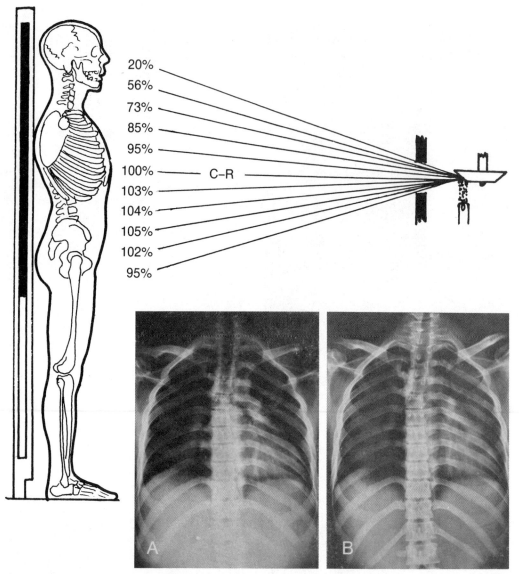

**Figure 4.16.** Anode heel effect illustrating greater intensity radiation projecting downward to the lumbopelvic area and lesser intensity radiation projecting upward to the cervicothoracic area; central ray being arbitrarily assigned 100% intensity. (Adapted from Eastman Kodak Co.)

which all patients will be required to conform, or (b) in an *individualized* attitude that a patient naturally assumes in accordance with their specific pelvic and spinal situation at the time the film is taken.

With regard to standardized positioning for all patients, it is generally accepted that any effort to impose a standard postural attitude on the patient during positioning will result in some degree of forced change in pelvic and spinal configuration; e.g. an appearance of aberrant biomechanical configuration which does not actually exist may be induced, or conditions which do exist may be eliminated.

Admittedly, there has been some degree of belief in the chiropractic profession that if a "subluxation" actually exists it will be evident regardless of how the patient is positioned—standardized or individualized

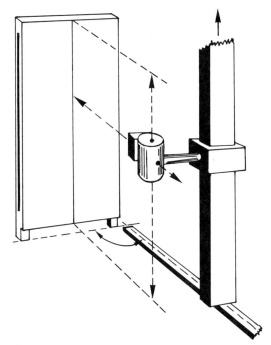

**Figure 4.17.** Installation alignment of Bucky-grid unit and floor-to-ceiling tubestand. Central ray should maintain a close-tolerance, 90° alignment to the center of the Bucky-grid unit through full ranges of horizontal and vertical travel.

posture; standing or reclining positions. Although there may be a degree of truth in this belief when a spinal subluxation is considered in its strict sense as a *fixed* misalignment, this is definitely not the case when considering it as a complex biomechanical event—*orthodysarthria*—which may encompass hypermobilities, hypomobilities and aberrant movement characteristics.

Consequently, the positioning concept whereby the patient assumes an individualized, natural, normal posture—as dictated by his/her vestibular and proprioceptive postural control senses—is preferred, regardless of whether the spinal column is relatively straight (on AP projection) or in a gross state of structural deviation. In fact, this normal positioning concept (along with equipment alignment) is the primary criterion by which diagnostic judgements may be made of a particular patient's pelvis and

spinal column. Expressed in terms of the equation, $A + B = C$; if $A$ represents the known of equipment alignment to gravity and the central x-ray beam, and $B$ represents the known of patient positioning relative to gravity and the dictates of their postural control senses, then $C$ is equal to the *difference* between the patient's actual pelvic and spinal configuration as compared to that which is considered ideal or correct—*normal*. Assuming, then, that this difference was not induced by equipment malalignment or patient malpositioning, its evaluation for evidence of biomechanical irregularities constitutes the objective of spinographic interpretation, which may be further explained by the following hypothetical examples:

1. If a patient assumes his/her natural posture between a properly aligned Bucky-grid unit and x-ray tube, and the resultant spinograph reveals a reasonably well aligned pelvis and spinal column as compared to that which is regarded as normal, it may be conjectured that there are no clinically significant biomechanical irregularities present at that point in time.
2. If a patient assumes his/her natural posture between a properly aligned Bucky-grid unit and x-ray tube, and the resultant spinograph reveals an abnormality of structural configuration as compared to that which is regarded as normal, it may be conjectured that there is a clinically significant biomechanical irregularity present at that point in time.
3. If the preceding patient undergoes an appropriate course of corrective therapy and again assumes a natural posture between a properly aligned Bucky-grid unit and x-ray tube, and the resultant spinograph reveals a return toward that which is regarded as normal, it may be conjectured that an improvement in the biomechanical status of the patient's pelvis and spinal column has occurred.

In order to affect the patient's natural posture (in accordance with the dictates of his/her vestibular and proprioceptive senses) after being placed in front of the Bucky-grid unit, the patient should be instructed to stand in that attitude which, under the circumstances of the patient's present clinical complaint, feels reasonably comfortable; *initially with eyes closed to cancel out visual interference to vestibular and proprioceptive senses.* The patient is then immobilized in that position, care being taken to avoid forcing any change in their natural posture.

## SPINOGRAPHIC POSITIONING PROCEDURES

The basic spinographic x-ray procedure is comprised of the *anteroposterior projection* (posteroanterior view) taken in the standing (or alternate, of sitting on a high stool if unable to stand without support) position in a single exposure at a 72-in (1.8-m) focal-film distance, and a *lateral projection* (left or right view as the case might be) taken in the standing (or alternate, sitting) position in two exposures at a 60-in (1.5-m) focal-film distance. The AP full spine projection may be supplemented by a *femoral head projection* taken at a 72-in (1.8-m) distance, a *sacral base projection* taken at a 40-in (1-m) distance, and an *upper cervical projection* taken at a 40-in (1-m) distance. In terms of this presentation, these five projections comprise a complete *full spine view series*; the objective of each view being as follows:

1. *Anteroposterior full spine view*—used to evaluate the lateral and rotational biomechanical characteristics of spinal vertebrae, and to make preliminary evaluations of the pelvic and upper cervical complexes.
2. *Lateral full spine view*—used to evaluate the AP (frontal plane) biomechanical characteristics of spinal vertebrae, and the pelvic and upper cervical complexes.
3. *Femoral head view*—used to determine actual femoral head level which is indicative of leg length inequality.
4. *Sacral base view*—used to evaluate the lumbosacral articulation from a projectional angle not provided by the AP full spine projection.
5. *Upper cervical view*—used to make a more precise evaluation of the upper cervical complex than is generally possible from the anteroposterior full spine view.

Ideally, all films should be taken in the patient's natural standing posture in order to demonstrate the effects of weight bearing on pelvic and spinal structures. However, in those cases where the patient may not be able to stand normally without support, taking the films with the patient in a semiseated position on a high stool is preferable to taking them in the reclining position. Although sitting on a high stool cancels out the effects of leg length inequality, the spinal column will still exhibit some degree of weight-bearing effects.

Additionally, the full spine series may be further supplemented by a specific upper cervical series taken in the seated position to make specific analyses of the upper cervical complex in accordance with certain *proprietary systems* of analysis, and various other *static* (regional views and spot films) and *kinetic* (cervical or lumbar stress films) procedures for general diagnostic purposes. However, since these procedures are highly individualized (according to a particular system of analysis or laboratory policy) and are generally covered adequately in other procedural manuals and texts, (15–17) they will not be included in this presentation.

### Positioning Criteria

The positioning for, and taking of, a full spine series is a complex procedure which must be carried out in a methodical, systematic, precise manner to insure proper results. In this context, it is very important that the technician have a clear understanding of the purpose of the films and an appreciation for the need to follow all procedures in an exacting manner. To this end, the attitude should be one which considers postural full spine radiography as a comprehensive radiological specialty in its own right; e.g. at least equivalent to such medical radiological procedures as neuroradiology, myelography, etc.

Although postural spinal radiographs are also used for general diagnostic purposes, their primary purpose is for the evaluation of biomechanical irregularities which may have clinical significance as health problems in themselves. Therefore, positioning becomes an important consideration insofar as these biomechanical impressions may be grossly varied by the manner in which the film, patient and x-ray tube are related to one another. If each are in a known position relative to one another at the time the spinograph is taken, the biomechanical impressions comprise a discernable pattern. Otherwise, the impressions will be ambiguous and of little or no value for any meaningful evaluation of biomechanical irregularities.

Previous discussion elaborated on the importance of equipment alignment and normal positioning posture. The final consideration is the technical procedures to be employed to position the patient so as to comprise a *positioning constant*. Although there may be some variation in such technical procedure between different x-ray facilities, the procedures given here have been generally recognized as the *standard* within the chiropractic profession.

## Preparatory Procedures

In consideration that full spine positioning and technical procedures is somewhat complex and time-consuming, all possible effort should be given to proper preparation so that the procedure may be carried out in a minimum period of time—the longer the time taken to position the patient the greater the possibility that fatigue will alter their normal posture. Preparation procedures include:

1. The general step-by-step procedure should be briefly explained to the patient in advance so that they may be as cooperative as possible. Ordinarily, most patients will not be aware of the nature of spinographic x-ray procedures and will be inclined to become confused unless they have some idea of what to expect.
2. The patient is provided with appropriate examination attire (gown, etc.) and instructed to remove all clothing and radiopaque objects—such objects being specifically mentioned if applicable; i.e. eyeglasses, dentures, hearing aids, hair pins, watches, necklaces, chains, orthopedic appliances, etc. Shoes are usually removed and slippers provided; if patient is fitted with orthopedic shoes this fact should be noted on the record since this information will have a bearing on inherent biomechanical and general clinical impressions.

3. The patient should be measured for all views in advance and the radiographic technics calibrated so that these factors may be set up quickly on the control panel during the positioning sequence.

## Positioning and Exposure Procedures

The following positioning and exposure procedures anticipates that the AP supplementary projections will be taken in their logical sequence following the AP full spine view. However, if they are to be omitted, the step-by-step process is picked up following AP full spine procedure, at that point which begins the lateral full spine procedure.

1. Turn on the control panel main switch and set exposure factors for the *anteroposterior full spine projection*; load 14 × 36-in (35.6 × 91.4-cm) cassette into the Bucky-grid unit; adjust focal-film distance to 72 in (1.8 m); align long axis of tubehead to vertical tube-stand column; attach required compensation filter and gonadal shield.
2. Instruct patient to: stand with his/her back toward, but not quite in contact with, the front of the Bucky-grid unit; step left or right to center hips (back of heels should be parallel with the Bucky and about 4 in apart; knees should be fully extended); close eyes and adjust body and head to a position that feels comfortable; and lean back against the Buck-grid unit. Instruct patient to hold that position while you set immobilization clamps to head, shoulders and hips, being careful not to force patient out of his/her normal posture. The patient may then be instructed to open eyes, but to hold the position.
3. Raise or lower cassette as required until horizontal center is level with the xiphoid process of the sternum; turn on collimator light and raise or lower x-ray tube until central ray is at the sternal xiphoid process; adjust horizontal shutters to include symphysis pubis and base of occiput; adjust lateral shutters to minimum area required; position compensating filter and gonadal shield using the collimator light as a guide; turn off collimator light and prepare to make exposure.
4. Instruct patient to open his/her mouth as wide as possible and *slowly* take a deep breath; make exposure at, or near, point of deepest inspiration (Fig. 4.18).

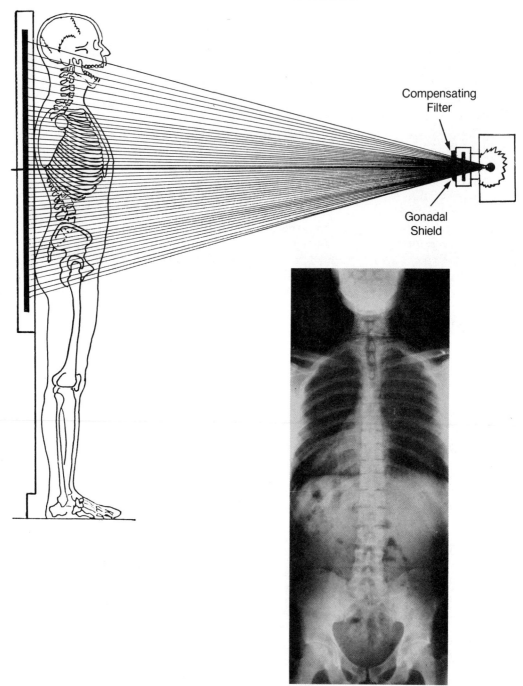

**Figure 4.18.** Anteroposterior full spine positioning and resulting posteroanterior view.

Immediately instruct patient to hold position and close mouth.

5. Set exposure factors for the *anteroposterior femoral head projection*; reload Bucky-grid unit with a 10 × 12-m (25.4 × 30.5-cm) cassette placed sideways and adjust horizontal center to approx-

imate level of the top of the femur heads; remove compensation filter from x-ray tube and readjust gonadal shield as required; collimate as required; and make exposure (Fig. 4.19). Immediately instruct patient to hold position.

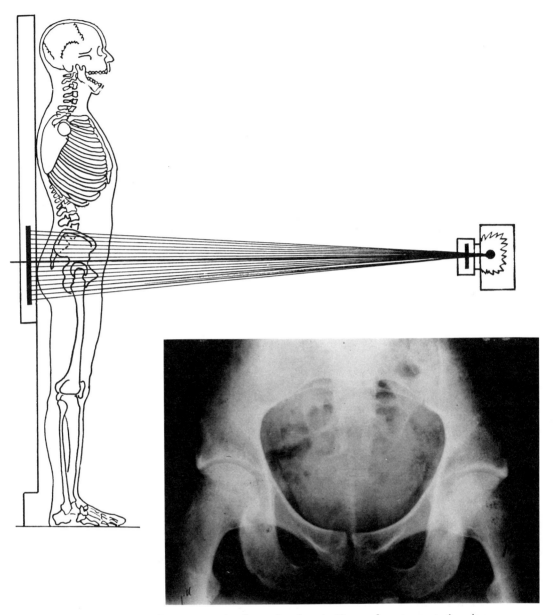

**Figure 4.19.** Anteroposterior femur head projection and posteroanterior view.

6. Set exposure factors for the *anteroposterior sacral base projection*; reload Bucky-grid with a 10 × 12-in (25.4 × 30.5-cm) cassette placed vertically and align horizontal center about 2 in (5.1 cm) above sacral base; adjust x-ray tube to a 40-in (1-m) focal-film distance at a 39° cephalic angle and lower until central ray projects approximately through lumbosacral interspace; collimate as required and readjust gonadal shield (Fig. 4.20); make

exposure and immediately instruct patient to hold position.

7. Set exposure factors for the *anteroposterior upper cervical projection*; reload Bucky-grid unit with an 8 × 10-in (20.3 × 25.4-cm) cassette placed vertically and align horizontal center 1-in (2.5-cm) above the occiput; if necessary, release immobilization clamps and have patient move feet left or right as may be required to center the midline of the head to the vertical center of the

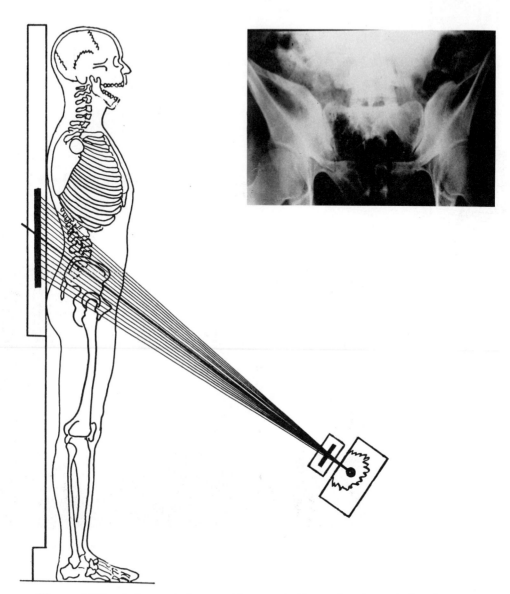

**Figure 4.20.** Anteroposterior sacral base projection and posteroanterior view.

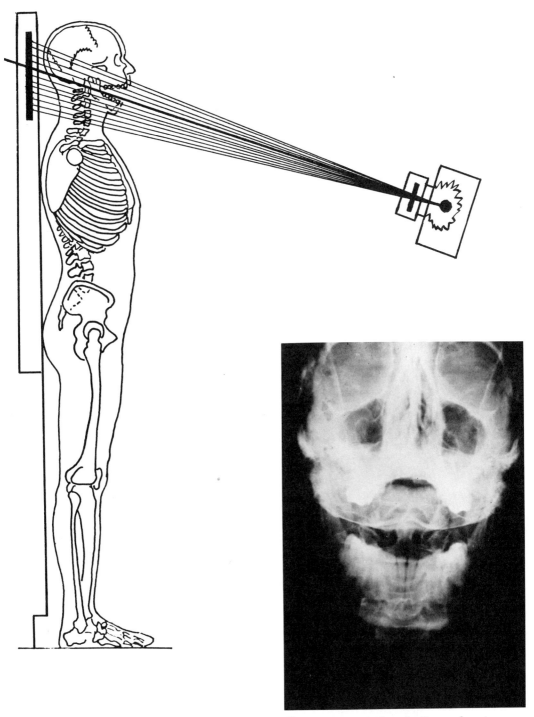

**Figure 4.21.** Anteroposterior supplementary standing upper cervical projection and posteroanterior view.

Bucky-grid unit, and reset head clamps; angle central ray about 12° cephalically and raise x-ray tube until central ray passes midpoint between the open mouth; remove gonadal shield and collimate as required; instruct patient to open mouth as wide as possible and make exposure (Fig. 4.21).

8. Set exposure factor for *thoracocervical section* of the *lateral full spine projection*; release patient from immobilization clamps; reload Bucky-grid unit with a 14 × 36-in (35.6-cm × 91.4-cm) cassette and align top edge to top of patient's ear; instruct patient to turn right or left side (whichever is most convenient for equipment installation) toward Bucky-grid unit; step forward or backward as required to center the midsagittal plane of body to vertical center of Bucky-grid unit; close eyes and adjust body and head to a comfortable position; place hands on opposite upper arms and raise away from body; set body and head immobilization clamps and instruct patient to hold position.

9. Adjust x-ray tube to a 60-in (1.5-m) focal-film distance and align long axis of x-ray tubehead to vertical tubestand column, and raise or lower as required to align central ray through 1st thoracic vertebral area; adjust the horizontal collimator shutters to include

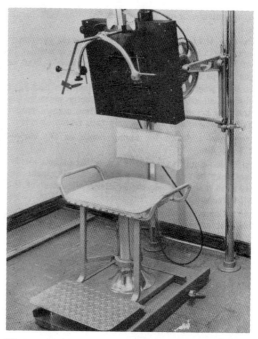

**Figure 4.23.** Upper cervical specific spinography positioning chair and tilting Bucky-grid unit.

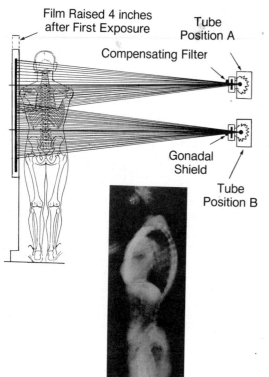

**Figure 4.22.** Right lateral two-exposure projection and left lateral view.

the occiput and the vertical shutters to minimum area as required; place compensating filter to accommodate cervical spine and make exposure; instruct patient to hold position.

10. Set exposure factors for the *lumbopelvic section* of the *lateral full spine projection*; raise cassette 4-in (10.2-cm) to allow for projectional overlap; lower x-ray tube 14-in (35.6-cm); remove compensating filters and place gonadal shield as required; adjust horizontal collimator shutters to include symphysis pubis; make exposure and release patient from immobilizaton clamps (Fig. 4.22).

## SPECIFIC UPPER CERVICAL SPINOGRAPHY

Throughout the years various specific upper cervical systems of spinography have been promoted, either as supplements to general full spine procedures or as enterpreneurial systems used as the sole application of x-ray to chiropractic biomechanical evaluations (14–16). These specific upper cervical procedures almost exclusively rely on minutely measured evaluations of

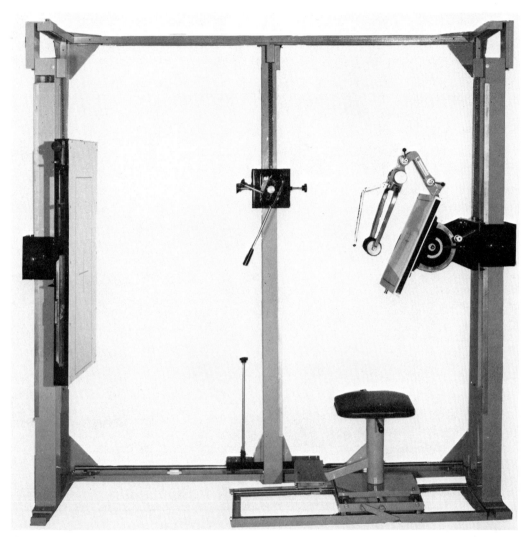

**Figure 4.24.** Constant-alignment chiropractic double L-frame spinography unit equipped for both upper cervical-specific and full spine procedures. (Courtesy of the American X-Ray Company, Inc.)

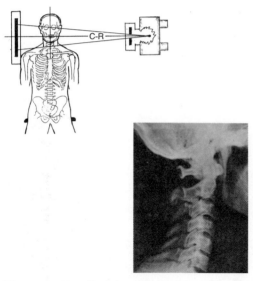

**Figure 4.25.** Left lateral specific upper cervical projection.

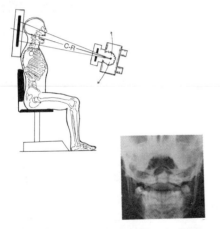

**Figure 4.26.** Anteroposterior open-mouth upper cervical specific projection and posteroanterior view.

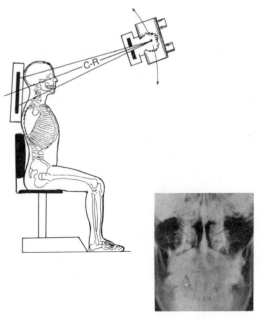

**Figure 4.27.** Anteroposterior nasium upper cervical projection and posteroanterior view.

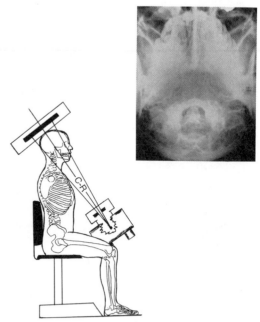

**Figure 4.28.** Inferosuperior base-posterior projection and superoinferior view.

the biomechanical relationships of the atlas relative to the occiput and/or axis, sometimes in terms of 1° or less of interarticular misalignments. Although these procedures are not included as a part of this present work, some mention of the specialized equipment used and technical procedures employed is presented here as an introduction to those who may wish to pursue further study of these methods.

Specific upper cervical procedure gener-

ally uses a specially designed positioning chair in which the patients sits and can be mechanically moved in various directions (forward, backward, sideways, and rota-

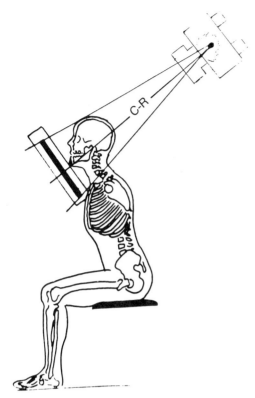

**Figure 4.29.** Upper cervical vertex projection sometimes used as an alternative to the base-posterior projection.

tionally) relative to an 8 × 10 or 10 × 12-in (20.3 × 25.4 or 25.4 × 30.5-cm) tilting Bucky-grid unit equipped with immobilizing headclamps (Figs. 4.23, 4.24). The basic procedures usually include a lateral cervical view (Fig. 4.25), a posteroanterior open mouth view (Fig. 4.26), a posteroanterior nasium view (Fig. 4.27), and a superoinferior (base posterior) view (Fig. 4.28), the latter sometimes being taken in a reverse direction as a vertex view (Fig. 4.29).

## References

1. Sportelli L: *The Wedge Filtration System: Concept and Use.* Palmerton, Penna, Sportelli, 1981.
2. Merkin JJ: *The Effect of Two New Compensating Filters on Patient Exposure in Full Spine Radiography.* Kenilworth, NJ, Bio-Med Associates, 1981.
3. Brown RF, Burnett B, Benary V: An acceptable gonadal shield. *Radiology* 99:264–269, 1971.
4. Church WW, Burnett BM: *The Clinical Testing of Male Gonad Shields, FDA 76-8025.* Washington, DC, Government Printing Office, 1975.
5. Hildebrandt RW: *Chiropractic Spinography: a Manual of Technology and Interpretation.* Des Plaines, Ill, Hilmark, 1977, pp 201–227.
6. Hoppenfeld S: *Scoliosis: a Manual of Concept and Treatment.* Philadelphia, Lippincott, 1967, pp 50–51.
7. Keim HA: Scoliosis. *Ciba Clin Symp* 30:22–24, 1978.
8. Cailliett R: *Scoliosis: Diagnosis and Management.* Philadelphia, Davis, 1975, pp 52–54.
9. Nolan JR: *Baulan Filtration System: Its Effectiveness in Patient Dose Control in Chiropractic Radiography.* Wanganui, New Zealand, Nolan, 1980.
10. Cartwright PH: The Baulan multiple filtration system: its effectiveness in patient dose control in chiropractic radiography. Christchurch, New Zealand, National Radiation Laboratory, Report NRL 1980/12, 1980.
11. Gray JE, Hoffman AD, Peterson HA: Reduction of radiation exposure during radiography for scoliosis. *J Bone Joint Surg* 65A:5–12, 1983.
12. Butler PF, Thomas AW, Gross RE: *Scoliosis Radiography: Better Images-Less Radiation.* Annual Conference of Radiation Control Program Directors. Des Moines, Iowa, Division of Intergovernmental Programs Center for Devices and Radiological Health, May 21–23, 1984.
13. Herbst RW: *Gonstead Chiropractic Science and Art.* Mt. Horeb, Wisconsin; Sci-Chi Publications, 1971.
14. Ritter EM, et al: Use of gradient intensifying screens for scoliosis radiography. *Radiology* 135:230–232, 1980.
15. Grostic JD, DeBoer KF: Roentgenographic measurement of atlas laterality: a retrospective pre- and postmanipulation study. *J Manipulative Physiol Ther* 5:63–71, 1982.
16. Pettibon BR: *Pettibon Method of Cervical X-Ray Analysis and Instrument Adjusting.* Tacoma, Wash, Pettibon, 1968.
17. Mears DB: *The Mears Technique.* St. Albans, Vt, Mears, 1976.

# PART 2

# ESSENTIALS OF SPINOGRAPHIC ANATOMY AND BIOMECHANICS

# CHAPTER 5

# Development of the Spinal Column and Pelvis

## GENERAL TOPOGRAPHY OF THE SPINAL COLUMN

The spinal column is the flexible *axial* support structure on the musculoskeletal system which initially consists of 33 vertebral segments distributed to five spinal column regions—7 cervical, 12 thoracic, 5 lumbar, 5 sacral and 4 coccygeal. With later fusion of the sacral and coccygeal segments into two composite units, the normal adult spinal column is comprised of 26 individual components (1–3).

During the fetal stage of development, the spinal column as viewed from the side describes a single posterior or *primary* curve and at the time of birth assumes a double posterior curve, one for the sacrum and one for the spine itself, with a sharp anterior or *secondary* curve at the lumbosacral junction. A second anterior curve develops in the cervical region at about 2–3 months after birth as the infant starts to hold its head erect. Finally, as the child begins to stand upright in the natural human bipedal attitude, an anterior lumbar curve begins to develop; after which the spinal column begins to assume its normal adult configuration of two primary (posterior) curves in the thoracic and sacral regions and two secondary (anterior) curves in the cervical and lumbar regions. The secondary or anterior spinal curves are also referred to as *compensatory* curves because of their development as a postural requirement of biped human beings (Figs. 5.1, 5.2).

When viewed from the anterior or posterior, the spinal column is relatively straight and progressively wider toward the caudal direction in order to sustain the increasing bilateral weight placed upon it in the postural or standing state. The sacrum, it will be noted, is a triangular-shaped structure which presents a *keystone wedge* between the ilia of the pelvic innominate bones and provides a somewhat level, stable base for the spine above.

The average length of the adult spinal column as a whole is approximately 28 in (71.1 cm) in the male and 25 in (63.5 cm) in the female, of which approximately one-fourth is taken up by the intervertebral disks (IVDs) which are fibrocartilaginous pads that separate the vertebrae and function as *shock absorbers*. These measurements will normally show morning-to-evening variations of as much as ¾ in (2 cm) due to postural compression of the IVDs. This decrease in length ordinarily corrects itself by the normal 6–8 h of nightly rest.

The overall length of the spinal column will also decrease with age; as much as 1 in (2.54 cm) due to what might be considered normal dehydration and thinning of the IVDs. Additional decreases of an indeterminant amount may also occur with age due to some actual compression of the vertebral bodies and increases in the magnitude of the normal anteroposterior spinal curves. These decreases of spinal column length with age, for all practical purposes, are permanent.

Relative to this topographical description of the spinal column, the chiropractic profession has generally held to certain distinctions in terminology which should be noted here for future reference. First, the

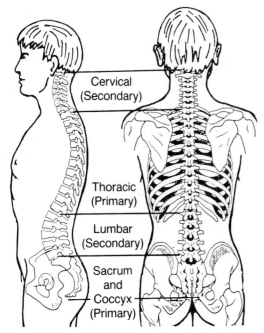

**Figure 5.1.** Lateral and posterior view of the spinal column illustrating major regional divisions.

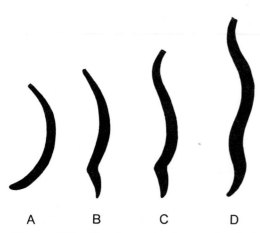

**Figure 5.2.** Development of normal spinal curves. *A*, single primary curve as appearing in the fetal stage; *B*, development of the lumbosacral secondary curve at time of birth; *C*, development of the cervical secondary curve at 1–2 yr; and *D*, adult configuration.

term *spine* is usually reserved for the 24 movable segments of the cervical, thoracic and lumbar regions (true vertebrae) while the term *spinal column* includes the sacrum and coccyx (false vertebrae). Second, the term *curve* is reserved to describe the nor-

mal anteroposterior deviations while the term *curvature* applies to abnormal deviations in any direction; i.e. *scoliosis* (left or right lateral), *kyphosis* (posterior) and *lordosis* (anterior) (4).

## CHIROPRACTIC CONCEPTS RELATED TO SPINAL DEVELOPMENT

The earliest musculoskeletal structures are recognized as dense concentrations of mesenchymal tissue cells which tend to take the shape of the bones they will become. Each mesenchymal *model* is converted to bone either directly or by first being converted into cartilage. Each unit develops most actively during specific periods and it is at such times that development is susceptible to external toxic influences, such as German measles contracted by the mother during pregnancy which may later result in developmental variations of the fetus.

Regardless of whether these developmental variations may manifest themselves as almost imperceptible bilateral asymmetries or gross malformations, it is accepted that each person develops individually and no two people are exactly alike. However, the role of such developmental variations as they may relate to the biomechanical efficiency of the spinal column in later life is a matter of some conjecture and difference of opinion in the chiropractic profession.

On one hand, there is a point of view that such developmental variations most certainly do have some detrimental effects on the structural and functional efficiency of the spinal column, the degree of effect depending proportionally on the magnitude of the anomaly. On the other hand, there is also a point of view that as a structural variation develops, the body also develops a *built-in* compensation to it and, therefore, does not result in a significant structural-biomechanical problem to that individual. As in many such divergent points of view, the truth probably lies at some point in between.

In any case, since such developmental variations do have a profound effect on spinographic analysis and interpretation procedure, it is important that some consideration be given here to the normal and abnormal development of the spinal column. Also, since this information may be new to some students of chiropractic x-ray procedure, a somewhat detailed introductory study of normal spinal anatomy is considered appropriate.

## MORPHOGENESIS OF THE SPINAL COLUMN

The musculoskeletal system in general develops from 38 pairs of mesenchymal tissue *somites* which lie posterolaterally to the *notochord*, which is a transient (temporary) axial support structure of embryonic mesodermal tissue located in the posteromedian line of the embryo between the *neural tube* and *primitive gut*, extending from the region of the future sphenoid bone of the skull to the coccygeal area. The somites, which appear at about the 4th week of fetal development, are distributed as follows: 1 pair for the occiput; 7 pair for the cervical vertebrae; 12 pair for the thoracic vertebrae; 5 pair for the lumbar vertebrae; 5 pair for the sacrum; and 8 pair for the coccyx, of which only 4 pair usually develop.

Each somite is composed of a *dermomyotome* which gives rise to the development of the musculature and connective tissue of

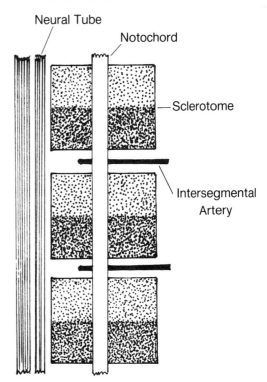

**Figure 5.4.** Initial stage of sclerotome development of vertebrae illustrating less dense cephalic portion and more dense caudal portion with intersegmental artery between anlage bodies.

the skin, and a *sclerotome* which gives rise to the development of the vertebrae and costal processes by a process of "migration" to surround the notochord from each side (Fig. 5.3). The migrated sclerotomes then undergo development into vertebrae by a three-phase process; the *mesodermal* (membranous) stage, the *chondrification* (cartilaginous) stage, and the *ossification* (bone-forming) stage.

### Mesodermal Stage of Vertebral Development

Initially, after migration to surround the notochord, the mesenchymal tissue cells of the sclerotomes undergo condensation and differentiate into a dense caudal and less dense cephalic portion separated by an intersegmental artery (Fig. 5.4). The sclerotomes then recombine, with the caudal portion of each uniting with the cephalic por-

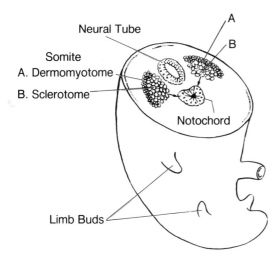

**Figure 5.3.** *Somite* development and migration of the *sclerotomes* to surround the *notochord* at the earliest stage of vertebral development.

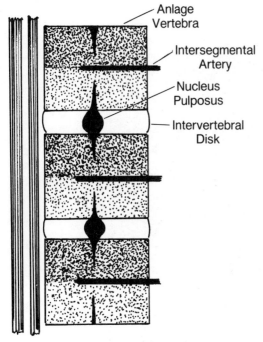

**Figure 5.5.** Recombined sclerotomes illustrating anlage vertebral bodies, rudimentary disk, and intersegmental artery now situated between the now more dense cephalic portion and now less dense caudal portion.

tion of the unit below; the intersegmental artery then being located between the now dense cephalic and less dense caudal portions (Fig. 5.5).

Following this recombination of the sclerotomes, a rapid growth of the mesoderm takes place in three directions: (*a*) medially around the notochord from the less dense caudal portion to begin formation of the vertebral body, (*b*) posteriorly around the neural tube from the more dense cephalic portion to begin formation of the neural arches composed of the pedicles and lamina, and (*c*) laterally from the more dense cephalic portion to begin formation of the costotransverse processes (Fig. 5.6).

As this development proceeds, the notochord becomes more and more compressed and squeezed between the two lateral halves of the anlage vertebral body, and begins displacement into the intervertebral spaces where remnants will persist as the nucleus pulposus of the IVD (Fig. 5.7).

## Chondrification Stage of Vertebral Development

Near the end of the 4th fetal week of development, the membranous vertebrae begin transformation into cartilage from four *centers of chondrification*; one in each half of the vertebral body lateral to the notochord, and one in each half of the neural arch. These four centers gradually enlarge and fuse about the 9–10th week of fetal development, but for a time a remnant of the notochord is left in the center of the body. This remnant is referred to as the *mucoid streak* and is continuous with those remnants that were forced into the IVD spaces.

During this same period of development the IVDs are supplied with blood vessels, some of which pass through the cartilaginous plates surrounding the nucleus pulposus, along with the notochordal remnants. These vessels and notochordal remnants regress shortly after birth; however, defects in chondrification are left in this area of the plates. These defects allow for a weakness that may persist throughout life, thus disposing to possible *herniation* of the nucleus pulposus into the vertebral

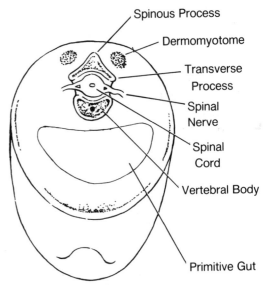

**Figure 5.6.** Membranous vertebra at about the end of the 4th fetal week of development.

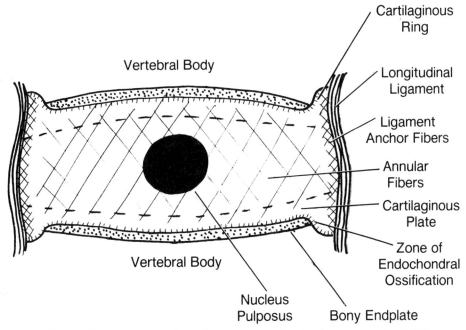

**Figure 5.7.** Cross-section of a completely developed intervertebral disk.

bodies creating cavities which are called *Schmorl's nodes*.

## Ossification Stage of Vertebral Development

Transformation of the cartilaginous vertebrae into bone begins typically by way of three *primary* centers of ossification; one in each vertebral body and one in each half of the neural arch which includes the pedicles, lamina and costal processes. The earliest primary ossification begins in the lower cervical region at about the 9–11th week of fetal development, by the 5th month have involved all but the sacral vertebrae and, by the time of birth, three distinct islands of primary ossification may be seen radiographically (Fig. 5.8). Full union of these primary centers is not complete until several years after birth.

At about the age of puberty, nine *secondary* centers of ossification appear; one at the caudal and cephalic aspects of each vertebral body, one in each half of the neural arches, and one in each articular process. These centers gradually close (unite with the primary centers to fuse the

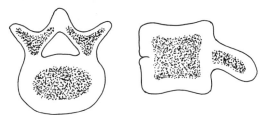

**Figure 5.8.** Primary centers of ossification which may be radiographically demonstrated at various stages between the 9th fetal week and birth.

cartilage plates to the vertebral bodies and complete the appendicular processes of the neural arches) at about the age of 19–25 yr; females about 1 yr earlier than males (Figs. 5.9–5.11).

## Development of the Skeletal Appendices

The spinal column and cranium are referred to as the *axial skeleton*; whereas the pectoral and pelvic girdles, along with the attached appendices (upper and lower extremities) are referred to as the *appendicular skeleton*. The appendicular skeleton is

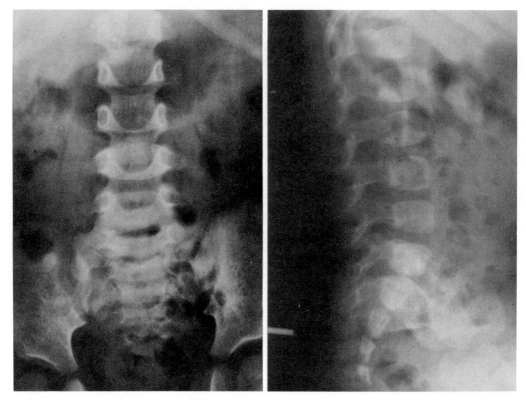

**Figure 5.9.** Radiographs illustrating appearance of primary centers at about the age of 2 yr.

derived directly from the unsegmented somatic mesenchyme. Definite masses are formed at the sites of the future pectoral and pelvic girdles and limb buds. This is followed by the sequence of bone development through cartilaginous and osseous stages (5).

The *clavicle* is the first bone of the appendicular skeleton to ossify. Before ossification a peculiar tissue resembling both membranous and cartilaginous tissue makes it difficult to classify the origin. Two primary centers of ossification appear.

The *scapula* is a single plate with two chief centers of ossification and several epiphyseal centers which appear later. An early primary center forms the body and spine of the scapula. The other, after birth, gives rise to the coracoid process.

The *humerus, radius* and *ulna* all ossify from a single primary center in the diaphysis and an epiphyseal center at each end. Additional epiphyseal centers are constant at the lower end of the humerus. Each

carpel bone ossifies from a single center. The *metacarpals* ossify from a single primary center and an epiphyseal center.

The *innominate bones* ossify from three main centers for each ilium, ischium and pubes. The three elements join at a cupshaped depression, the *acetabulum*, which is the articulation for the head of the femur. At first, the cartilaginous plate of the pelvis lies perpendicular to the vertebral column; later it rotates to a position parallel with the vertebral column and in relation to the first three sacral vertebrae, at which point the *sacroiliac articulations* are formed.

### Development of Joints

Articulations or joints are the functional interconnections between the different bones of the skeleton. In some of the articulations the bones are held together by *immovable* attachments, as in the sutures or articulations between practically all bones of the skull, in which case the bones

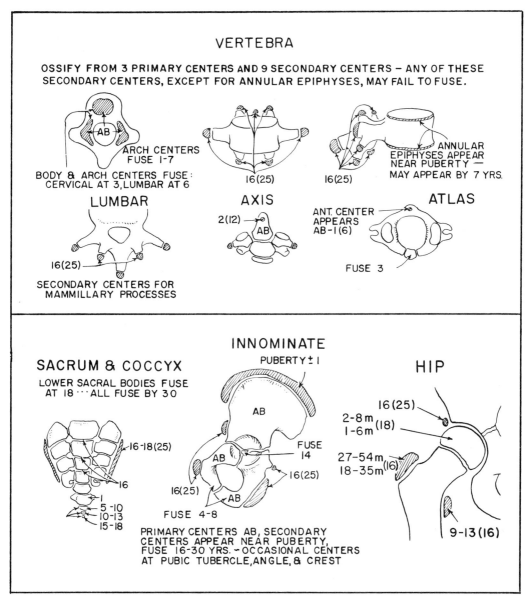

**Figure 5.10.**  Age in years of appearance and closure (in parens) of the secondary centers of ossification. (Adapted from Girdany and Golden; *American Journal of Roentgenology* 68:922–923, 1952.)

are separated merely by a thin layer of fibrous membrane called the suture ligament. Where *slight movement* combined with great strength is required, the osseous surfaces are united by tough and elastic fibrocartilages, as in the joints between the vertebral bodies (intervertebral disks) and the interpubic bodies of the pelvic innominate bones. In the *freely movable* joints the bony surfaces are completely separated; the bones forming the articulation are ex-

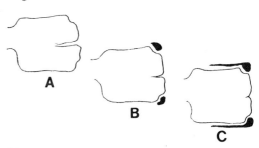

**Figure 5.11.**  Normal radiographic appearance of secondary centers of ossification. *A*, under 6 yr; *B*, 6–9 yr; *C*, 9–15 yr.

panded for greater convenience of mutual connection, covered by cartilage and enveloped by capsules of fibrous tissue which are lined with a lubricating synovia fluid-secreting membrane. These freely movable joints are strengthened by strong fibrous bands called ligaments. An immovable joint is called a *synarthrosis*; a slightly movable joint is called a *diarthrosis*; a freely movable joint is called an *amphiarthrosis*.

The mesoderm from which the different parts of the skeleton are formed shows no initial differentiation into masses corresponding with the individual bones; the continuous cores of mesoderm form the axes of the limb buds and a continuous column of mesoderm form the future vertebral column. The intervening noncondensed portions consist at first of undifferentiated mesoderm, which may develop in one of three directions—converted into fibrous tissue, as with the sutures of the skull; converted into cartilage, as with the joints between the vertebral bodies; or converted into membrane (synovia), as with the articulations between the spinal articular facets.

## TYPICAL AND ATYPICAL DEVELOPMENT OF VERTEBRAE

Although there are, of course, a number of variations in the development of vertebrae between the different spinal regions and of specific vertebrae within those regions, all vertebrae do have certain common characteristics which may or may not similarly develop; i.e. all vertebrae have one body (or centrum), two pedicles, two lamina, four articular processes, two costal-transverse processes, and one spinous process. These components of a composite vertebra are schematically described as follows (Fig. 5.12):

1. The *vertebral body* (centrum, corpus vertebrae) is a columnar structure somewhat representative of a long bone in that it is concave on its sides (except at its dorsal aspect which is flattened to form the ventral or anterior border of the neural canal) and supports an epiphyseal plate on its caudal and cephalic ends. The vertebral body is generally wider than it is deep, and constitutes the weight-bearing portion of the vertebra when the spinal column is in the upright standing posture.

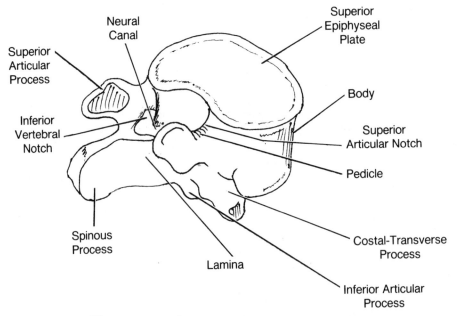

**Figure 5.12.**   Components of a composite vertebra.

2. The *pedicles* (roots, radices arci vertebrae) are two short columns of bone which project dorsally from each side of the body to form the lateral aspect of the neural canal on each side. Each pedicle has a groove on its caudal and cephalic aspects—the vertebral notch—which form the caudal and cephalic borders of the intervertebral foramen when two vertebrae are in articulated relation to one another. The caudal vertebral notches are generally deeper than the ones on the cephalic aspects of the pedicles.

3. The *lamina* are two plates of bone extending dorsomedially from the pedicles to join in the posterior midline—the junction of the lamina. The lamina are generally longer than the pedicles, form the dorsomedial border of the neural canal, and are somewhat more flattened.

4. The *articular processes* arise from the caudal and cephalic aspects of the lamina-pedicle junctions on each side and constitute support structures for the articular facets or zygapothyses. The cephalic facets (prezygapothyses) generally face dorsally and the caudal facets (postzygapothyses) generally face ventrally.

5. The *costal-transverse processes* are extensions of bone projecting laterally from the neurocentral junction of the vertebral bodies and pedicles. In the cervical, lumbar and sacral regions the costal processes are united to the transverse processes, while in the thoracic region the costal processes are separated from the transverse processes to form the ribs (Fig. 5.13).

As a whole, the human spinal column is designed to allow the body to function in an upright standing, bipedal, attitude and each specific region within it is differentially developed in accordance with the role it will eventually play in that effort; i.e. the *cervical spine* to give support and mobility to the head, the *thoracic spine* to give rigidity to the upper trunk and fulcrum attachment for the ribs, the *lumbar spine* to give strong but mobile support to the spine above and to play a principal role in the bipedalism of man, and the *sacrum* to provide a balanced foundation for the lumbar spine. Since the coccyx does not contribute to any significant function in man, his bipedalism or otherwise, it accordingly does not develop to any significant degree.

For the most part, each spinal segment

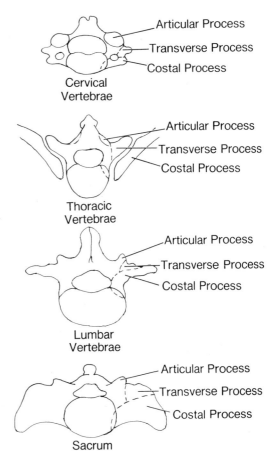

**Figure 5.13.** Homologous parts of cervical, thoracic, lumbar, and sacral vertebra.

develops similarly in accordance with the structural and functional characteristics of the particular region it occupies, and for this reason are referred to as *typical* vertebrae. On the other hand, the vertebrae located in the transitional areas of the spinal column (occipitocervical, thoracocervical, thoracolumbar and lumbosacral) are for the most part considered *atypical* in that they either tend to take on characteristics of both regions or develop peculiarly to fulfill a specific purpose beyond that of the regions they occupy. Consequently, the following discussion of specific vertebral topography is so organized.

### Development of the Cervical Vertebrae

The *typical* cervical vertebrae are the third through the sixth which develop from

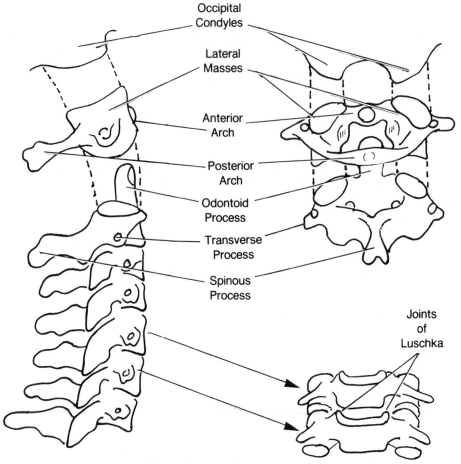

**Figure 5.14.**   Cervical spine.

three primary and nine secondary centers of ossification. The principal anatomic features of the completely developed typical cervical vertebrae are as follows (Fig. 5.14):

1. The *bodies* are elongated laterally (about twice as wide as they are deep); slope caudoventrally, and present lateral ridges on their cephalic surfaces (uncinate processes) which overlap the bodies below to form the uncovertebral joints or joints of Luschka.
2. The *pedicles* are short, while the *lamina* are relatively long, which provides a somewhat triangular-shaped neural canal in this area of the cervical spine.
3. The *articular processes* are somewhat pillar-like when viewed from the side. The facet surfaces are rounded and present a shallow angle of incline which allows for the free movement characteristic of the cervical spine.

4. The *costotransverse processes* are short and present a foramen (foramen transversarium) for the passage of the vertebral artery.
5. The *spinous processes* are caudally inclined at an angle of about 30–35°, and are bifurcated (bifid) at their tip.

The *atypical* cervical vertebrae are the first (atlas), the second (axis or epistropheus) and the seventh. Their principal distinguishing characteristics are as follows:

1. The *atlas* has no body, but instead is comprised of two lateral masses (articular support structures) connected together by an anterior and posterior arch. The lateral masses and posterior arch ossify from one primary center in each lateral mass which appear about the 7th week of fetal development and, except for the center of the posterior arch, is complete at the time of

birth. The anterior arch ossifies from one primary center which appears in the center of the arch at about the time of birth and closes with the lateral masses at about the 7th year of life. The superior articular surfaces (fovea) are kidney shaped to conform to the shape of the occipital condyles; the inferior fovea are rounded to conform to the superior articular surface of the second cervical vertebra, and a fifth articular surface (fovea dentalis) is present on the center of the inner surface of the anterior arch for articulation with the odontoid process of the second cervical vertebra. The costotransverse processes present a transverse foramen, and the rudimentary spinous process is represented by a small tubercle on the center of the posterior arch.

2. The *axis* essentially develops in the same manner as the typical cervical vertebrae, with the exception of an odontoid process (dens) which appears as a peglike structure on the cephalic aspect of the body, and is actually the displaced body of the atlas. The odontoid process ossifies from two primary centers located in its base which appears at about the 6th week of fetal development, and two secondary centers (in the base and apex) which appear at about the 2nd yr of life and close at about the age of 12 yr. The odontoid finally fuses with the body of axis by a rudimentary intervertebral disk at about the 18th year of life.

3. The *seventh* cervical vertebra is considered atypical due to the presence of an extra primary center of ossification in the costal processes which sometimes result in the formation of a "cervical rib." The spinous process is not bifurcated, but begins to take on the characteristic of the upper thoracic vertebral spinous processes.

## Development of the Thoracic Vertebrae

The *typical* thoracic vertebrae are the second through the eighth and develop typically from three primary centers and nine secondary centers of ossification. Their principal features are as follows (Fig. 5.15):

1. The bodies are more uniform in their lateral and dorsoventral dimensions than in the cervical region; somewhat heart shaped when viewed from above or below, and present two pair of "demifacets" (half costovertebral articular fovea) for articulation of the ribs: half with the body above and half with the body below.

2. The *pedicles* are short while the lamina are only slightly longer, thus forming a somewhat circular neural canal in this region. The vertebral notches are considerably deeper on the caudal aspect of the pedicles than on the cephalic aspect.

3. The *articular facets* are steeply inclined and their facet surfaces are more or less aligned to the coronal plane of the bodies.

4. The *transverse processes* are relatively long, angled dorsolaterally at about 45° relative to the midsagittal plane of the body, and present costotransverse facets on their ventrolateral surfaces for articulation with the ribs.

5. The *spinous processes* are long, slender and triangular on cross-section. They are caudally inclined at about 35° in the upper thoracic area and about 45° in the lower thoracic area.

The *atypical* thoracic vertebrae are the first, ninth, tenth, eleventh, and twelfth. Their principal features are as follows:

1. The *first* thoracic vertebral body is shaped similar to the lower cervical bodies, being transversely broad and presenting uncinate processes on its cephalic surface. There is one pair of full costal fovea on the cephalic aspect of the body for articulation with the first pair of ribs, and one pair of demifacets on the caudal aspects for articulation with half of the second pair of ribs. The spinous process is similar to that of the seventh cervical, being relatively long and protruding—when longer than the seventh cervical, it is referred to as "vertebrae prominens."

2. The *ninth* thoracic vertebra is similar to the eighth with the exception of the arrangement of the costal facets—generally one pair of demifacets, but may have two pair of demifacets and is also designated as typical.

3. The *tenth* thoracic vertebra generally has one complete pair of costal facets on the cephalic aspect of the body, but in some cases may have one pair of demifacets in those cases where the ninth has two pair of demifacets.

4. The *eleventh* thoracic vertebra is characterized by the presence of one complete pair of costal facets on the upper lateral aspects of the body and no facets on the ventrolateral aspects of the transverse processes.

5. The *twelfth* thoracic vertebra is considered a transitional segment in that it takes on

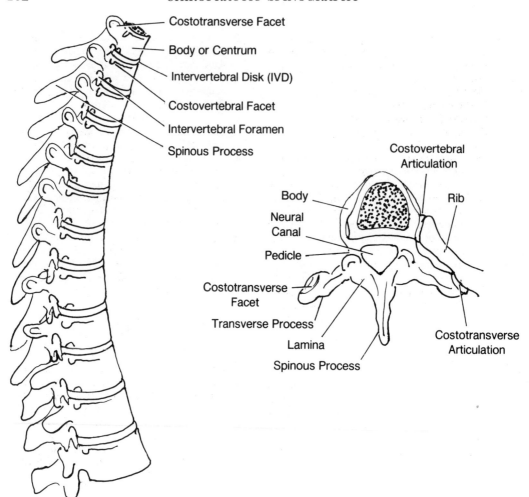

**Figure 5.15.** Thoracic spine.

some of the characteristics of both the thoracic and lumbar areas. However, its principal distinguishing features are one complete pair of costal facets on the body for articulation with the twelfth pair of ribs, no transverse facets and presence of a protuberance on the distal aspect of the transverse processes similar to the mammillary processes of the lumbar vertebrae.

## Development of the Lumbar Vertebrae

The lumbar vertebrae are ossified from five primary centers (the two additional being for the development of the "mammillary processes" peculiar to the lumbar area) and nine secondary centers. All lumbar vertebrae are relatively typical for that region

as a whole, with the possible exception of the fifth which is sometimes considered atypical because of its sacral transitional nature. The principal distinguishing features of the lumbar vertebrae are as follows (Fig. 5.16):

1. The *bodies* are heavily constructed, somewhat thicker at their ventral aspects (particularly the fifth) and are kidney shaped when viewed from above or below.
2. The *pedicles* are short, with the lamina being relatively longer, thus providing a somewhat triangular shape to the neural canal similar to the cervical region.
3. The *articular processes* are heavily constructed with the facets being nearly vertical and more or less aligned to the sagittal plane of the body: i.e. coronally faced.
4. The *mammillary processes* are heavy,

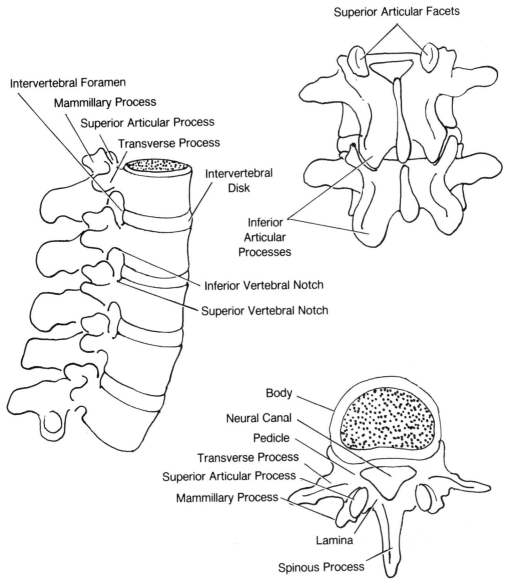

**Figure 5.16.**  Lumbar spine.

strong and clublike projections arising from the dorsolateral aspects of the articular processes.

5. The *spinous processes* are heavy, strong and clublike at their tips.

### Development of the Sacrum and Coccyx

Each of the five sacral segments initially ossify from five primary centers, one in each body and two in each neural arch. The primary centers in the cephalic three seg-

ments appear at about the 8th fetal week and those in the caudal two segments at about the 6–8th fetal month. The two primary centers in the neural arches appear at about the 6th fetal month and finally unite with the bodies at about the 2nd yr of life. Additional primary centers in the ventrolateral aspects of the cephalic three segments appear at about the 6th fetal month and correspond to the costal elements of the true vertebrae.

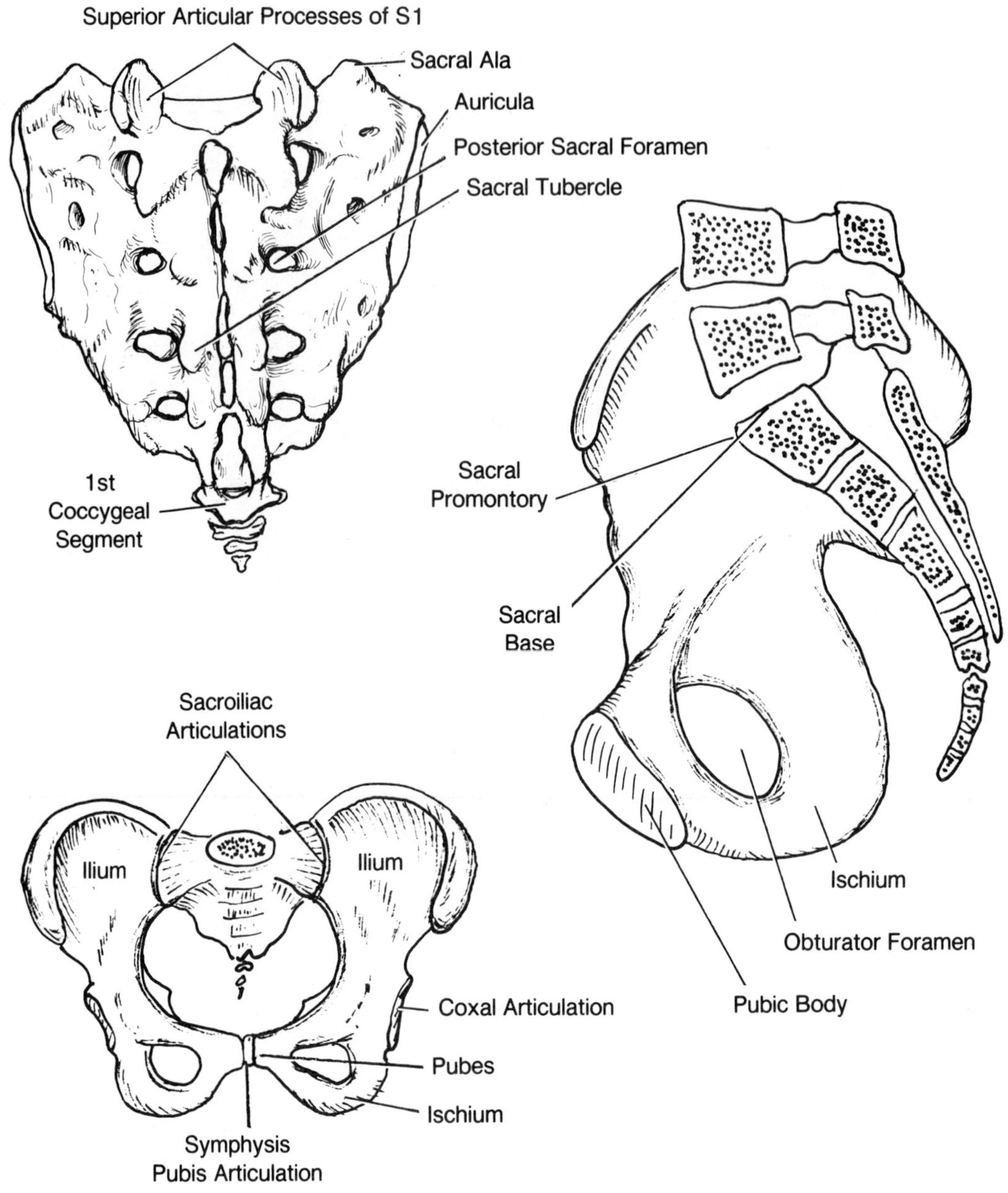

**Figure 5.17.**　Sacrum, coccyx, and innominate bones.

At about the age of 18 yr, secondary centers appear at the caudal and cephalic aspects of each sacral segment body and on the lateral aspects of the three cephalic costotransverse elements. On closure, the secondary centers unit the sacral segments into one solid structure and form the auricular facets on the lateral aspects of the cephalic three segments for articulation with the auricular facets of the ilia (Fig. 5.17).

The coccyx ossifies from one primary center in each of the four segments, all of which appear after birth. Ossification begins in the first (most cephalic) segment and gradually moves caudally until the coccyx is complete and all segments are fused into one solid unit by about the 18–25th yr of life. The coccyx often fuses with the sacrum in later life.

# DEVELOPMENTAL ANOMALIES OF THE SPINAL COLUMN

From the chiropractic point of view, developmental anomalies of the spinal column are considered from the dual aspect of those relatively minor variations from the *anatomically correct* (which are generally significant only insofar as they may adversely affect spinal biomechanics and/or spinographic interpretation), and those more gross congenital aberrations which may have added clinical significance in themselves. For purposes of this discussion, the distinction between these minor and gross structural alterations will be classified as *normal developmental variants* and *congenital anomalies* (6, 7).

## Normal Developmental Variants

Because major concern of this discussion is for the effects of normal developmental variants on static and dynamic function of the spinal column, and on postural spinographic evaluation of such function, it is most appropriate to discuss these considerations in relation to the three body planes (coronal, sagittal and transverse) in the upright standing posture.

1. Coronal plane variants are those dissimilarities that may be present bilaterally (over, under or asymmetrical development of one side relative to the other side) which may result in some degree of scoliosis and/or may cause difficulties in spinographic analysis procedure to the extent that standard methodology is inappropriate. The most common coronal plane variants encountered are: inequality of leg length, asymmetrical development of pelvic components, unilateral sacral agenesis, asymmetrical facets (coronal on one side and sagittal on the other side) and bilateral asymmetries of the vertebral bodies or disks.
2. Sagittal plane developmental variants are those subtle anomalies which may be present anteroposteriorly, resulting in increase or decrease of normal spinal curves and/or general biomechanical inadequacies. The most common sagittal plane variants are: variations in the vertical attitude of the pelvis, sacral anomalies which displace the base to a greater or lesser degree of normal angulation, and variations in the vertical dimensions of the bodies or disks.
3. Transverse plane variants are those developmental alterations which may be present around the vertical axis of the body, resulting mainly in functional disturbances of the spinal column; i.e. asymmetrical flexion, extension, lateral flexion, or rotation. The most common transverse plane variants are: unequal anterolateral flaring of the innominate bones, rotational malposition of the sacrum within the innominate bones, asymmetrical facet alignment, and circumferential variation of vertebral body or disk symmetry.

## Congenital Anomalies of the Spinal Column

Congenital anomalies of the spinal column may occur at any stage in the developmental process and may vary from minimal to extremely gross. If a defect originates during the period of initial sclerotome development, complete absence of a part of a segment, or an entire segment, may result. If a defect originates during later stages of development, an almost endless variety of anomalies may result. For an overview of developmental anomalies, the following outline [modified from Meschan (8)] is of perspective value.

## ABNORMALITIES OF SEGMENTATION

  A. Extravertebral bodies
  B. Extra-apophyses

## ABNORMALITIES OF FUSION

  A. Excessive fusion
   1. Fused transverse processes, as in sacralization and lumbarization
   2. Superficial and deep accessory sacroiliac articulations
   3. Fusion of the spinous processes
   4. Fusion of the vertebral bodies
     a. Block vertebrae
     b. Klippel-Feil syndrome
     c. Occipitalization of atlas

B. Nonfusion
   1. Cleft vertebrae
   2. Spina bifida
      a. Meningocele
      b. Myelocele
   3. Spina bifida oculta
   4. Spondylolisthesis

## ABNORMALITIES OF CHONDRIFICATION

A. Ochronosis
B. Defective intervertebral disks
C. Persistent notochord
D. Hemivertebrae
E. Failure of chondrification and ossification of portions of the neural arch
F. Basilar invagination

## ABNORMALITIES OF OSSIFICATION

A. Hemivertebra
B. Spina bifida
C. Diastematomyelia
D. Congenital systemic disorders affecting developmental processes
   1. Congenital stippled epiphysis
   2. Morquio's and Pfaundler-Hurler syndrome
   3. Achondroplasia
   4. Osteogenesis imperfecta
   5. Fibrous dysplasia
   6. Osteopathia striata
   7. Engelmann's disease
   8. Mongolism
E. Diminution of size of the spinal canal
   1. Achondroplasia

2. Fibrous dysplasia
3. Paget's disease

## ABNORMALITIES OF ALIGNMENT (CONGENITAL)

A. Idiopathic scoliosis and kyphoscoliosis
B. Subluxation of the atlas and axis
C. Kyphosis due to congenital systemic disease, such as Morquio's and Hurler's syndrome
D. Spondylolisthesis

The foregoing outline of congenital anomalies is not intended to represent a complete categorization of all such conditions that may occur, but is given mainly to illustrate the nature and relationship of such disorders to the developmental process—further reading on the subject is recommended.

### References

1. Meschan I: *An Atlas of Anatomy Basic to Radiology.* Philadelphia, Saunders, 1975, pp 36–63.
2. Aegerter E, Kirkpatrick JA: *Orthopaedic Diseases.* Philadelphia, Saunders, 1963, pp 3–30.
3. Schmorl G, Junghams H: *The Human Spine in Health and Disease,* Am ed 2. New York, Grune & Stratton, 1977, pp 2–30.
4. Pharaoh DO: *Chiropractic Orthopedy.* Davenport, Iowa, Palmer School of Chiropractic, 1956.
5. Turek SL: *Orthopaedics: Principles and Their Application.* Philadelphia, Lippincott, 1950, pp 3–56.
6. Hadley LA: *Anatomico-Roentgenographic Studies of the Spine.* Springfield, Ill, Charles C Thomas, 1964, pp 3–29.
7. Epstein BS: *The Spine: A Radiological Text and Atlas.* Philadelphia, Lea & Febiger, 1976, pp 13–42.
8. Meschan I: *Roentgen Signs in Clinical Practice,* Philadelphia, Saunders, vol 1, 1966.

# CHAPTER 6

# Postural Complex of the Human Body

## EVOLUTION OF HUMAN POSTURE

Human posture is specially *adapted to* (rather than as some would say, designed for) the upright *bipedal* posture. It has been proposed by Jones, (1) Brennan (2) and Farfan (3) that the human skeletal system in general, and the pelvis and lower extremities in particular, are today the product of an evolutionary adaptative process that has been ongoing since man first appeared on earth over one million years ago.

On the basis of geological examination of the earth's layers, and other evidence, the *theory of evolution* sets forth the hypothesis that some 250 million years ago all vertebrates were cold-blooded, water-based animals. These vertebrates, it is contended, evolved over the next 150 million years, passing through various stages of development—*amphibians, reptiles and mammals*—until the *primates* appeared. At that point, the primates branched off into the *simian-anthropoid division* and the *humanoid* (ape man, Neanderthal man and modern man) *division.*

Although this theory of the evolutionary development of man has been opposed by a "creationism" concept, scientific evidence today overwhelmingly supports the hypothesis that man is the product of an evolutionary process and that over the past million years has adapted at an ever-increasing pace to reach its present-day, specialized, unique and distinct form. This ongoing process of man fitting himself to his environment by successive, accelerating stages of improvement is aptly summarized by Jones (1) as follows:

"A study of the entire picture in relation to the time element, leaves one with the inescapable conclusion that the rate of evolutionary progression is increasing at a rapidly accelerating pace. It was slow in the long ancient history phase, picked up speed in the middle ages, and has become kaleidoscopic in the modern era. Consequently, the human of only a few thousand years hence may well consider our appearance as incongruous as modern man finds that of the ape-man remains from South Africa. All of this serves only to throw into sharper perspective the fact that, while the earth is very old, the human race is very young." (From Jones L: *The Postural Complex: Observations as to Cause Diagnosis and Treatment.* Springfield, Ill, Charles C Thomas, 1955, pp 5–32.)

At this point in evolutionary time, the human postural complex is still in the process of adapting to its specialized erect-standing attitude. However, it cannot be denied that it is already well suited to the requirements placed on it by man's bipedalism, and that the distinctions between it and that of the quadripeds is profound. Conversely, because of the complexities of the human postural complex it is subject to structural distortions that may create clinically significant health problems, particularly within the pelvis and spinal column.

According to Jones (1), postural distortions throughout the *skeletal super-structure* (pelvis and spinal column) begin with the most inferior element in the postural chain—the feet. This belief is expressed by Jones as follows:

"For more than a decade it has gradually become apparent that postural imbalance has assumed a vital and ever-increasing importance. This viewpoint is a result of observations that accompanied radically different approaches to the manifold problems of diagnosis and treatment. This presentation will differ sharply from present-day majority opinion which largely considers that each symptom (of musculoskeletal distortion) arises from a defect of local origin. Conversely, evidence will be presented to show that postural deviation regularly gives rise to a generalized pattern of symptoms, and that cause and effect are an indivisible unit. Great emphasis will be placed on the key that opened the door—the observation that deviations in foot planes cause corresponding serial changes in the superstructure. Indeed, whereas most standard texts consider the foot almost as if it were a separate structure, here it will be repeatedly demonstrated that the foot is not only an integral part, but is actually the foundation of the body." (From Jones L: The Postural Complex: Observations as to Cause Diagnosis and Treatment. Springfield, Ill, Charles C Thomas, 1955, pp 5–32.)

According to Jones, the *primary trigger mechanism* is an internal rotation of the lower extremity, beginning with the foot, which is in essence a holdover evolutionary characteristic of prehistoric primates.

## POSTURAL MECHANICS OF THE AXIAL SKELETON

Understanding of the role of the human spinal column in health and disease necessitates that its function as the *axial organ* of the human body be recognized and appreciated. As such, it is charged with the responsibility of allowing man to function in his environment as a biped—to allow him to stand in almost effortless equilibrium (whether in the erect attitude or in compensation to standing on an unlevel surface) and to allow him to kinetically perform the myriad activities of work or play. These functions or duties of the spinal column (and its pelvic support structure) are most admirably met, in spite of its presently ongoing evolutionary state, by its general structural design and intersegmental functional characteristics.

## Static Posture of the Axial Skeleton

In the static standing postural attitude, the general structural design of the spinal column and pelvic support structure is such that the gravitational forces exerted on the body are equalized, three-dimensionally, around a *vertical central axis* (VCA) located at the intersection of the midsagittal and midcoronal (frontal) body planes (Fig. 6.1). This VCA originates as a point midway between the vestibular apparatuses of the inner ear (center of gravity of the head) (4, pp 146–152; 5) passes downward through the spinal column to a point of bisection between the femur heads (center of gravity of the pelvis), (4, pp 124–127) and further descends to distribute the body weight equally on both feet on the sagittal body plane and on the apexes of the arches of the feet on the coronal body plane (Figs. 6.2, 6.3).

## Dynamic Posture of the Axial Skeleton

Whether standing in a statically erect postural attitude or in compensation to standing on an unlevel surface, the maintenance of equilibrium is not completely effortless on the part of the axial skeleton. Rather, this maintenance of equilibrium in a so-called "static" state, is a *dynamic* process whereby associated musculature are "kept" in a low level state of contraction (tonus) by an interplay of motor/sensory neurological impulses. This "dynamic" concept of postural equilibrium control (which will be discussed more fully later in this chapter) has been described by Illi (6) as the "dynamostatics" of the human body, which may be conceptually thought of as the "motor of the body" being kept in a constant state of *idle* in preparation for movement; i.e. kinetic action.

## PELVIC POSTURAL FOUNDATION UNIT

The human pelvis constitutes a biomechanically organized support structure for

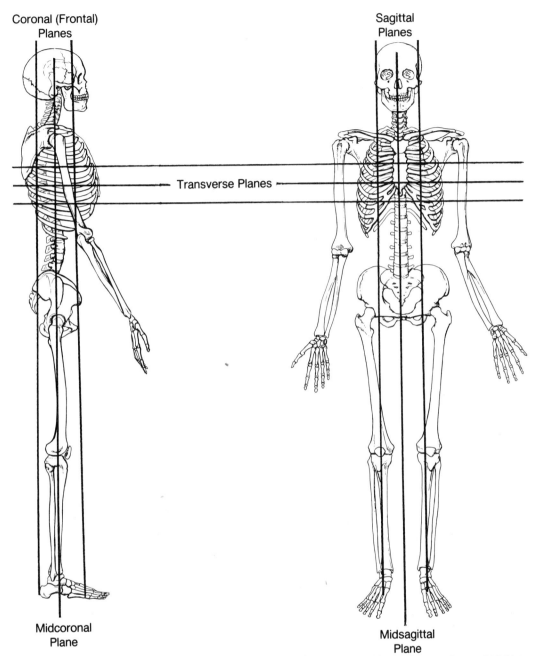

**Figure 6.1.** Planes of the human body in erect-standing position. Vertical central axis (VCA) is the vertical intersection of the midcoronal and midsagittal planes.

the body trunk and spinal column. Anatomically, the pelvis is a closed bony ring supported bilaterally by the femur heads and comprised of the *sacrum* and *innominate bones*—the innominate bones are each, in turn, comprised of the *ilium, ischium* and

*pubes.* In the static-standing posture, the pelvis tends to seek a balance around its *center of gravity* (intersection of the midsagittal and coronal plane lines at a level with the top of the femur heads); such center of gravity being considered the point

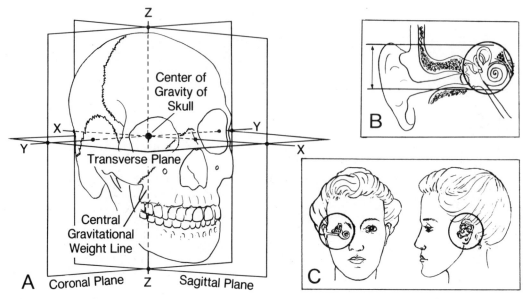

**Figure 6.2.** Center of gravity of the head as proposed by Hildebrandt and Seeman. [From Seeman DC, *Journal of Manipulative* and *Physiological Therapeutics* 4:15–18, 1981 (5).]

of geographic orientation of all movements of the pelvis and its individual component parts (Fig. 6.4) (4, pp 124–127).

### Articulations of the Pelvis

The bilateral junction of the iliac portion of the innominate bones and the sacrum comprises the *sacroiliac articulations.* The median-caudal junction of the pubic bodies comprises the *symphysis pubes articulation.* The junction of the ischial portion of the innominate bones with the femur heads comprises the *coxal articulations.* The character of these articulations, along with the design of the bones themselves, determines the manner of normal movements of the pelvis and the nature of the subluxations that may occur within the pelvic unit as a whole.

## SACROILIAC ARTICULATIONS

The nature of the sacroiliac articulations have been a source of much debate since the time of Hippocrates (460–377 B.C.) when the pelvis was considered a rigid bony ring in which the articulations were classi-fied as "immovable synchondroses," except during pregnancy when they supposedly became very loose to allow for passage of the fetus (7, 8). This idea has persisted even in more recent times; *Gray's Anatomy* states (9): "*The sacroiliac articulation is a synchondrosis . . . a temporary form of joint, for the cartilage is converted into bone in later life."* *Gray's* further compounds the confusion by then stating: "*In a considerable part of their extent, especially in advanced life, they are separated by a space containing a synovia-like fluid, hence the joint presents the characteristics of diarthroidal gliding joint."*

In an effort to resolve this controversy, because of its importance to chiropractic concepts of interpelvic subluxations, the chiropractic profession conducted a number of investigations to determine the nature of the sacroiliac articulations. The first of these investigations was conducted by Illi and Janse in 1940 wherein they examined a number of cadaveric pelvises (6). These studies provided some rather conclusive evidence that although the sacroiliac articulations are only slightly movable (amphiarthrodial) at the time of birth, they do

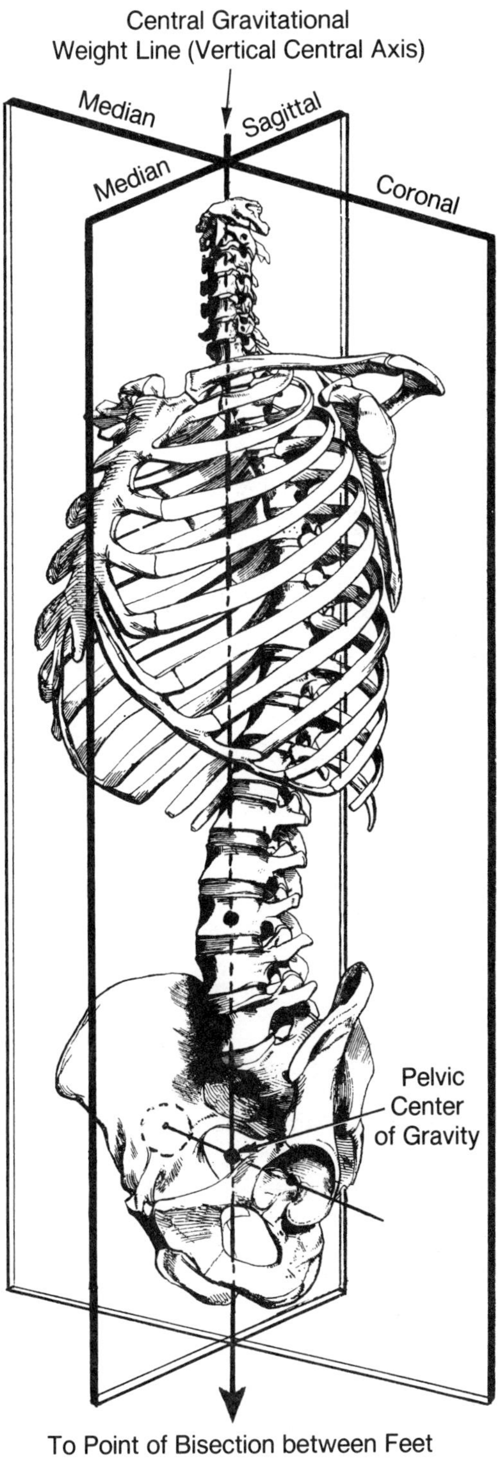

Central Gravitational
Weight Line (Vertical Central Axis)

Median    Sagittal

Median    Coronal

Pelvic
Center
of Gravity

To Point of Bisection between Feet

**Figure 6.3.** Vertical central axis of the body as it passes downward through the pelvic center of gravity (PCG) to a point of bisection between the two feet.

take on freely movable (diarthrodial) characteristics later in life by the development of a "synovia-like" membrane—a fact that is suggested by *Gray's Anatomy* but paradoxically dismissed by its classification as a synchondrosis.

Since that time, many others within the medical and osteopathic professions have agreed with the Illi-Janse findings (8, 10–19) and a more recent chiropractically based study provides further confirmation (20). Consequently, it must at this time be concluded that the human sacroiliac articulations, at least in adult life, are *diarthrodial* (synovial) articulations of the *arthrodial* (gliding) variety which are held in proximate integrity by four primary ligaments; the *anterior* sacroiliac, the *long posterior* sacroiliac, the *short posterior* iliac, and the *interosseous.*

With regard to the unique transitional nature of the sacroiliac articulation (slightly movable at birth to freely movable in later life) this author holds to a rather provocative theory that this transition is consistent with the evolutionary progression of the human body to higher levels of development to suit the environmental demands placed on the bipedal human being. The synchondrosis-amphiarthroidal nature of the sacroiliac articulations in early human embryonic development is characteristic of the quadripedal origin of the human body. However, by virtue of the body's capacity to evolve itself to meet environmental demands, the sacroiliac articulation takes on freely movable characteristics (develops a synovia-like membrane) at such time as the infant/child begins to stand, walk and run. This theory is not regarded, incidently, as being inconsistent with the *creationist* concept of the origin of man— although it seems that all animals were created according to some sort of a "master plan," man was created uniquely in many ways; not the least of which is the development of the sacroiliac articulations to allow for his bipedalism, a characteristic which is not inherent within the evolutionary progression of lower types of animals.

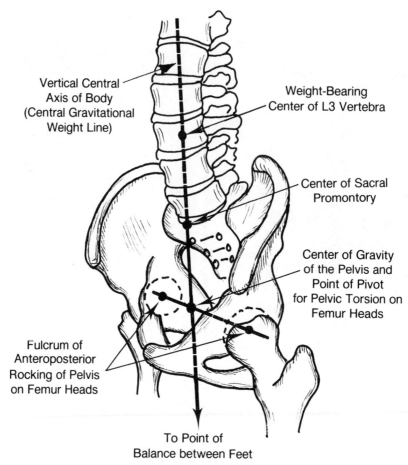

**Figure 6.4.** Biomechanical relationship of the pelvis to its center of gravity—the point of fulcrum for all pelvic movements, as a whole and of its component parts.

## SYMPHYSIS PUBIS ARTICULATION

The symphysis pubis articulation is classified as amphiarthrodial and is believed to have only limited movement capability, at least in certain directions. The ligaments of the symphysis pubis articulation are: the *superior* pubic, the *inferior* pubic, and the *interpubic fibrocartilaginous lamina* or interpubic disk (Fig. 6.5).

Although there may be some significant rotatory or torsional movement capability, it is unlikely that any significant shearing (anteroposterior/superoinferior) movement activity is possible between the pubic bones because of the nature of the interpubic disk (7, 21–23). In support of this

contention, it has been shown by the *Technique of Chamberlain* (x-raying the symphysis pubis while the patient stands with a block placed alternately under each foot) (24) that the normal range of pubic shear is 0–0.5 mm in the male and 0–1.5 mm in the female (Fig. 6.6). However, it is generally accepted that when the interpubic disk is traumatically or pathologically damaged, considerable shear is possible to the extent that instability of the entire pelvis is evident (Fig. 6.7). In cases where the interpubic disk has been surgically severed (to supposedly offer a wider birth canal during labor) the patients were left virtually crippled due to the low back and pelvic pain

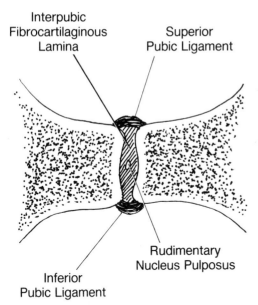

Interpubic
Fibrocartilaginous
Lamina

Superior
Pubic Ligament

Rudimentary
Nucleus Pulposus

Inferior
Pubic Ligament

**Figure 6.5.** Symphysis pubis articulation illustrating its firm but elastic ligamentous attachments which contraindicates any significant shearing action proposed by certain proprietary chiropractic technique procedures; particularly the Gonstead concept of interpelvic biomechanics.

brought on by the concomitant sacroiliac and symphyseal instability (24).

## COXAL ARTICULATIONS

The articulations of the femur heads with the ischial portions of the innominate bones are diarthroidal, freely movable, ball and socket joints.

### Normal Pelvic Mechanics

Normal pelvic mechanics concerns those movements of the pelvis as a unit and by its individual component parts relative to each other, as they may be allowed in bipedal posture, in accordance with the nature of the coxal, sacroiliac and symphysis pubis articulations. Although these movements of the pelvis as a unit are to some extent three-dimensional, these movements are discussed here in relation to single body planes for explanatory purposes.

## GROSS PELVIC MOVEMENTS

As a composite unit (without consideration of possible interpelvic movements), gross movements of the pelvis on the femur heads (at the coxal articulations) may be described as follows (Fig. 6.8).

A. On the *transverse body plane*, the pelvis may move rotationally around its center of gravity, with the femur heads being the points of bilateral pivot.
B. On the *coronal body plane*, the pelvis may shift laterally on the femur heads. In the

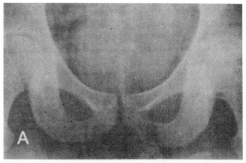

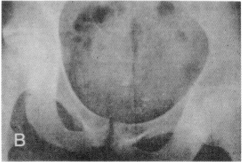

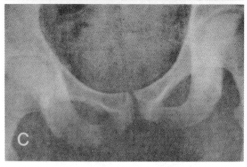

**Figure 6.6.** Technique of Chamberlain—x-rays of patient's pelvis in the *A*, neutral position; *B*, with a block under the left leg; and *C*, with a block under the right leg. Note no noticeable shearing action present in the case of a normal symphysis.

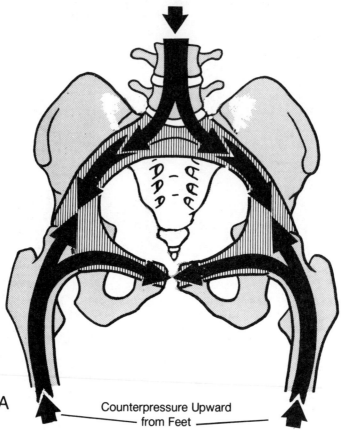

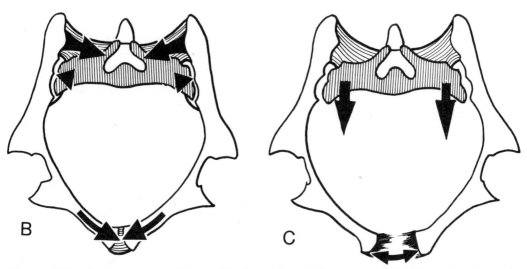

**Figure 6.7.** Counter pressure forces of body weight which act to stabilize the pelvis when the body is in a relaxed postural state. *A*, anterior view of counter pressure forces. *B*, superior view showing stabilizing forces to the symphysis pubis and sacroiliac articulations. *C*, severe unstabilizing action of the pelvic girdle with rupture of the symphyseal interpubic fibrocartilaginous lamina. [Adapted from Kapandji (31).]

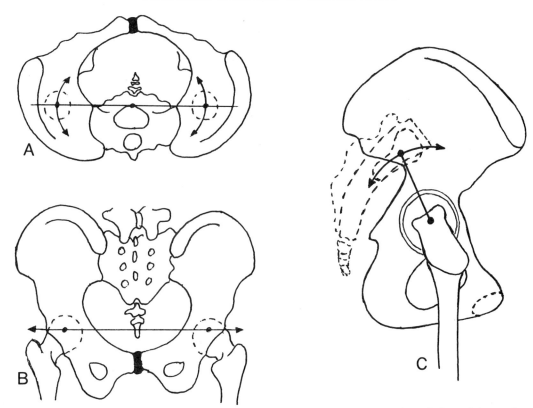

**Figure 6.8.** Gross movements of the pelvis. *A*, transverse plane rotation of the pelvis on the femur heads around the pelvic center of gravity. *B*, lateral shifting of the pelvis—normally without pelvic unleveling when femur heads are directly over the feet. *C*, anteroposterior rocking of the pelvis on the sagittal plane on a femur head pivot.

normal stance, with the femur heads directly over the feet, lateral shift is not accompanied by any pelvic unleveling. However, if the feet are placed farther apart than the femur heads, the pelvis will lower on the side of lateral shift; if the feet are placed closer together than the femur heads, the pelvis will raise on the side of lateral shift.
C. On the *sagittal body plane*, the pelvis may rock (flex and extend) anterior or posterior on a coronal axis through the femur heads.

## INDEPENDENT MOVEMENT OF THE INNOMINATE BONES

The independent movement of the innominate bones (relative to each other) are in an opposed anteroposterior direction. However, the exact mechanism of this anteroposterior movement of the innominate bones in opposed directions to each other (as a normal action or an abnormal sublux-

ation action) has been a source of some debate in the chiropractic profession—the primary consideration in the debate being the point of pivot or fulcrum between the opposed-moving innominate bones (4).

On one hand, one particular proprietary procedure of spinographic analysis has contended that the point of pivot or fulcrum between the opposed-moving innominate bones is at the femur heads (25). This procedure maintains that while one innominate bone moves anterior and superior (AS) at the ilium, the opposite innominate will move posterior and inferior (PI) at the ilium (Fig. 6.9). However, with the exception of those cases where there may be severe looseness of the symphysis pubis due to trauma or pathology of the pubic disk, anteroposterior movement of the innominate bones on a femur head pivot are not possible to any significant degree.

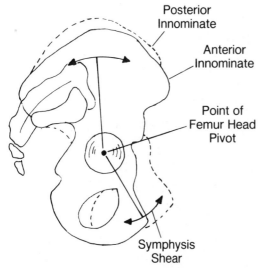

**Figure 6.9.** Gonstead theory of independent movement of the opposed innominate bones, relative to each other, on a femur head pivot. This concept is highly unlikely to occur in cases where interpubic ligaments are intact.

On the other hand, this author has proposed the more plausible concept that opposed anteroposterior movement of the innominate bones (as a normal action in postural compensation and locomotion or an abnormal action in sacroiliac subluxation) takes place at a symphyseal pivot or fulcrum (Fig. 6.10) (4). Although the intact interpubic disk will not allow for any significant shearing action between the pubic bodies, considerable torsion at the symphysis is possible. This concept has been verified by the work of Frigerio et al. (20).

With regard to this distinction, it is important that the reader accept the fact that opposed anteroposterior movement of the innominate bones does take place on a symphyseal point of pivot, rather than on a femur head pivot—spinographic interpretive impressions and manipulative corrective procedure requires that one have a clear understanding of the related biomechanics.

## INDEPENDENT MOVEMENTS OF THE SACRUM

Movements of the sacrum relative to the ilia, independent of the aforedescribed in-

nominate bone movements, are possible as a normal action in postural compensation and locomotion or as a criterion of sacroiliac subluxation. Although there is some difference of opinion regarding the exact mechanics involved, the following are considered primary possibilities (Fig. 6.11) (4, 26).

1. On the *sagittal body plane* the sacrum can flex (rock anteriorly) or extend (rock posteriorly) which results in the increase or decrease of the angle of the sacral base relative to a horizontal plane. These flexion/extension movements of the sacrum within the ilium are considered a mechanism of postural accommodation by their effect of increasing or decreasing the normal lumbar lordotic curve. When these movements extend beyond the normal range allowable by the sacroiliac articulations, subluxation is manifest (Fig. 6.11*A*).
2. On the *transverse body plane* the sacrum can rotate within the ilia on its normal incline plane of 35–42° (Fig. 6.11*B*). This anteroinferior/posterosuperior rotatory action, combined with the inferior flexion/posterior extension movements on the sagittal body plane, provides a compound "variable pitch" control of lumbar spine curve compensation—lumbar spine movements are three-dimensional; lateral flexion, rotation and anterior flexion/posterior extension are concomitant actions.
3. On the *coronal body plane* the sacrum can laterally flex to some degree, but this does not appear to be as free an action as rotation and flexion/extension due to the buffering action of opposing postural forces (Fig. 6.8*A*).

## SPINAL AXIAL ORGAN UNIT

As the so-called "axial organ" of the musculoskeletal system, the spinal column is comprised of a series of articular complexes, referred to by various authors as the *vertebral motor units* (27), the *functional units* (28, pp 1–23), and the *motion segments* (29, 30). By whatever term, these functional components of the spinal column have been described as "*a biomechanical concept which confers a quantity and quality of motoricity to the relationship of two vertebrae, firmly but elastically interconnected by the intervertebral disk and re-*

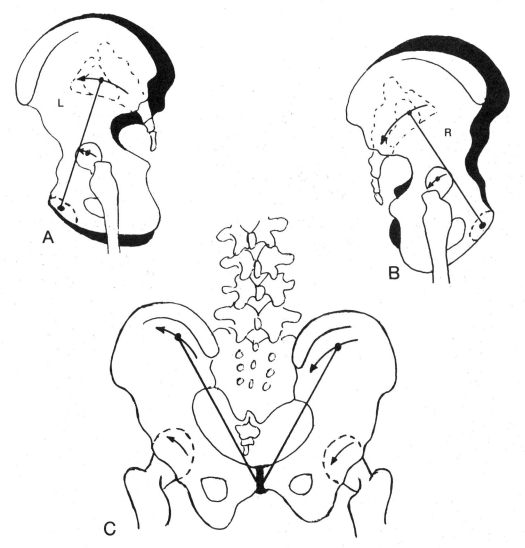

**Figure 6.10.** Hildebrandt theory of independent movement of the innominate bones in opposed directions to each other—point of pivot is depicted at the symphysis which, although not allowing for significant shearing action, may permit significant torque action. *A*, left side illustrating anterior movement of the ilia and retraction (physiological shortening) of the left leg. *B*, right side illustrating posterior movement of the ilia and extension (physiological lengthening) of the right leg. *C*, illustration of combined action of a left anterior-right posterior innominate (ilia) on a symphysis pivot.

*straining ligaments, which is activated to purposeful function by muscles which are respondent to a controlled interplay of sensory and motor nerve supply"* (4) (Fig. 6.12).

The spinal column as a whole consists of 25 such functional components and the kinetic efficiency of the total spinal column is herein described as *"that condition of the vertebral functional units—individually and collectively—in which each gravitationally dependent segment above is free to seek its normal resting position in relation to its supporting segment below; is free to move efficiently through its normal ranges of motion on the composite of all three body planes (flexion-extension, lateral flexion and rota-*

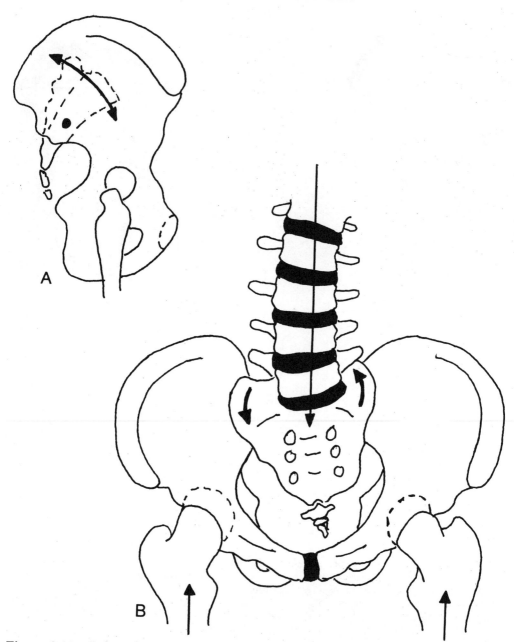

**Figure 6.11.** Independent movements of the sacrum within the ilia. *A*, anteroposterior rocking on a sagittal plane on a transverse axis of pivot at the lower aspect of the sacroiliac articulation. *B*, transverse plane rotation of the sacrum, on a 35–42° incline, within the ilia. Note how rotation of the sacrum (the degree being influenced by the amount of sagittal plane rocking) affects a mechanical action of the lumbar spine functional units resulting in a combined rotation-lateral flexion action.

*tion), and is free to return to its normal resting position after movement*" (4) (Fig. 6.13).

In consideration of the traditional chiropractic term, "normal vertebral alignment," which is used to designate the cor-

rect position of one vertebra relative to its supporting structure below, here the term "normal resting position" is preferred insofar as it more appropriately describes the kinetic properties of the spinal articular complex.

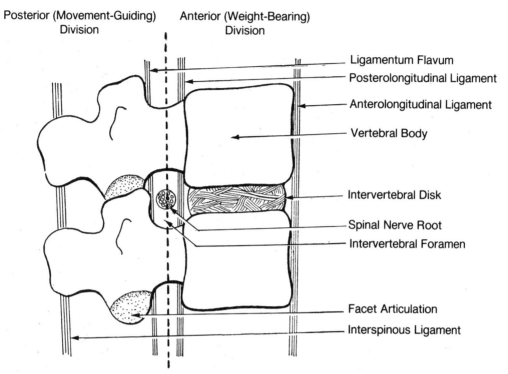

**Figure 6.12.** Spinal functional unit illustrating major osseous and soft tissue components [Adapted from Cailliet (28).]

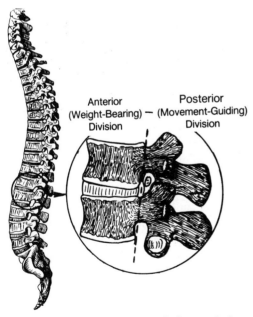

**Figure 6.13.** The spine as a whole, consisting of 25 interconnected functional units.

### Movement of Individual Vertebra

Normal movements of a vertebral segment relative to its supporting structure below may be described in accordance with its ability to laterally flex on the coronal body plane, rotate on the transverse body plane, and anteroflex-retroextend on the sagittal body plane. To some extent all vertebra are able to function in all three body planes, however, the magnitude and character of such movement varies to some degree between the various spinal regions and their transitional areas. In fact, it may be considered that each articular complex in the spinal column is unique within itself as it individually contributes to spinal function as a whole.

### CONTROLLING FACTORS OF VERTEBRAL MOVEMENT

Conjecturally, the primary factor determining the *character* of vertebral movement relative to its supporting structure below, is the particular design of the vertebral structures themselves—the bodies and articular processes. The primary factor in determining *magnitude* of vertebral movement relative to its supporting structure below, is the nature of its interconnecting ligaments—particularly the intervertebral disk (IVD).

Although it probably has little to do with the actual character or magnitude of movement of one vertebra relative to its supporting structure below, there has been some debate regarding two differing theories of IVD dynamics which should be mentioned. On one hand, Cailliet (28, pp 4–6) and Kapandji (31) contend that the nucleus pulposus of the IVD displaces toward the side of intervertebral convexity (i.e. is "squeezed" away from the side of concavity). White and Panjabi (32), on the other hand, contend that the opposite is true—that the nucleus pulposus of the IVD is displaced toward the side of intervertebral concavity (Fig. 6.14).

Each of these theories seem to have their good and bad points of reference which, until more definitive knowledge of IVD dynamics is available, leaves the reader with his or her own choice based on the manner by which these differing decisions were made—Cailliet (28) and Kapandji (31) on the basis of theoretical logic; White and Panjabi (32) on the basis of cadaveric studies which does not take the living dynamics of the human body into consideration.

## DIRECTIONAL LISTINGS OF VERTEBRAL MOVEMENT

Specific movement characteristics of spinal vertebrae have traditionally been designated in chiropractic procedure relative to their "subluxation" configurations (i.e. *listings* and/or *classifications*) rather than their normal movement characteristics; this concept having been subjectively arrived at on the basis of early day consideration of the spinal subluxation from a static point of view. In other words, since the correct relationship of two vertebrae was "perfect alignment," any deviation from that position was a subluxation which was "listed" according to its direction of malposition. These vertebral subluxation listings (which will be discussed in detail in Chapter 7) have been divided into two basic

concepts according to "schools of thought." These are:

A. The *Palmer-Gonstead-Firth* classification wherein the direction of subluxation displacement is listed according to spinous process deviation.
B. The *National-Diversified* classification which lists the direction of subluxation displacement according to body displacement.

Additionally, a method of subluxation designation in accordance with their relationship to functional characteristics (which will also be discussed in more detail in Chapter 7) has been offered under the heading of "radiological classifications"; namely, the flexion-extension, lateral flexion, rotation, and aberrant movements of vertebrae on an individual or sectional basis (33).

More recently, an *international method* of vertebral movement and subluxation classification has been proposed by White and Panjabi (29, 32, pp 12–20); the *Right-Handed Cartesian Orthogonal Coordinate System*, which has been further evolved by Jerow (34) in an effort to coordinate the Palmer-Gonstead-Firth/National-Diversified concepts of spinal subluxation (Fig. 6.15).

### Kinematics of the Spine

With the introduction of their book on *Clinical Biomechanics of the Spine*, White and Panjabi (32) have set forth certain new concepts of spinal mechanics which the chiropractic profession has viewed with considerable interest. For more complete consideration of all pertinent knowledge relating to this discussion of "The Spinal Axial Organ Unit," the information which summarizes these concepts (32, pp 61–65), is paraphrased as follows:

## TERMS AND DEFINITIONS

**Kinematics**—that phase of mechanics concerned with the study of motion of rigid bodies, with no consideration of the forces involved (Table 6.1).

**Central coordinate system**—a method

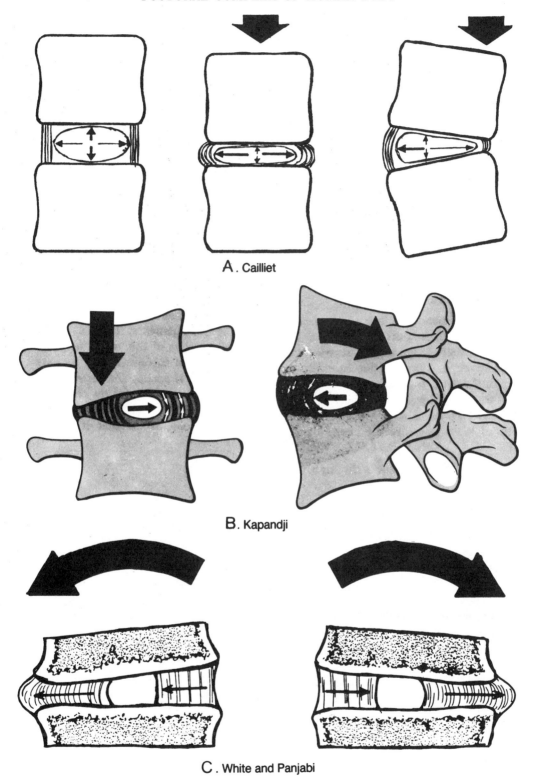

A. Cailliet

B. Kapandji

C. White and Panjabi

**Figure 6.14.** Intervertebral disk dynamics as considered by A, Cailliet (28), (B), Kapandji (31), and C, White and Panjabi (32).

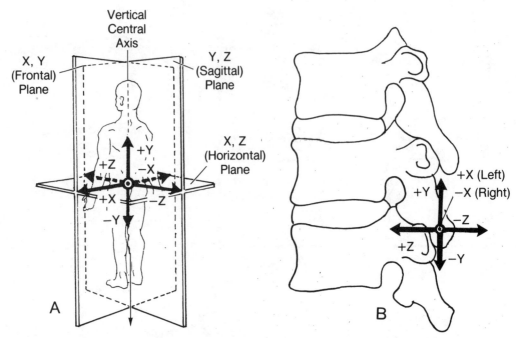

**Figure 6.15.** Right-handed cartesian orthogonal method of White and Panjabi (29, 32). *A*, relationship of system to the body planes. *B*, application of the system to vertebral movement through the six degrees of freedom. [Adapted from White and Panjabi (29, 32).

**Table 6.1.**
**Comprehensive description of kinematics of the spine[a]**

The important basic and clinical aspects of kinematics of the spine are as follows:

Range of motion for all six degrees of freedom

  Rotations
  Translations

Traditional physiologic patterns of motion

  Flexion/extension
  Lateral bending
  Axial rotation

Coupling characteristics and ratios (Instantaneous axes of rotation of motion segments in each of the traditional planes);

  Sagittal plane (y, z)
  Frontal plane (y, x)
  Horizontal plane (x, z)

Helical axes of motion located throughout the range of motion; functions of anatomic elements; description of roles played by various anatomic elements in determining kinematic characteristics; analysis of cephalocaudal variations within the regions; analysis and comparison of regional variations:
  Occipito-atlanto-axial
  Thoracic
  Lumbar

[a] From AA White and MM Panjobi: *Clinical Biomechanics of the Spine.* Philadelphia, Lippincott, 1978, pp 61–65.

of describing spatial relationships and movement of vertebrae in relation to the three body planes.

**Motion segment**—the traditional unit of study in spinal kinematics, constituted by two adjacent vertebrae and their intervening soft tissues—motion is described in terms relative to the subjacent vertebra.

**Rotation**—a body (any piece of matter) is said to be in rotation when movement is such that all particles along some straight line in the body or a hypothetical extension of it have zero velocity relative to a fixed point. Rotation is a spinning or angular displacement of a body about some axis—the axis may be located outside the rotating body or inside it.

**Translation**—a body is said to be in translation when movement is such that all particles in the body at a given time have the same direction of motion relative to a fixed point.

**Degrees of freedom**—one degree of freedom is motion in which a rigid body may translate back and forth along a straight line or may rotate back and forth about a particular axis—vertebrae have six degrees of freedom, translation along, and rotation about, each of the three orthogonal axes.

**Range of motion (ROM)**—the difference between the two points of physiologic extremes of movement is the range of motion; translation is expressed in meters or inches and rotation in degrees; the range of motion can be expressed for each of the six degrees of freedom.

**Coupling**—refers to motion in which rotation or translation of a body about or along one axis is consistently associated with simultaneous rotation or translation about another axis.

**Pattern of motion**—defined by the configuration of a path that the geometric center of the body describes as it moves through its ranges of motion.

**Instantaneous axes of motion (IAR)**—at every instance, for a rigid body in plane motion there is a line in the body or a hypothetical extension of this line which does not move; the instantaneous axis of rotation is this line; plane motion is fully defined by the position of the instantaneous axis of rotation and the magnitude of rotation about it.

**Helical axis of motion (HAM)**—screw motion; a superimposition of rotation and translation about and along the same axis; has the same direction as the resultant of the three rotations about the x, y and z axes; for a given, moving, rigid body in space; the location of this axis and the designation of numerical values for rotation and translation constitute a complete, precise, three-dimensional description of the motion.

## KINETICS AND MUSCLE ACTIVITY

"Kinematics has been defined as that phase of mechanics concerned with the study of movement of rigid bodies, with no consideration of what has caused the motion. *Kinematics* includes the study of the forces responsible for the motion. The muscles are the primary source of force resulting in motion of the vertebrae. This extremely complex topic is one that has been studied least from the viewpoint of biomechanics ... The muscles which may produce motion of the spine include the anterior, posterior and lateral muscles (Table 6.2). The anterior muscles include the abdominal and illiopsoas, which flex the spine; if an anterior muscle runs obliquely and contracts independently of the muscle on the opposite side it will rotate the spine as well as flex it. Similarly, a posterior muscle in the back extends the spine when it contracts; if the muscle runs obliquely and contracts independently of its counterpart on the opposite side, it will axially rotate and bend the spine laterally. If the lateral muscles contract, they will bend the spine laterally ..." (32, pp 61–65).

## OCCIPITOCERVICAL COMPLEX

The occipitocervical complex (occiput, atlas and axis) is intricately designed to

**Table 6.2.**
**Vertebral muscles and their motor functions**

---

### ANTERIOR

Anterior muscles flex the spine. If the muscle runs more or less obliquely and contracts independently of the corresponding muscle on the opposite side, it rotates and bends the spine.

| | |
|---|---|
| Longus colli[a] | Obliquus internus abdominis[a] |
| Longus capitus | Psoas major[b] |
| Rectus capitus anterior | Psoas minor[b] |
| Rectus capitus lateralis[b] | Iliacus |
| Obliquus externus abdominis[a] | Quadratus lumborum |

### POSTERIOR

Posterior muscles extend the spine. If the muscle runs more or less obliquely and contracts independently of the corresponding anterior muscle, it rotates and bends the spine laterally as well as extending it.

| *Superficial stratum* | *Deep stratum* |
|---|---|
| Splenius capitus[a, b] | Semispinalis |
| Splenius capitus[a, b] |   Thoracic[a] |
| Erector spinae (sacrospinalis) |   Cervicis[a] |
| Iliocostalis[a, b] |   Capitis[a] |
| Longissimus[a, b] | Multifidi[a] |
| Spinalis[a, b] | Rotores[a] |
| | Interspinalis |
| | Intertransversarii[a] |

### LATERAL

Muscles on the side bend the spine laterally. If muscle runs more or less obliquely and contracts independently of the corresponding muscle on the opposite side, it rotates and bends the spine as well as laterally flexing it.

| | |
|---|---|
| Trapezius | Scalenus[a] |
| Sternocleidomastoid[a] | Anterior |
| Quadratus lumborum | Medial |
| | Posterior |

---

[a] Muscles with axial rotation function.
[b] Muscles with lateral bending function.

function as a balance mechanism for the head in static postural accommodation and in locomotion; such design being oriented to the objectives of the vestibular apparatuses in their efforts to maintain the head in balance around its center of gravity (Fig. 6.3). This center of gravity of the head constitutes a *point of vector* around which all movements of the head on the atlas and axis seemingly takes place. These movements, on the three body planes, are described as follows (28, pp 4–6; 31; 32, pp 1–7):

A. Occipitoatlanto articulation
  1. On the *sagittal body plane* (Figs. 6.16, 6.17) the head may anteroflex and retroextend on an axis of pivot transversely through the vestibular apparatuses of the inner ear. This is allowed by the occipital condyles *rocking* and *gliding* posteriorly on the atlas lateral masses in flexion and by *rocking* and *sinking* anteriorly on the axis lateral masses in extension, this later "sinking" action being effected as a result of the posteriorly divergent angle of the condyles and lateral masses.
  2. On the *coronal body plane* (Fig. 6.18) the head may laterally flex on a sagittal axis through the point of bisection between the vestibular apparatuses, this action being allowed by the lateral incline of the condyles and lateral masses. As the head is flexed laterally, the condyles on the side of flexion "sink"

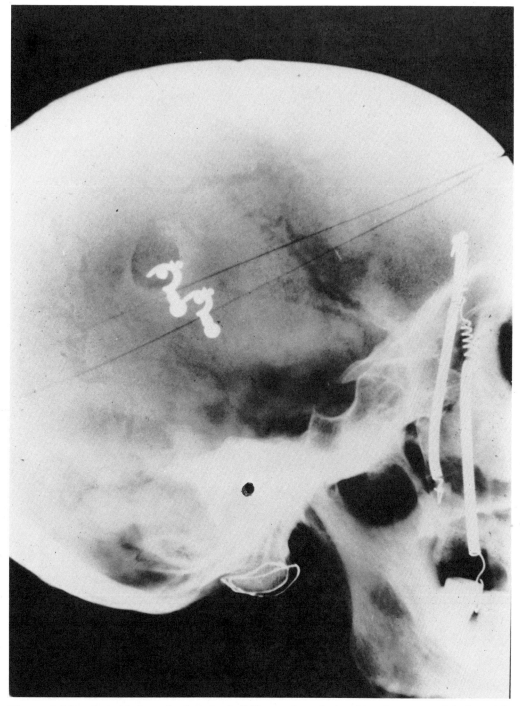

**Figure 6.16.** Lateral view of cadaveric skull illustrating relationship of convex occipital condyles to vestibular apparatuses.

downward into the corresponding lateral mass, and on the opposite side the condyle rides upward on its corresponding lateral mass.

3. On the *transverse body plane*, in spite of some contention to the contrary by proponents of certain upper cervical spinographic analysis systems, there is

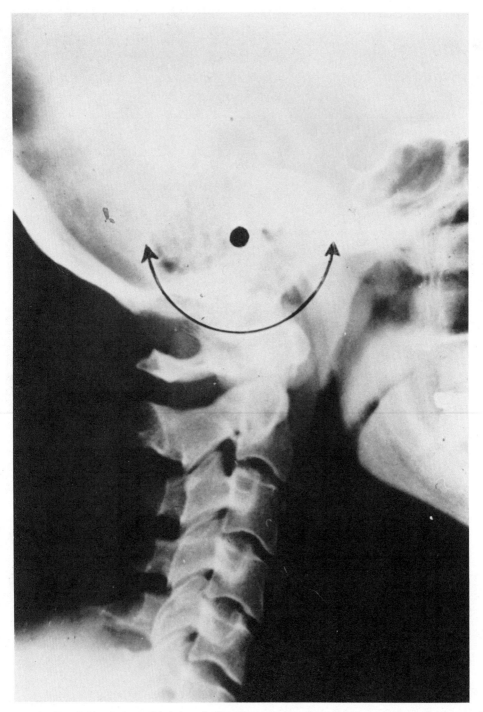

**Figure 6.17.**   Lateral view of in vivo skull with articulated cervical spine. Note obvious arch of occipital condyles, on the atlas lateral masses, around a point of pivot at the vestibular apparatuses.

no true rotation between the condyles and atlas lateral masses, this being due to the effect of their convex/concave

design (Fig. 6.19A). However, when the combined sagittal and coronal plane movements are considered on a three-

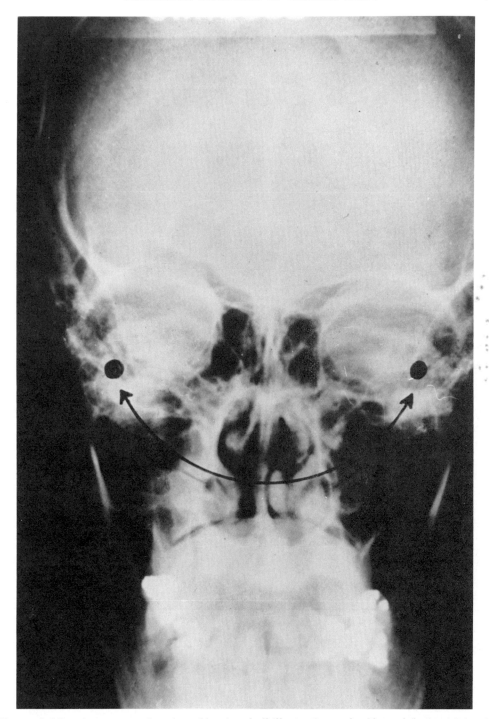

**Figure 6.18.** Anteroposterior view of in vivo skull illustrating arch of lateral flexion of the skull on the atlas lateral masses around a point of pivot midway between the vestibular apparatuses.

dimensional basis, a *screwlike* movement is allowed around a vector at the center of the head—the head (rather than rotating on the atlas) may move in a screwlike action on the atlas while maintaining its point of vector at the center of gravity of the head (Fig. 6.19*B*).

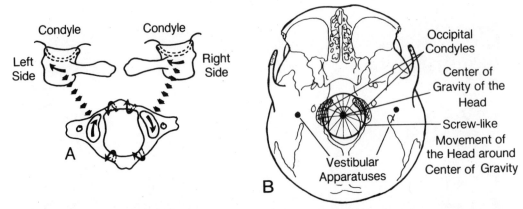

**Figure 6.19.** *A*, torsion of the anterior and posterior arches which would preclude any normal rotation of the atlanto-occipital articulation beyond that allowed by the synovial joint spacing. *B*, combined three-dimensional flexion-extension/lateral flexion movements of the occiput and atlas, thus allowing for a "screwlike" movement around the center of gravity of the skull located midway between, and on a level with, the vestibular apparatuses.

In order to completely accomplish its objective as a balance control mechanism for the head, the atlas requires the biomechanical support of the axis, on which it rests and on which it depends for certain "complimentary" movements. These movements between the atlas and axis may be described as follows (Fig. 6.20):

    B. Atlantoaxial articulation
        1. On the *sagittal body plane* the atlas may anteroflex and retroextend on a transverse axis at the upper aspect of the odontoid process, with the inferior articular processes of the atlas gliding anteriorly in extension and posteriorly in flexion on the superior articular processes of the axis. Since the integrity of this movement is critically dependent upon the integrity of the atlas transverse ligament, any laxity of this ligament due to trauma or pathology can severely upset the normal function of the entire occipitocervical complex.
        2. On the *coronal body plane* the atlas may laterally flex on the axis, in an arc, with its axis of pivot located at some point in the lower cervical area. This movement is characterized by the atlas sliding downward on the side of flexion and upward on the side of extension due to the laterally inclined design of the atlas-axis articulations.
        3. On the *transverse body plane* the atlas can freely rotate (up to 90° in each direction) on the axis, the point of pivot being around the odontoid.

## NEUROMUSCULOSKELETAL INTEGRATION OF SPINAL FUNCTION

The activation of the spinal functional units in postural accommodation and locomotion is a mechanically initiated muscular action which is neurologically integrated with the vestibular apparatuses of the inner ear, the eyes and the proprioceptive postural control reflexes from throughout the body (30, 35–43), but most importantly from the functional units themselves. Cailliet (28) explains this mechanism as follows:

"A constant attempt is made by antigravity forces to maintain balance against gravity by initiating proprioceptively stimulated righting reflexes . . . Movement is initiated by muscular action exerting its traction effects on the functional units . . . The functional units are the component operational units of the entire spinal column and, as the units individually move, so moves the total column."

Consequently, it can be seen that the spinal functional units are not only initiated to function by proprioceptively controlled neuromuscular action, but once initiated such action is constantly *monitored* and *dampered* to effect purposeful movement of each functional unit individually and all functional units collectively.

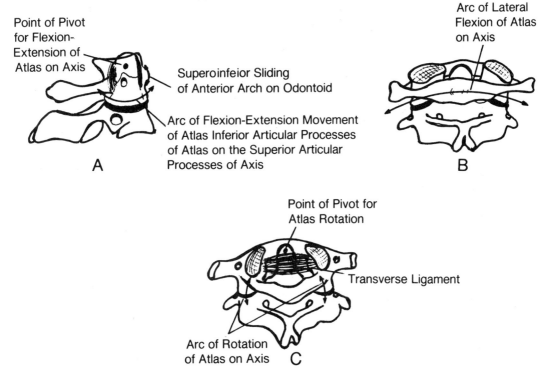

**Figure 6.20.**   Normal movements of atlas on axis. *A*, sagittal plane movement. *B*, coronal plane movement. *C*, rotational movement.

## Unitized Control of Spinal Function

When the body is in a static, erect-standing position, all spinal functional units may be said to be in their "normal resting positions" for the particular individual. On the sagittal body plane the spinal column will be relatively straight with the body weight distributed equally on each side. On the coronal body plane the normal spinal curves will be adjusted (kinetically compensated) so that the body weight will be equally distributed to the front and back. The "vertical central axis" of the body will be gravitationally erect with the "center of gravity of the head" in vertical alignment over the "center of gravity of the pelvis," and body weight will be equally distributed on both feet—bilaterally and anteroposteriorly. Thus, the body will be maintained in an erect, balanced state of postural equilibrium with minimal muscular effort. Grice (40) and Johnson (44) have depicted this balance state of postural equilibrium of the body by a series of inverted pyramids representing the head, trunk and lower extremities (Fig. 6.21).

Whenever the body is then required to shift balance to compensate to changes in the gravitational forces being exerted on it (statically as in compensation to standing on an unlevel surface or kinetically as in walking) the spinal functional units are activated to function by appropriate musculature responding to an *interplay* of sensory (vestibuloproprioceptive) and motor nerve supply. In this manner, the spinal column laterally flexes, rotates, anteroflexes, and extends in exactly the correct manner and degree to readjust the body to a posturally compensated state.

## LATERAL FLEXION AND ROTATION OF THE SPINAL COLUMN IN POSTURAL COMPENSATION

In the normally erect postural state the sacrum (on the coronal plane) serves as a

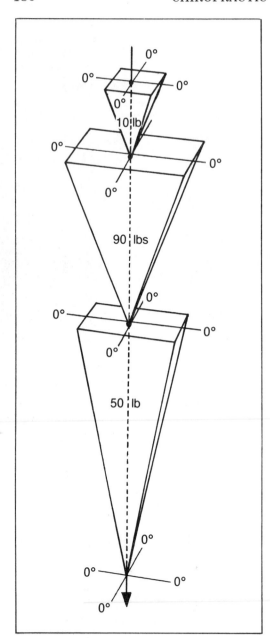

**Figure 6.21.** Grice (40) and Johnson (44) inverted pyramid depiction of the body in a static state of postural equilibrium.

level base for the spine above (Fig. 6.22A). When the sacral base is unleveled for any reason (as an independent action or in response to unleveling of the entire pelvis) the spine above will initially follow, thus tending to shift the body off balance toward the side of the lowered sacrum (Fig. 6.22B).

However, sensing this imbalance through the action of the proprioceptive and vestibular righting reflexes, the central nervous system dispatches motor signals to the appropriate muscles which activate the spinal functional units to affect a compensated spinal curvature (functional scoliosis to bring the body back to a state of balance.

The normal configuration of a compensated spinal curvature is a long Ŝ-Shaped functional scoliosis. The lumbar spine curvature will normally convex toward the side of the lowered sacral base, and the vertebral bodies will rotate *posterior* on the side of the convexity (Fig. 6.23). The thoracic spine will be maintained in a relatively straight configuration due mainly to the stability imposed on it by the ribs. The cervical spine will normally convex in the direction opposite that of the lumbar spine curvature, and the vertebral bodies will rotate *anterior* on the side of the convexity (Fig. 6.24). Thus, the body will be compensatorily balanced with the center of gravity of the head directly over the center of gravity of the pelvis.

## ANTEROPOSTERIOR FLEXION AND EXTENSION OF THE SPINAL COLUMN IN POSTURAL COMPENSATION

When viewed from the side, the posturally erect spinal column presents four normal curves. Those of the cervical, thoracic and lumbar regions are designated as "physiological curves" insofar as they are comprised of spinal functional units and are actively involved in spinal kinetic activities. The sacrococcygeal curve, which is not comprised of functional units and is not intrinsicly involved in spinal kinetic activities (as far as the curve itself is concerned), is designated as an "anatomic curve." However, the sacrum as a unit serves an important function as a support structure for the spine above and a control mechanism for spinal postural compensation—a kinetic control which is mandatory for man's bipedal posture.

Normally, the base of the sacrum slopes

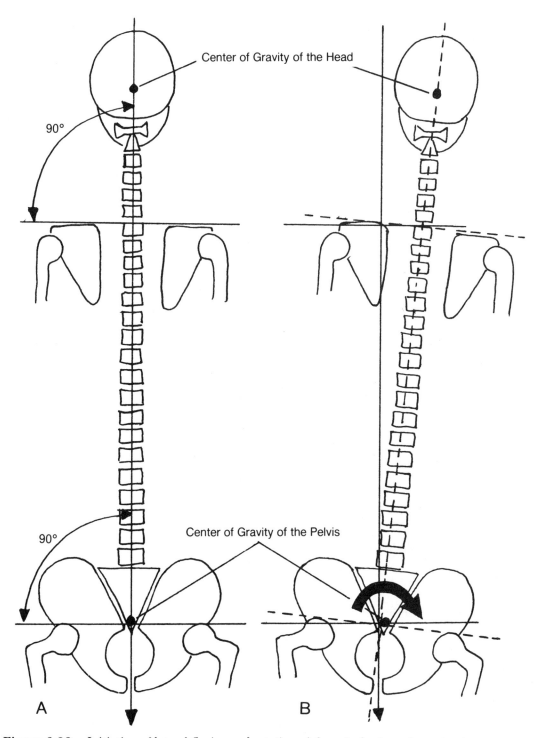

**Figure 6.22.**   Initiation of lateral flexion and rotation of the spinal column in postural compensation. *A*, ideal/normal erect spinal column in postural equilibrium; muscles in a minimal state of tonus under the control of the proprioceptive/vestibular righting reflexes. *B*, unleveling of the sacropelvis initially results in the spine deviating off center of gravity as a rigid column.

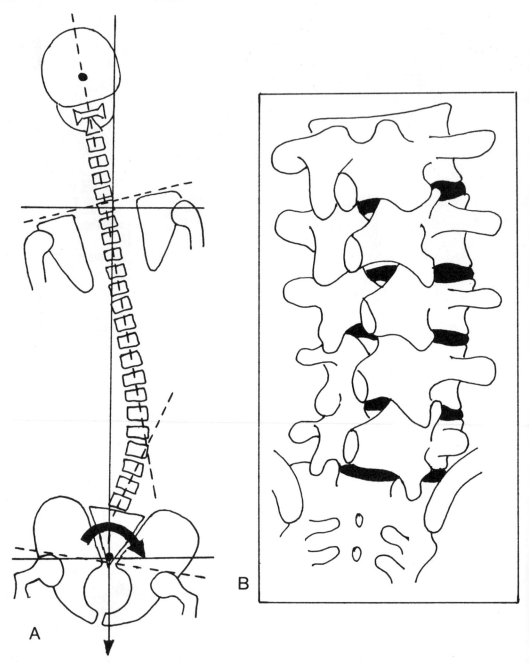

**Figure 6.23.** Deviation of the spine off center of gravity results in an instantaneous stimulation of sensory proprioceptive/vestibular righting reflex contraction of muscles to affect a compensatory curvature of the lumbar spine in an effort to restore body equilibrium; the lumbar vertebrae will laterally flex and rotate *posterior* on the side of the lowered sacropelvic base. *A*, gross spinal response. *B*, specific response of lumbar spine. Note that although the lumbar spine has affected compensatory response, the head is now off balance in the opposite direction.

anteriorly and inferiorly at an angle of about 39° (35–42° range) and establishes the magnitude of the spinal physiological curves. All three physiological curves, in their ascent, ordinarily must intersect at the midcoronal plane of the body to antero-

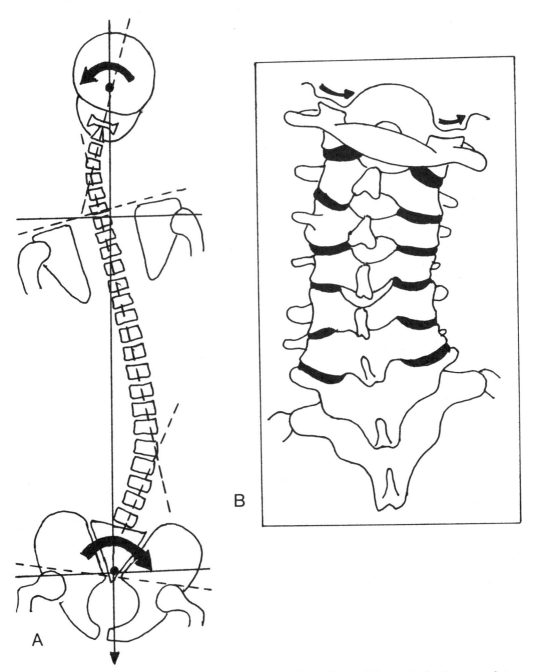

**Figure 6.24.** Stimulation of the proprioceptive righting reflexes of the cervical spine musculature results in the development of a reverse (from the direction of the lumbar spine curvature) curvature of the cervical spine. *A*, gross postural compensation of the entire spine in an effort to restore equilibrium; the cervical spine vertebrae laterally flexing and rotating anterior on the side of convexity, opposite to that of the lumbar spine. *B*, with the head now off balance, the vestibular apparatuses will attempt to level it to gravity, a situation that could result in articular jamming at the atlanto-occipital junction—theoretically this is the mechanism that could cause a *compensatory* occipitoatlanto subluxation as a result of a *primary* sacroiliac subluxation.

posteriorly balance the body to gravity (Fig. 6.25A). Although the slope of the sacral base and configuration of the spinal curves are probably established genetically (according to body build; i.e. muscular = mesomorphic, heavy = endomorphic, lean = ectomorphic), environment also plays a significant role in modifying individual configurations.

The action of the physiological spinal curves in compensating to changes in the gravitational forces being exerted on the body on the anteroposterior (sagittal) plane, as in the lateral (coronal) plane, are intimately respondent to sacral balance control biomechanics. For example, when the pelvis and sacrum, or the sacrum independently of the innominate bones, is caused to increase or decrease relative to gravity, the spine will kinetically compensate by activation of the functional units which then regulate the magnitude of the physiological curves (Fig. 6.25B).

## CRANIOSACRAL MECHANISM

The *craniosacral mechanism* is a unique and somewhat controversial biomechanical activity originally promoted by members of the osteopathic profession (11, 19, 45). This concept was originally proposed by Sutherland (19) and is described by Ward and Sprafka (46) as follows:

> "'Craniosacral mechanism' is a term used by W. G. Sutherland, D.O., to describe the synchronous movement of the sacral base with the cranial base. This synchrony is accomplished by the attachment of the dural tube to the foramen magnum and sacral canal, and probably is aided by cerebrospinal fluid fluctuation. It is thought that the foramen magnum moves forward and upward during flexion of the sphenobasilar articulation which through the dural tube pulls the sacral base superior and posterior around a transverse axis at the articular processes posterior to the canal and through the second sacral segment."

Inherent within this craniosacral mechanism theory, are the following explanations (46):

1. **Cerebrospinal fluid fluctuations**—a description of the hypothesized action of cerebrospinal fluid with regard to the craniosacral mechanism which is thought to be the result of the inherent motility of the central nervous system. These changes in pressure are thought to produce motion of the osseous cranium along with movement of the falx cerebri and tentorium cerebelli.

2. **Cranial concept**—relates the anatomical and physiological mechanisms of the skull that are purported to represent the action of the primary respiratory mechanism as the motivating force relevant to the craniosacral mechanism expressed through the cranial rhythmic impulse. The cranial concept represents the application of the concept of somatic dysfunction to the craniosacral mechanism. Study of the diagnosis and management of the somatic dysfunction as extended to the craniosacral mechanism embraces: (a) introduction and maintenance of somatic dysfunction; (b) the pathological effects of somatic dysfunction; (c) specific methods for palpatory diagnosis and manipulative therapy.

3. **Cranial rhythmic impulse**—the result of minute rhythmic (cyclic) changes in the primary respiratory mechanism. The cumulative effect of these cyclic changes is expressed as a palpably perceived wave of variable intensity thought to be the consequence of rhythmic fluctuations of cerebrospinal fluid. The impulse occurs throughout the craniosacral mechanism. Rhythmic changes thought to be driven by the primary respiratory mechanism can be palpated throughout the body.

4. **Primary respiratory mechanism**—a term used to describe the interdependent function of several anatomic and physiologic components of the central nervous system. This primary respiratory function is purported to have remote effects on the entire body. Usually refers specifically to the inherent pulsating movements of the brain and spinal cord (8–12 cycles/min); a rhythmic fluctuation of cerebrospinal fluid and circulation independent of pulmonary respiration and heart rate; the articular mobility of the cranial bones; and the involuntary movement of the sacrum between the ilia seemingly correlated and interdependent with rhythmic cerebrospinal fluid fluctuations. Elements of the term are justified as follows:
   a. Primary—refers to the internal tissue respiratory process.
   b. Respiratory—refers to the process of internal respiration; i.e. the exchange of respiratory gases between tissue cells and their internal environment constituted of the fluids bathing the cells.

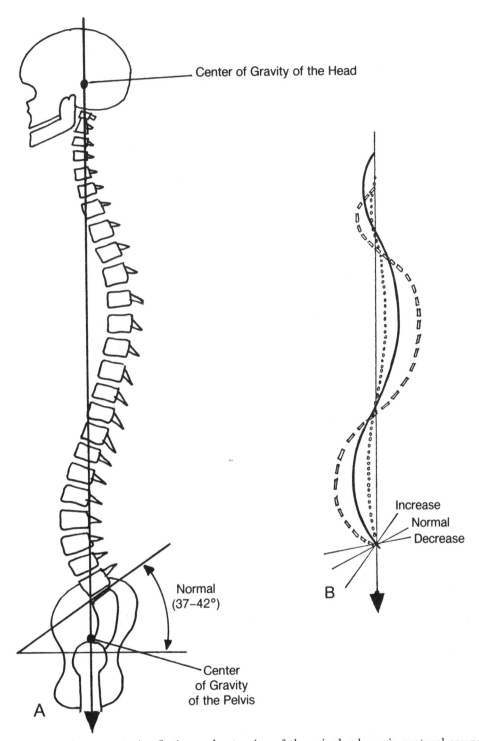

Center of Gravity of the Head

Normal
(37–42°)

Center
of Gravity
of the Pelvis

A

Increase
Normal
Decrease

B

**Figure 6.25.** Anteroposterior flexion and extension of the spinal column in postural compensation. *A*, normal erect attitude of the spinal column on the sagittal plane in consideration of a normal 35–42° sacral-base angle. *B*, theoretical response of compensating spine to increase or decrease in sacral-base angle beyond normals. [Adapted from Cailliet (28).]

  c. Mechanism—refers to the interdependent movement of tissue, bones and fluid.

5. **Extension, craniosacral**—anterior movement of the sacral base around a transverse axis in relation to the ilia, occurring during sphenobasilar extension.
6. **Flexion, craniosacral**—posterior movement of the sacral base around a transverse axis in relation to the ilia, occurring during sphenobasilar flexion.
7. *Sacral motion, respiratory*—the hypothetical transverse axis around which the sacrum moves during the respiratory cycle; passes from side to side through the articular processes of the second sacral segment. Also called the "superior transverse axis."

# RANGES OF SPINAL MOVEMENT

As a whole, the spinal column from sacrum to skull is, in a sense, equivalent to a joint with *three degrees of freedom*; it allows flexion and extension, right and left lateral flexion, and right and left rotation. The ranges of these elementary movements at each vertebral level is relatively minute, but in view of the number of joints involved the cumulative effect is considerable.

## Flexion and Extension

Flexion (forward bending) and extension (backward bending) takes place on the sagittal body plane. Kapandji (31) measures the total range of spinal sagittal plane movement at 250° in a very supple individual; the reference of movement being the *plane of bite* (as if a sheet of cardboard were held between the teeth) and the sacral base. This range is considerable when compared to the 180° maximum for all composite joints as has been reported. The segmental contributions to the total range of spinal movement is as follows:

**Lumbar spine**—flexion, 60°; extension, 35°.
**Thoracolumbar**—flexion, 105°; extension, 60°.
**Cervical**—flexion, 40°; extension, 60°.
    **Total range**—flexion to extension, 110–140°.

All figures are approximations as there is little agreement among authors regarding the normal range of movement at various levels; moreover, these values vary considerably with age. Therefore, only the maximum values as given by Kapandji are presented here (31).

## Lateral Flexion

Lateral flexion occurs on the frontal or coronal body plane and these values are relatively easy to measure and are, therefore, reasonably accurate. Reference planes are either the axis of the vertebrae or the orientation of the superior plateau of a particular vertebra. At the skull level the intermastoid line (the line joining the two mastoid processes of the skull) is used.

**Lumbar spine lateral flexion**—20°.
**Thoracic spine lateral flexion**—20°.
**Cervical spine lateral flexion**—35–45°.
    **Total range from sacrum to skull**—75–85°.

## Rotation

The ranges of axial rotation of the spinal column from the fixed pelvis to the skull are as follows

**Lumbar**—5°.
**Thoracic**—35°.
**Cervical**—50°.
    **Total range from sacrum to skull**—90–95°.

Additionally, it has been theorized that rotation of the sacrum within the ilia of the innominate bones is approximately 2–3°.

### References

1. Jones L: *The Postural Complex: Observations as to Cause, Diagnosis and Treatment.* Springfield, Ill, Charles C Thomas, 1955, pp 5–32.
2. Brennan MJ: Adaptation to bipedalism. *ACA J Chiropractic* 17:24–33, 1980.
3. Farfan HF: The biomechanical advantage of lordosis and hip extension for upright activity: man as compared to other anthropoids. *Spine* 3:336–342, 1978.
4. Hildebrandt RW: *Chiropractic Spinography: A Manual of Technology and Interpretation.* Des Plaines, Ill, Hilmark, 1977.
5. Seeman DC: Center of gravity of the skull: a review of theories and a pilot study to determine location. *J Manipulative Physiol Ther* 4:15–18, 1981.
6. Illi FW, Janse J: *The Vertebral Column: Lifeline*

of the Body—Supplemental Edition. Lombard, Ill, National College of Chiropractic, 1975.

7. Heyman J, Lundqvist A: The symphysis pubis in pregnancy and parturition. Acta Obstet Gynecol Scand, 12:191–226, 1932.

8. Colachis SC, Worden RE, Bechtol CO, Strohm BR: Movement of the sacroiliac in the adult male: a preliminary report. Arch Phys Med Rehail Sept:490–498, 1963.

9. Gray H: Anatomy of the Human Body, 29. Goss CM (ed). Philadelphia, Lea & Febiger, 1973, p 312.

10. Don Tigny RL: Dysfunction of the sacroiliac joint and its treatment. J Orthop Sports Phys Ther Summer:23–25, 1979.

11. Greenman PE: Roentgen findings in the craniosacral mechanism. J Am Osteopath Assoc 70:60–71, 1970.

12. Grieve E: Lumbopelvic rhythm and mechanical dysfunction of the sacroiliac joint. Phys Ther 67:171–173, 1981.

13. Nicholas AS: Dysfunction of the innominate complex. Osteopath Med Jan:65–67, 1979.

14. Travel W, Travel J: Technic for reduction and ambulatory treatment of sacroiliac displacement. Mod Med July:66–67, 1942.

15. Weismantel A: Evaluation and treatment of sacroiliac joint problems. Bull Orthop Am Phys Ther 3:5–20, 1978.

16. Wilder DG, Pope MH, Frymoyer JW: The functional topography of the sacroiliac joint. Spine, 5:575–579, 1980.

17. Slatter P: Sacroiliac pain and lumbar instability. Osteopath Ann 9:52–54, 1981.

18. Strachan WF, Bechwith CG, Larson NJ, Grant JH: A study of the mechanics of the sacroiliac joint. J Am Osteopath Assoc 37:576–578, 1938.

19. Wales AL: The work of William Garner Sutherland. J Am Osteopath Assoc 71:788–793, 1972.

20. Frigerio NA, Stowe RS, Howe JW: Movement of the sacroiliac joint. Clin Orthop 100:370–377, 1974.

21. Olerud S, Grevsten S: Chronic pubic symphysiolysis. J Bone Joint Surg 56A:799–802, 1974.

22. LaBan MM, Meerschaert JR, Taylor RS, Tabor HD: Symphyseal and sacroiliac joint pain associated with pubic symphysis instability. Arch Phys Med Rehabil 59:470–475, 1978.

23. Gaucher PL: Pathology of the symphysis pubis. Chiropraxis (French). June:25–41, 1978.

24. Percy-Lancaster R: Pelvic arthropathy. S. Afr Med J 10:551–557, 1969.

25. Herbst RW: Gonstead Chiropractic Science and Art. Mt. Horeb, Wisc, Sci-Chi Publications, 1971, pp 1–11.

26. Illi FW, Janse J: The Spinal Column: Lifeline of the Body. Lombard, Ill, National College of Chiropractic, 1975.

27. Drum DC: The intervertebral motor unit and the intervertebral foramen. In The Research Status of

Spinal Manipulative Therapy. NINCDS Monograph No. 15. Washington DC NIH 76-998, 1975, pp 63–75.

28. Cailliet R: Low back pain syndrome, ed 2. Philadelphia, FA Davis, 1968, pp 1–23.

29. White AA, Panjabi MM: The basic kinematics of the human spine: a review of past and current knowledge. Spine 3:12–30, 1978.

30. Schmorl G, Junghams H: The human spine in health and disease, Am ed 2. New York, Grune & Stratton, 1971 pp 30–41.

31. Kapandji IA: The Physiology of Joints, vol 3, The Trunk and Vertebral Column. London, Churchill-Livingstone, 1974, pp 10–51.

32. White AA, Panjabi MM: Clinical Biomechanics of the Spine. Philadelphia, Lippincott, 1978, vol 3, pp 12–20.

33. Basic Chiropractic Procedural Manual: Des Moines, Iowa, American Chiropractic Association, 1973, vol 1.

34. Jerow G: Osseous configurations of the axial skeleton: specific application to spatial relationships of vertebrae. J Manipulative Physiol Ther 7:35–40, 1984.

35. Weeks ZR: Effects of the vestibular system on human development: overview of function and effects of stimulation. Am J Occup Ther 33:376–381, 1979.

36. Stejskal L: Postural reflexes in man. Am J Phys Med 58:1–25, 1979.

37. Seliktar R, Susak Z, Najenson T, Solzi P: Dynamic features of standing and their correlation with neurological disorders. Scand J Rehabil Med 10:59–64, 1978.

38. Ferni GR, Holiday PE, Holiday PJ: Postural sway in amputees and normal subjects. J Bone Joint Surg 60A:895–898, 1978.

39. Plummer JP: Acupuncture and homeostasis: physiological, physical (postural) and psychological. Am J Chin Med 1–14, 1981.

40. Grice AS: Posture and postural mechanics. J Can Chiropractic Assoc July:12–17, 1970.

41. Bailey HW: Theoretical significance of postural imbalance, especially the "short leg." J Am Osteopath Assoc 77:452–455, 1978.

42. Terekhov YV: Instrumentation for automatic measurement and real-time evaluation of man's postural equilibrium. J Med Eng Technol 2:182–186, 1978.

43. Sahlstrand T, Ortengren R, Nachemson A: Postural equilibrium in adolescent idiopathic scoliosis. Acta Orthop Scand 49:354–365, 1978.

44. Johnson LC: The gravity line relation to AP posture. J Can Chiropractic Assoc 6, 1962.

45. Morey LW: Uses of cranial manipulative therapy. Osteopath Med July:48–52, 1978.

46. Ward RC, Sprafka S: Glossary of osteopathic terminology. J Am Osteopath Assoc 80:552–566, 1981.

# CHAPTER 7

# Biomechanical Disorders of the Spinal Column

## ORIGIN OF CHIROPRACTIC THEORY

Following a period of some 8–10 yr of independent study of therapeutic manipulation, on September 18, 1895 Daniel David (D.D.) Palmer announced the formal existence of *Chiropractic* as a new and specialized approach to the diagnosis and treatment of health problems. This announcement followed the reported successful outcome of a "test case" in which Palmer had relieved a case of deafness by the *specific* manipulation (adjustment) of a patient's 4th thoracic vertebra, which he believed to be in a *subluxated* (minute biomechanical misalignment) state, which in turn he believed was causing an *impingement* of nerves (autonomic) leading to the hearing apparatuses. Palmer then *described* his new concept of health care as follows (1).

> "... Chiropractic is the name of a systematized knowledge of the science of life—biology, and a methodical comprehension and application of adjusting anatomical displacements, the cause of biological abnormalities; also an explanation of the methods used to relieve humanity of suffering and the prolonging of life ..."

By virtue of his studies, Palmer had reached a conclusion which the biological sciences is only coming to appreciate today—that "the human body is a self-contained biological unit which inherently possesses all the necessary requisites to maintain itself in physiological equilibrium (biological homeostasis), within itself and within its environment, and when so maintained has a reasonable expectation of good health as a natural condition." With this thought as the basic premise of his theory, Palmer then hypothesized essentially as follows:

1. The primary component charged with the responsibility of maintaining physiological equilibrium of the body is the *nervous system*, which directly or indirectly controls all other systems.
2. Malfunction of the nervous system may result in physiological disturbances, within itself and ultimately within all other body systems, which in turn may render the individual *susceptible* to the development of disease conditions; e.g. disordered physiology always precedes pathology.
3. A major cause for malfunction of the nervous system (in a body in which normal function was originally present) is some form of *physical insult* within the confines of the spinal column, or in close proximity to it; i.e. the spinal cord, spinal nerves, autonomic nerves, etc.
4. The nature of the physical insulting factor to the nervous system—within or in close proximity to the spinal column—is frequently a biomechanical aberration between two contiguous vertebrae; e.g. *subluxation.*
5. Identification and manipulative management of such biomechanical aberrations of the spinal column *anticipates* relief of attendant neurological dysfunction and its concomittant disturbances of physiological equilibrium, thus providing an *optimal medium* for alleviation of related disease states by reactivation of the body's inherent healing processes.
6. Return of normal health following the correction of such subluxations and their concomittant neurological deficits by a specifically applied manipulation—*adjustment*—of the offending vertebra, is to some extent dependent upon the *residual healing*

*capacity* of the individual and it was accepted that related pathophysiological states may advance to a degree beyond which the body's own healing resources may be inadequate to sufficiently cope. In this case, other methods of health care may be required.

Initially, Palmer's overall theory for the basis of chiropractic was astute and worthy of further scientific study. However, later efforts of others (2) to refine his theory by reducing it to *dogma-like* definitions resulted in a severe loss of its scientific credibility. For example, chiropractic was defined as "*a philosophy, science and art of things natural; a system of adjusting the segments of the spinal column by hand only, for correction of the cause of dis-ease*"; the vertebral subluxation was defined as "*the condition of a vertebra that has lost its proper juxtaposition with the one above or the one below, or both; to an extent less than a luxation—complete dislocation—which impinges nerves and interferes with the transmission of mental impulses.*"

It is not the purpose of this discussion to go into any drawn-out explanations of the inaccuracies and inadequacies of these definitions as a preface to spinographic evaluation of spinal biomechanical integrities—we will leave the reader to make their own analysis of the dichotomy between Palmer's original concept and the definitions of his followers. Suffice it to say at this point that the chiropractic profession as a whole is attempting to reconstruct its basic theory, with strong emphasis on the original concepts put forth by Palmer (1), and are generally attempting to repudiate the unscientific claims of his followers which still plague the profession today (3).

## CHIROPRACTIC SUBLUXATION SYNDROME

Stated more in terms of present day knowledge of the subject, rather than the aforementioned definition of a *chiropractic subluxation*, chiropractic clinical concern is to a significant extent directed toward a *cause*-and-*effect* relationship between dis-ordered biomechanical integrities of the spinal column (orthodysarthrias) and the development of pathophysiology anywhere in the body. In its entirety, this cause-and-effect relationship is a complex biological syndrome which may be further clarified by the following component-part outline of the *chiropractic subluxation syndrome* (4):

1. Biomechanical Cause
   a. *Direct*
      A direct biomechanical cause is that condition in which a loss of biomechanical integrity (static or functional) of the spinal column is precipitated by the direct effects of trauma or postural stresses; such condition reflecting clinically identifiable signs of spinal functional unit malfunction.
   b. *Indirect*
      An indirect biomechanical cause is that condition in which a loss of biomechanical integrity of the spinal column is precipitated by the indirect effects of muscular dystonia (possibly due to muscular injury or aberrant somatospinal reflexes); such conditions reflecting clinically identifiable signs of spinal functional unit malfunction.
2. Pathophysiological effects
   a. *Primary*
      Primary pathophysiological effects are those conditions which may occur within the confines of a malfunctioning spinal functional unit, itself, as a result of attendant tissue irritation; such as, inflammation, swelling, etc.
   b. *Secondary*
      Secondary pathophysiological effects are those conditions which may occur in outlying areas of the body (extraspinal) as an extension of the primary effects of a malfunctioning spinal functional unit.
   (1) Biomechanical
      The secondary effects of spinal orthodysarthrias may be biomechanically transmitted to outlying areas of the body by their influence in the induction of spinal curvatures (scolioses, kyphoses, lordoses) or other disseminated stress effects of spinal functional unit malfunction.
   (2) Neurological
      The secondary effects of spinal orthodysarthrias may be neurologically transmitted to outlying areas of the body (extraspinal) by their influence in the induction of aberrant patholog-

ical, spinosomatic-spinovisceral, reflexes.

With respect to the primary pathophysiological effects and those secondary effects which are biomechanically related, there is little or no dispute that such conditions do constitute clinically significant concerns. However, in the case of the secondary effects which are neurologically related, the situation is not as yet so clear cut, although considerable evidence has been compiled in recent years to support the contention that neurovascular insult at the site of a spinal orthodysarthria may result in the development of outlying pathophysiology due to aberrant spinosomatic/spinovisceral reflexes (3–7).

In consideration of the chiropractic spinal subluxation as such a complex cause-and-effect clinical syndrome, it may be conjectured that once initiated, a spinal orthodysarthria may effect an etiologic *vicious cycle* from cause to effect and from effect back to cause which, if not interrupted by corrective effort, may carry on to an ultimate (perhaps fatal) conclusion. With respect to this possibility, the following by Janse (8) is an appropriate illustrative statement:

> ". . . The mechanical lesion referred to by chiropractors as a subluxation is an attending complication of those chemical, mechanical and/or environmental irritations of the nervous system which in man, the biped, produce muscle contraction sufficient to cause articular dysfunction. Once produced, the lesion becomes a focus of sustained irritation. It irritates proprioceptors in the articular capsules, ligaments, tendons, and muscles of the involved spinal segment. A barrage of impulses stream into the spinal cord where interneurons receive them and relay them to motor pathways for conduction to muscles and glands, initially in excessive amounts. *The contraction which provoked the subluxation in the first place is thereby reinforced, thus perpetuating both the subluxation and the pathological process it engenders.*"

Although this concept represents a thought-provoking hypothesis, it is emphasized that in chiropractic spinography the principal objective is to evaluate the *bio-mechanical* status of the spinal column for evidence of structural deviations which may have clinical significance. The exact nature of the clinical implications, however, is not discernable on the basis of radiographic impressions alone, but must be correlated with other clinical impressions; i.e orthopedic and neurological tests, etc. In other words, the chiropractic subluxation in its entirety is not discernable by radiographic impression alone, only the biomechanical element of it is.

## CLASSIFICATION OF SUBLUXATIONS AS ORTHODYSARTHRIC LESIONS

Traditionally, the term "alignment" (proper juxtaposition) has been used chiropractically to designate the correct relation of two vertebrae and the term "misalignment" has been used to designate the biomechanical element of the chiropractic subluxation. However, in terms of present day knowledge of the subject, which considers the *dynamics* involved, these designations are inadequate.

In this presentation, normal or abnormal (proper relationship of vertebrae to each other or subluxation) considers the biomechanical efficiency of the spinal functional units. Therefore, the term *normal resting position* is given to designate the proper biomechanical attitude of one vertebra relative to its supporting structure below and, thus, the structural aspect of the spinal subluxation syndrome is defined as: "the inability of a vertebra to *move from* its normal resting position, to *move through* its normal ranges of motion, or to *move back* to its normal resting position after it has been biomechanically activated." These three types of spinal functional unit *orthodysarthrias* are then classified as follows (9):

Type A: The inability of a spinal functional unit to allow a vertebra to *move from* its normal resting position in relation to its supporting structure below; i.e. a vertebra *fixed* in its so-called normal alignment position due to bilateral muscle spasm, facet jamming, disk degeneration, etc. This type of spinal orthodysarthria is biomechanically significant primarily because of loss of movement contribution of the offending vertebra to spinal column function as a whole and the hypermobile stresses that will occur in the spinal functional units above and/or below when the spinal column is kinetically activated in body locomotion.

**Type B:** The inability of a vertebra to *move properly through* its normal ranges of movement; i.e. a vertebra partially fixed in or out of its so-called normal alignment due to unilateral muscle spasm, unilateral facet jamming, etc. This type of spinal orthodysarthria is biomechanically significant primarily because it will result in aberrant or erratic movement and unilateral hypermobile stresses within the involved spinal functional unit, as well as hypermobile compensatory stresses above and/or below when the spinal column is kinetically activated in body locomotion.

**Type C:** The inability of a vertebra to *move back* to its normal resting position after movement; i.e. a vertebra completely fixed out of its so-called normal alignment (off-centered but within its normal movement range) due to bilateral muscle spasm, facet jamming, etc. This type of spinal orthodysarthria is the traditional fixed subluxation and is biomechanically significant because it will result in static stresses within the involved spinal functional unit, as well as extended spinal distortions above and/or below when the spinal column is kinetically activated in body locomotion.

# CLASSIFICATION OF SUBLUXATIONS FOR CLAIM-REPORTING PURPOSES

In 1972, Public Law 92-603 was passed by the Congress of the United States which, in part, authorized payment for chiropractic services under Medicare. Insofar as there was not at that time a uniform agreement within the profession as to classification of subluxations, the following was adopted by representatives of the profession's academic, clinical and organizational communities for that purpose (10):

## General Considerations
### DEFINITION OF SUBLUXATION

A spinal subluxation is any alteration of the biomechanical and physiological dy-

namics of contiguous structures which can cause neuronal disturbances.

## MANIFESTATIONS OF SUBLUXATION

In evaluation of this complex phenomenon, we find that it has or may have biomechanical, pathophysiological, clinical, radiologic, or other manifestations.

## SIGNIFICANCE OF SUBLUXATIONS

Subluxations are of clinical significance as they are affected by or evoke abnormal physiological responses in neuromuscular structures and/or other body systems.

### Radiological Manifestations

In considering the possible radiological manifestations of subluxations, it is important to emphasize that clinical judgement is required to determine the necessity of exposing a patient to the potential hazards of ionizing radiations. An important purpose of exposure, besides the evaluation of subluxations, is the determination of the evidence of other pathologies. The radiologic procedures necessary to determine possible fractures, malignancies, etc., may not be the specific views needed to evaluate the possible radiological manifestations of subluxation. When subluxation can be evaluated by other means, it may be prudent to avoid radiation exposure.

## STATIC INTERSEGMENTAL SUBLUXATIONS

1. Flexion malposition (Fig. 7.1A)
2. Extension malposition (Fig. 7.1B)
3. Lateral flexion malposition (Fig. 7.1C)
4. Rotational malposition—left or right (Fig. 7.1D)
5. Anterolisthesis and/or spondylolisthesis (Fig. 7.1E)
6. Retrolisthesis (Fig. 7.1F)
7. Lateralisthesis—left or right (Fig. 7.2A)

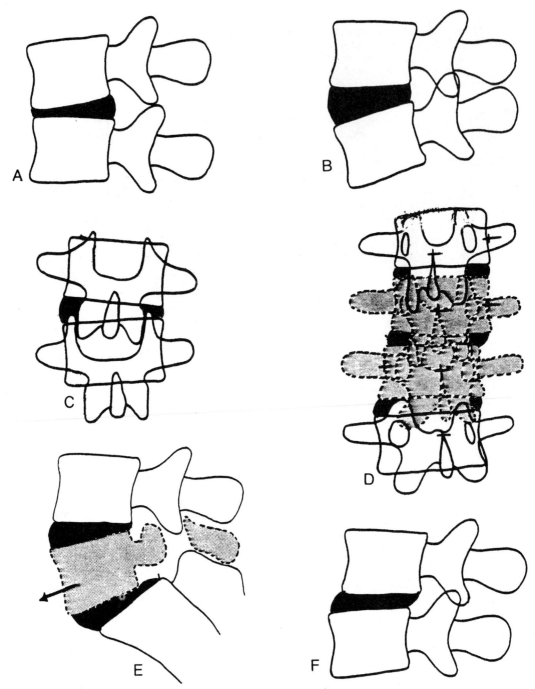

**Figure 7.1.** A, flexion malposition (A1); B, extension malposition (A2); C, lateral flexion malposition (A3); D, rotational malposition (A4); E, anterolisthesis-spondylolisthesis (A5); F, retrolisthesis (A6).

8. Altered interosseous spacing—decreased or increased (Fig. 7.2B)
9. Osseous foraminal encroachment (Fig. 7.2C)

KINETIC INTERSEGMENTAL SUBLUXATIONS

1. Hypomobility—fixation subluxation (Fig. 7.2D)

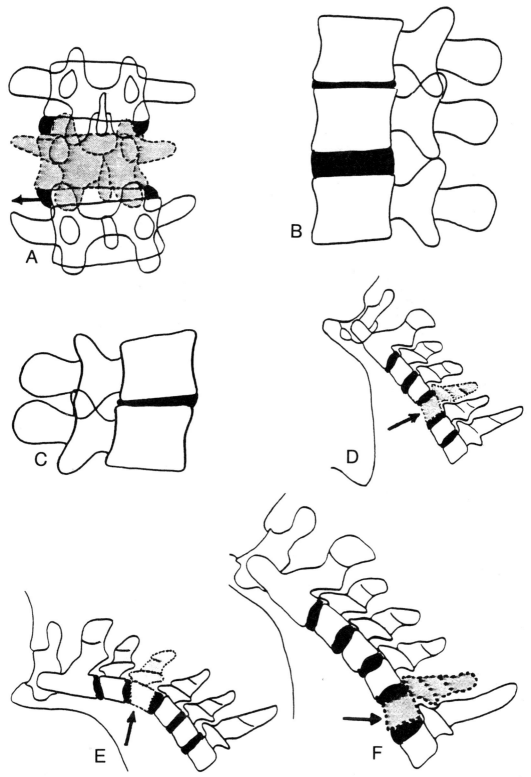

**Figure 7.2.** *A*, laterallisthesis (A7); *B*, altered interossseous spacing—decreased above, increased below (A8); *C*, osseous foraminal encroachment (A9); *D*, hypomobility subluxation (B1); *E*, hypermobility subluxation (B2); *F*, aberrant motion subluxation (B3).

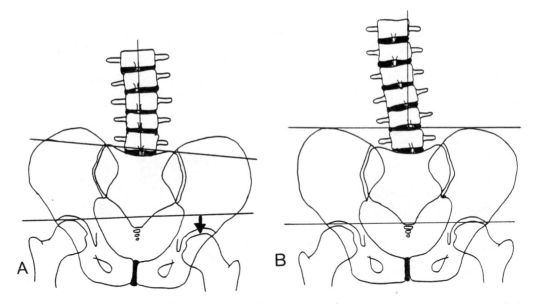

**Figure 7.3.** *A*, scoliosis and/or alterations of curves secondary to structural asymmetries (C1); *B*, scoliosis and/or alterations of curves secondary to muscular imbalance (C2).

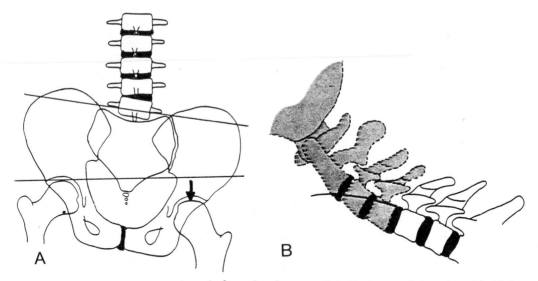

**Figure 7.4.** *A*, decompensation of adaptational curves (C3); *B*, abnormalities of motion (C4).

2. Hypermobility—loosened vertebral motor unit (Fig. 7.2*E*)
3. Aberrant motion (Fig. 7.2 *F*)

## SECTIONAL SUBLUXATIONS

1. Scoliosis and/or alteration of antero-posterior curves secondary to structural asymmetries (Fig. 7.3 *A*)
2. Scoliosis and/or alteration of antero-posterior curves secondary to muscular imbalance (Fig. 7.3*B*)
3. Decompensation of adaptational curves (Fig. 7.4*A*)
4. Abnormalities of motion (Fig. 7.4*B*)

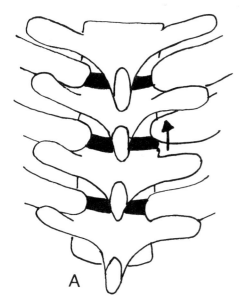 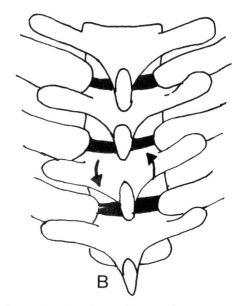

**Figure 7.5.**   Costovertebral-costotransverse subluxation. *A*, primary; *B*, secondary.

## PARAVERTEBRAL SUBLUXATIONS*

1. Costovertebral/costotransverse disrelationship—primary or secondary (Fig. 7.5)
2. Sacroiliac subluxation—primary or secondary (Fig. 7.6)

## CLASSIFICATION OF SPINAL SCOLIOSIS

Traditionally, both the chiropractic and medical professions have recognized certain concepts of scoliosis classification. To

---

* The costovertebral/costotransverse disrelationship subluxations have been further subdivided by the author (beyond that of the original classifications agreed upon by the chiropractic profession at the Houston Conference in 1972) to allow for the biomechanical etiology distinction of whether the disrelationship is *primary* to a rib disrelationship with otherwise correctly aligned vertebrae, or *secondary* to a vertebral subluxation. For the same reason, the sacroiliac subluxation classification has been further subdivided by the author to allow for the biomechanical etiology distinction of whether the disrelationship is *primary* to a sacral disrelationship within properly aligned innominate bones, or *secondary* to ilia disrelationship due to opposed anterior-posterior movement of the innominate bones at a symphysis pubis point of pivot. These distinctions were considered important to the determination of corrective procedure (particularly manual manipulation) to be employed if costovertebral/costotransverse or sacroiliac subluxation is spinographically diagnosed).

some extent these classifications were included in the preceding *Medicare Claim Reporting Classifications* of sectional subluxations. However, since certain elements of these traditional classifications include both etiological as well as clinical considerations they are included here for a more comprehensive understanding of scoliosis, as well as to attempt to illustrate a correlation between that knowledge of the subject which is peculiar to the chiropractic profession and that knowledge which is universal within the various health care professions.

### General Classification of Scoliosis

The following classification of scoliosis is that which is generally accepted within the health care professions at large and constitutes the standardized description on an etiological basis (11–13):

### FUNCTIONAL SCOLIOSIS

Functional scoliosis is a lateral curvature with elements of rotation which occurs in normal spinal function without alteration (fracture, pathology, developmental anomaly) of structural configuration of component spinal parts (Fig. 7.7A).

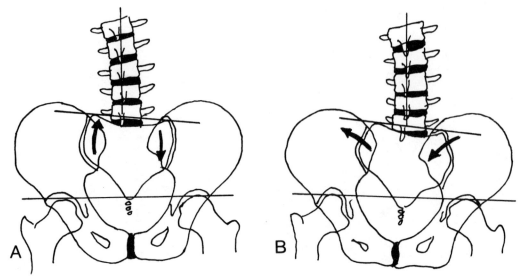

**Figure 7.6.** Sacroiliac subluxation. *A*, primary, *B*, secondary.

Although there is no structural asymmetry present, the function of the spinal column may be considered asymmetrical. The functional scoliosis is reducible by prone or supine position, and is correctible by leveling the base of spinal support which is responsible for the curvature by the use of heel/sole lifts, manipulation, elimination of muscle distony, etc.

## STRUCTURAL SCOLIOSIS

Structural scoliosis is a combination of lateral bending and rotation of the spinal column (or sections thereof) due to anatomic changes of spinal or pelvic configuration as a result of pathology, trauma or abnormal development (Fig. 7.7*B*). Specific etiologies of structural scoliosis are almost infinite—congenital variations, infections, tumors, trauma, surgery, erosive diseases, radiation retardation of spinal growth asymmetry, etc.

## IDIOPATHIC SCOLIOSIS

Idiopathic (unknown etiology) scoliosis is generally classified as follows (14):
1. Infantile
   a. Progressive
   b. Resolving
2. Juvenile
3. Adolescent

Idiopathic scoliosis (of the juvenile/adolescent types) usually begin as a functional scoliosis during the later part of the juvenile stage of development (8–10 yr of age) and progresses to a structural stage at the end of puberty. It is thought to be related to a congenital or hereditary defect of muscle development, it is seen more often in females than males, and may reach severe life-threatening proportions (15). Early detection is an important consideration in treatment and in recent years there has been increased effort given to school *scoliosis screening programs* (16–23).

Early treatment often requires concentrated use of orthopedic appliances, such as the Milwaukee brace (24), and late treatment may require surgery to relieve cardiopulmonary distress. Although therapeutic manipulation has not yet been proven to be directly effective in the treatment of adolescent idiopathic scoliosis, anecdotal evidence suggests that it may be helpful in minimizing progression during the early stages, particularly when used in conjunction with therapeutic exercises to strengthen weak muscles. Recent experiments with electrical muscle stimulation

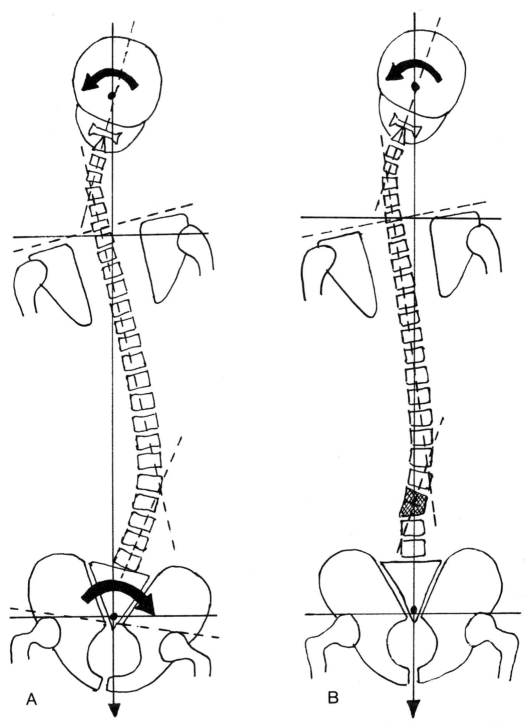

**Figure 7.7.** *A*, functional scoliosis due to pelvic unleveling compensation; *B*, structural scoliosis due to pathological, traumatic or developmental asymmetry of a vertebral body.

procedures have also shown some promise in minimizing progression of the scoliotic curvatures by strengthening muscles through intermittant contraction, and by replacing the use of braces by sustained contraction (24, 25).

### Lovett Classification of Scolioses

The Lovett concept of curvature evaluation is an early day method of classifying lumbar spine scolioses in accordance with their functional/structural characteristics and clinical significance (26). Six types have been described:

### LOVETT POSITIVE

The vertebral bodies rotate compensatorily toward the side of the scoliosis convexity, which is on the low side of a deviated sacral base. The angle of the vertebral plane at both ends of the scoliosis is in conformity with that of the sacrum. This type is a competently developed compensation to an unleveling of the sacral base and is generally asymptomatic (Fig. 7.8A).

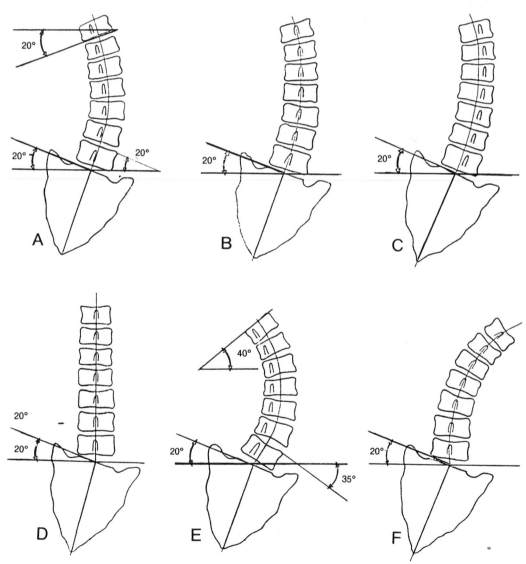

**Figure 7.8.** *A,* Lovett positive; *B,* Lovett static; *C,* Lovett negative; *D,* Lovett failure; *E,* Lovett excess; *F,* reverse.

## LOVETT STATIC

Convexity of scoliotic deviation is toward the low side of an unleveled sacral base, but without body rotation. This type is usually symptomatic and suggests moderate spasm of the psoas and multifidous muscles on the side of scoliotic convexity (Fig. 7.8B).

## LOVETT NEGATIVE

There is a scoliotic deviation to the low side of an unleveled sacral base, but vertebral body rotation is toward the side of scoliotic concavity. This type tends to be acutely symptomatic and suggests severe spasm of psoas and multifidous muscles on the convex side of the scoliosis (Fig. 7.8C).

## LOVETT FAILURE

The sacrum is deviated low on one side or the other but the lumbar spine remains straight—without scoliotic deviation or compensations. This situation suggests bilateral psoas and multifidous muscle spasm and is said to be frequently associated with disk disorder (Fig. 7.8D).

## LOVETT EXCESS

There is a scoliotic deviation with the vertebral bodies rotated toward the side of a low sacral base, but the degree of vertebral body deviation and scoliotic deviation are in excess to that which would be suggested by the degree of sacral base lowering. This type suggests: (a) an undue spasm of the psoas and multifidous muscles on the high side of the sacral base, (b) a possible wedging of the L5 vertebra on the low side of sacral deviation and/or (c) a loosening of the disk and ligamentous restraining structures (Fig. 7.8E).

## LOVETT REVERSE

There is a scoliotic deviation to the high side of the sacral base due to marked wedging of L4 or L5, or severe spasm of the psoas and multifidous muscles on the low side of the sacral base. Marked hypolasia of the lumbosacral facets may also be suspect on the side of the high sacral base and side of atypical scoliotic convexity (Fig. 7.8F).

# PELVIC AND SPINAL LISTINGS

In chiropractic procedure it is a frequent practice to assign a *listing* to those pelvic or spinal structures that are believed to be in a state of subluxation, the primary purpose being for manipulative correction orientation. The following are those most commonly used (27):

**Pelvic Listings** (Torsion of the total pelvic unit on the femur heads)

RAP-LAP (Right Anterior Pelvis/Left Anterior Pelvis)

**Innominate Listings** (Direction of ilia movement)

RPIN-LPIN (Right Posterior Innominate/Left Posterior Innominate)
RAIN-LAIN (Right Anterior Innominate/Left Anterior Innominate)

**Sacral Listings** (Relative to sacral base)

AS (Anterior Sacrum)
PS (Posterior Sacrum)
ARS-ALS (Anterior Right Sacrum/Anterior Left Sacrum)†
PRS-PLS (Posterior Right Sacrum/Posterior Left Sacrum)†

**Vertebral Listings**

The listings given here are in accordance with what has been designated as the National-Diversified System which lists misalignments according to direction of vertebral body movement. The Palmer-Gonstead-Firth System (another popular method) designates misalignment of vertebrae with reference to the spinous process, therefore designations are opposite; e.g. a Right-Posterior (RP) National-Diversified listing would be a Left Posterior (LP) Palmer-Gonstead-Firth listing.

RP-LP (Right Posterior/Left Posterior)
RL-LL (Right Lateral/Left Lateral)
RI-LI (Right Inferior/Left Inferior)
AI-PI (Anteroinferior/Posteroinferior)

**Occipital Listings**

RPO-LPO (Right Posterior Occiput/Left Posterior Occiput)

---

† Denotes rotation of sacrum within the ilia.

RLO-LLO (Right Lateral Occiput/Left Lateral Occiput)

AIO-PSO (Anteroinferior Occiput/Posterosuperior Occiput)

## References

1. Palmer DD: *The Science, Art and Philosophy of Chiropractic.* Portland, Portland Printing House, 1910, p 1.
2. Stephenson RW: *Chiropractic Textbook.* Davenport, Iowa, Palmer School of Chiropractic, 1942, p 2.
3. Goldstein M (ed): *The Research Status of Spinal Manipulative Therapy. NINCDS Monograph No. 15.* Washington, DC, DHEW Publication No. (NIH) 76-998, 1975.
4. Hildebrandt RW: *Synopsis of Chiropractic Postural Roentgenology.* Lombard, Ill, National College of Chiropractic, 1974, pp 32-34.
5. Korr IM (ed): *The Neurobiologic Mechanisms in Manipulative Therapy.* New York, Plenum, 1977.
6. Buerger A, Tobis J (eds): *Approaches to the Validation of Manipulative Therapy.* Springfield, Ill, Charles C Thomas, 1977.
7. Haldeman S (ed): *Modern Developments in the Principles and Practice of Chiropractic.* New York, Appleton-Century-Crofts, 1980.
8. Hildebrandt R (ed): *J. Janse Principles and Practice of Chiropractic.* Lombard, Ill, National College of Chiropractic, 1976.
9. Hildebrandt RW: *Chiropractic Spinography: Manual of Technology and Interpretation,* ed 1. Des Plaines, Ill, Hilmark, 1977, pp 10-13.
10. *Basic Chiropractic Procedural Manual,* Des Moines, Iowa, American Chiropractic Association, 1973.
11. Hoppenfeld R: *Scoliosis: a Manual of Concept and Treatment.* Philadelphia, Lippincott, 1967.
12. Keim HA: Scoliosis. *Ciba Clin Symp* 30:22-24, 1978.
13. Cailliet R: *Scoliosis: Diagnosis and Management.* Philadelphia, FA Davis, 1975.
14. Hildebrandt RW: Adolescent idiopathic scoliosis: a review of current concepts of etiology, incidence, pathophysiology and treatment. *J Manipulative Physiol Ther* 1:170-175, 1978.
15. Levine DB: Pulmonary function in scoliosis. *Orthop Clin North Am* 10:761-768, 1979.
16. Belstead JS, Edgar MA: Early detection of scoliosis. *Br Med J* September:937-938, 1978.
17. Drummond DS: Spinal deformity: natural history and role of school screening. *Orthop Clin North Am* 10:751-759, 1979.
18. Smyrnis PN, Valavaris J, Alexopoulos A, Siderakis G, Giannestrass NJ: School screening for scoliosis in Athens. *J Bone Joint Surg* 61B:215-217, 1979.
19. Dendy JM, Chase S, Determann P: School screening for scoliosis. Physiotherapy 69:272-276, 1983.
20. Connolly BH, Michael BT: Early detection of scoliosis: a neurological approach using the asymmetrical tonic neck reflex. *Phys Ther* 64:304-307, 1984.
21. Kane WJ, Brown JC, Hensinger RN, Keller RB: Scoliosis and school screening for spinal deformity. *Am Fam Physician* 17:123-127, 1978.
22. Dickson RA, Stamper P, Sharp A, Harker H: School screening for scoliosis: a cohort study of clinical course. *Br Med J* July 26:265-267, 1980.
23. Low WD, Mok CK, Leong JCY, Uau AC, Liskowski FP: The development of Southern Chinese girls with idiopathic scoliosis. *Spine* 3:152-156, 1978.
24. Bobechko WP, Herbert MA, Friedman HG: Electrospinal instrumentation for scoliosis: current status. *Orthop Clin North Am* 10:927-940, 1979.
25. Eckerson LF, Axelgaard J: Lateral electrical surface stimulation as an alternative to bracing in the treatment of idiopathic scoliosis: treatment protocol and patient acceptance. *Phys Ther* 64:483-490, 1984.
26. Lovett R: The mechanism of the normal spine and its relation to scoliosis (an archival classic) *Boston Med Surg J.* 153-349, 1905.
27. States AE: Pelvic and spinal technics. Lombard, Ill, National College of Chiropractic, 1970.

# PART 3

# PRINCIPLES OF SPINOGRAPHIC INTERPRETATION

# CHAPTER 8

# Spinographic Evaluation of Diagnostic Signs

## OVERVIEW OF ROENTGEN DIAGNOSIS

It is generally accepted that a confirmed diagnosis of bone pathologies on the basis of roentgen studies alone are limited in many cases and frequently requires the combined efforts of the attending doctor, radiologist, orthopedist, pathologist and others depending upon the nature of the problem that is suspect. However, since the process of diagnosis usually begins with the attending doctor, he or she has the initial responsibility to at least make a reasonably thorough *survey* of the films for *possible* pathological involvements which may constitute clinically significant conditions in need of referral and/or may qualify biomechanical evaluations. Accordingly, the following classic approach from Greenfield (1) appropriately sets the stage:

"The basic approach should be simple. The roentgen pattern should be accurately and objectively analyzed with respect to approximately 30 distinct, independent features. On the basis of this objective analysis, a list of differential diagnoses can be prepared. This list should be broad, so as not to exclude the correct diagnosis. The differential diagnoses are then applied to the particular case. The age of the patient is of prime importance, and the possibilities for the presence of many disease entities can be eliminated on this basis alone. The sex and race of the patient are also important. These factors are correlated with the total clinical picture, and the biochemical values are determined. This effectively reduces the list to a few possibilities... The objective analysis should be made before clinical influences prevail, so as not to prejudice an accurate description.

"The clinical correlation of objective radi- ological patterns is an exercise in statistics. However, bone has a limited response to disease processes. There are many more diseases than avenues of bone response, so it should not be surprising that the different lesions can give similar patterns. In addition, many lesions distinguished by a typical characteristic on roentgen films often present an atypical appearance. To these atypical lesions that may lack one or more distinctive features (e.g. the 'sunburst' appearance in osteosarcoma, or laminated periosteum in Ewing's sarcoma), an old adage seems applicable: 'a three-legged dog is still a dog.'

"Only about a dozen primary bone tumors occur with appreciable frequency, of which most are readily diagnosable radiologically in their typical forms. A definitive diagnosis of certain asymptomatic benign entities, such as cortical defect of nonossifying fibroma, may be made on radiological grounds.

"The statistical correlation for a solitary atypical lesion can be no better than a guess, which may be valid when applied on a percentage basis to a large population, but which is inadequate when applied to the individual patient. Thus, definitive procedures such as amputation must never be performed on the basis of the roentgen picture alone, but only after adequate tissue sections have first been studied. The roentgen findings alone, isolated from clinical and pathologic reality, should be considered insufficient information in themselves for a definitive diagnosis." [From Greenfield GB: *Radiology of Bone Disease*. Philadelphia, JB Lippincott, 1969 (1).]

## CLINICAL WORK-UP IN THE DIAGNOSIS OF BONE DISORDERS

Seemingly, since the first use of x-rays for the diagnosis of human ailments, there have been opposing points of view regarding whether roentgen studies should precede other indicated clinical evaluations (physical examination, laboratory tests, etc.) or whether these general clinical studies should precede the roentgen studies. The consensus in the radiological specialties generally favors the former for the reason that evaluation of the x-ray films, as stated by Greenfield (1), should be "objective" and all possible effort should be expended to avoid being subjectively influenced by preconceived ideas gained through advanced knowledge of what the clinical studies may have revealed. However, this "objective approach" does not ordinarily apply to the primary (patient first contact) physician who must initially justify the exposure of patients to x-rays, but, rather, only to the referral (secondary physician) radiologist or roentgenologist who is attempting to provide the primary physician with objectively gained information by which he or she may make a definitive diagnosis. Consequently, since the doctor of chiropractic generally functions as a primary physician (under the above definition), the following clinical work-up is considered essential prior to making a decision to take spinographic x-ray films, whether or not they are to be taken directly by the doctor or on a referral basis:

1. History of trauma, surgery, systemic disease, radiation exposure, etc.
2. Family history
3. Physical signs of deformity
4. Vital signs
5. Onset of present complaint—acute or insidious
6. Duration of symptoms, severity, mode of relief, previous diagnosis and treatment
7. Extent of involvement
8. Inflammatory signs
9. Orthopedic and neurological tests

Additionally, in the case of suspected bone disorders (other than biomechanical), the following laboratory studies are considered minimal supporting data requirements (Table 8.1):

1. Complete blood count (CBC)
2. Serum calcium
3. Serum phosphorus
4. Serum alkaline phosphatase

Additional laboratory studies for confirmation of roentgen impressions may also include the following:

1. Urine studies for calcium, phosphorus and abnormal constituents
2. Serum uric acid
3. Serum uric phosphatase
4. Calcium balance
5. Renal function tests
6. Hematological studies
7. Electrophoretic studies
8. Other (studies which may be specifically indicated in cases where bone disorders may be secondary to general constitutional conditions)

## ROENTGEN SIGNS IN BONE DISORDERS

It is an accepted fact that the single most important clinical skill leading to the diagnosis of bone disorders is that relating to one's ability to roentgenologically differentiate between normal and abnormal tissue densities, changes in contour and size of bone, architectural alterations, and the impairment of function. Although one may not know the precise diagnosis, being able to detect that an abnormality exists is a good start.

The second most important requisite is that of approaching the films in a methodical, organized, systematic manner in order that no significant finding is missed and/or improperly considered. The following outline of roentgen signs in bone disorders is given to assist in the development of these skills and to serve as a guideline for further study (2):

### Alteration in Bone Density

NORMAL RADIOGRAPHIC DENSITIES

Air Density

Air is the most radiolucent (radiographically penetrable) of all body tissues: as seen in the lungs and gas in the bowels. Abnormally, air density may be seen in subcutaneous emphysema, gas gangrene, etc.

**Table 8.1.**
**Differential diagnosis of bone diseases from laboratory findings[a]. [Adapted from Meschan (3).]**

| Condition | Serum Calcium | Serum Inorganic phosphorus | Serum Alkaline phosphatase | Urine Calcium | Urine Phosphorus |
|---|---|---|---|---|---|
| Hyperparathyroidism: primary | | | | | |
|   Early | ↑ | N | S ↑ | ↑ | N |
|   Advanced | ↑ | ↓ | ↑ | ↑ | ↑ |
|   Terminal | ↑ | ↑ | ↑ | ↑ | ↓ |
| Hyperparathyroidism: secondary | N–↓ | ↑ | R ↑ | ↑ | ↓ |
| Hypoparathyroidism (Seabright Bantam) | ↓ | ↑ | N–↓ | ↓ | ↓ |
| Pseudohypoparathyroidism | ↓ | ↑ | N–↓ | ↓ | ↓ |
| Pseudo-pseudohypoparathyroidism[b] | N | N | N | N | N |
| Hyperthyroidism, marked | N | N | ↑ | ↑ | ↑ |
| Hypothyroidism | N | N | N | N | N |
| Hypercortisonism (Cushing's disease or syndrome) | N | N | N | ↑ | ↑ |
| Senile osteoporosis | N | N–O ↓ | N | N | N |
| Fracture healing (multiple and severe disuse atrophy) | ↑ | ↑ | ↑ | ↑ | N |
| Hypovitaminosis D | | | | | |
|   Child rickets, active | ↓ | ↓ | ↑ | N | N |
|   Adult osteomalacia | N–↓ | ↓ | ↑ | N | N |
| Hypervitaminosis D | ↑ | N–↑ | ↑ | ↑ | N |
| Hypovitaminosis C | | | | | |
|   Untreated | N | N | ↓ | N | N |
|   Healing | N | N | ↑ | N | N |
| Osteitis deformans (Paget's) | | | | | |
|   Mild—few bones | N | N | S–↑ | N | N |
|   Generalized and active | R ↑ | R ↓ | ↑ | N | N |
| Multiple myeloma | | | | | |
|   Uncomplicated | ↑ | N–↑ | R ↑ | ↑ | ↑ |
|   With renal involvement | ↑ | ↑ | R ↑ | ↑ | ↓ |
| Osteosarcoma | N | N–↑ | ↑ | N | N |
| Tumor, metastic to bone | N–↑ | N | O ↑ | N | N |
| Polyostotic fibrous dysplasia | O ↑ | N | O ↑ | N | N |

[a] Code: ↑, increased; N, normal; S, slight; ↓, decreased; R, rarely; O, occasionally.
[b] May ultimately prove to be congenital abnormality with sex chromosomal aberration.

## Fat Density

Fat is less radiolucent than air, but more radiolucent than soft tissue. Some soft tissues may be visible roentgenologically only when outlined by the fat around them; such as in the retroperitoneal structures, joint capsules, etc. Pathologically, fatty tumors (lipomas) may show such increased radiolucency over soft tissues.

## Water Density

All major components of soft tissue, organs and blood are of water density. Pathologically, tumors composed of ordinary soft tissue will not ordinarily be detected roent-genologically when located within normal soft tissue.

## Calcific Density

The calcific density of bone is the least radiolucent of all normal body tissues. Normal bone can be recognized by its organization into cortical and trabecular patterns. Although of the same relative density, normal bone should not be confused with calcification. Pathologically, calcific density may be encountered in calcified vessels, sclerosis of soft tissue, tumors composed of new bone formation, etc. Small amounts of new bone in fibrous tissue lesions gives a "ground glass" appearance.

## Metallic Density

Metallic objects are very radiopaque (resistant to x-ray penetration) and cast a white shadow due to lack of penetration. Metallic compounds (such as gold and sodium chloride injected for treatment of syphilis) may be mistaken for calcifications in the muscle tissues. Metallic radioactive implants may be mistaken for undigested calcium tablets or needles in the body cavities.

## ALTERATIONS IN NORMAL DENSITIES OF BONE

### Decreased Bone Density

May be due to disturbances in osteoid production or mineralization of normal or near-normal presence of osteoid material. Osteoporosis is an example of decreased bone density due to lack of osteoid material in which mineralization of bone takes place. Rickets and osteomalacia are examples of defective osteoid mineralization. Specific factors relative to age and disease processes may be summarized as follows:

1. In young growing bone, an increased radiolucency will be mainly produced by disturbance of normal calcium or protein metabolism, or osteoblastic function. Since most active portions of growing bone is at the epiphyseal line, the manifestations will tend to be most evident in the related zones of provisional ossification and calcification.
2. In the adult, increased radiolucency of bone is more likely to be widespread throughout the entire bone. The condition will be variably related to an increased osteoblastic activity or deficient calcification.
3. In inflammatory conditions of bone, the appearance will be somewhat variable depending upon the primary site of involvement. In congenital syphilis the involvement will generally be distributed throughout the entire bone. In the mycoses it will be predominantly localized in the diaphysis. In osteomyelitis it will be distributed distally to the nutrient channels. In tuberculosis the condition will tend to be generalized, often including the joints. The process in all cases is generally one of bone destruction, damage to the blood supply and interruption of the bone formation process.
4. In tumors, the process is primarily one of stimulated osteoclastic activity, rather than by direct action of tumor cells. Practically, a complete absence of bone matrix and calcium results—or only spicules of bone may remain scattered throughout the tumor area. The extent of such spiculization within a tumor depends largely upon the degree of the malignancy and the rapidity of growth. Benign tumors tend to be more sharply demarcated and localized, whereas malignant tumors are more widespread within the bone as well as in the soft tissues.

### Increased Bone Density

Increased bone density, or osteosclerosis, may be due to increased calcium deposition within the bone (as in osteopetrosis) or to increased bone formation of normal composition, which can be classified according to three general types:

1. Periosteal bone proliferation which is subclassified as layer-like or laminated, lace-like or irregular, and spiculated. Periosteal bone proliferation may be caused by trauma, toxic agents, chronic cardiopulmonary disorders, chronic inflammations, subperiosteal hemorrhage, or tumors.
2. Endosteal new bone formation may accompany any periosteal proliferation, but is most frequently seen in myelophthisic anemias and may proceed to actual closure of the marrow cavity of tubular bones.

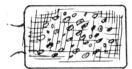

Moth-eaten osteolytic foci characteristic of metastatic carcinoma, multiple myeloma, and hyperparathyroidism

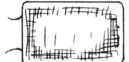

Homogenous sclerosis characteristic of prostatic carcinoma

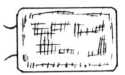

Framed sclerosis with coarse trabeculation characteristic of Paget's disease

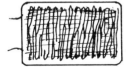

Vertical striped trabeculation characteristic of hemangioma

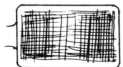

Diffuse osteoporosis characteristic of senility and nutritional deficiency diseases

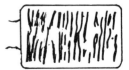

Patchy sclerosis and osteoporosis characteristic of lymphomas and leukemias

**Figure 8.1.**   Differential diagnosis of skeletal disorders from vertebral bone density alterations. [Adapted from Meschan (3).]

3. Spongiosclerotic new bone formation may be either generalized as in hypoparathyroidism, or localized as in osteitis condensans ilii and localized metastatic carcinoma of the prostate. In the localized variety of osteosclerosis the increase in bone density may be compact and fairly regular in shape, as with secondary metastasis from carcinoma of the prostate, or irregular as with Paget's disease.

## Mixed Increased and Decreased Densities

In some cases, combined osteoblastic and osteoclastic activity results in mixed osteoporosis and osteosclerosis. This is sometimes the case with certain neoplasms; particularly lymphomata and metastatic carcinoma of the prostate. In such cases the combined appearance is caused by the dual elements of bone proliferation and bone destruction with replacement by the tumor cells.*

---

*Although the process of osteoporosis and osteosclerosis are relatively simple to understand, the range of disorders in which they may be characteristic is extremely wide and constitutes a veritable differential diagnostic nightmare. For example, Teplick and Haskin (2) list over 50 conditions in which osteoporosis may be found and 25 for osteosclerosis. Consequently, the general practitioner is cautioned against making any rigid judgments of specific diagnoses without proper consultation.

## Architectural Alterations of Bone

The architecture of each type of bone is somewhat distinctive and there are some gender and racial differences, but, in general, present similar characteristics. The calvarium of the skull is comprised of three layers; an outer and inner layer of compact bone with a layer of loose, spongy bone in between. The long bones (including the vertebrae) are composed of an outer shell of compact bone with an inner shaft of spongy bone in the metaphysis; the spongy bone presenting an organized arrangment of trabeculae. Architectural alterations of bone relates to disturbances of this organized design by the effects of disease processes.

In the reparative stage of chronic inflammations, degenerative processes, or in other conditions, such as Paget's disease, osteoid may be laid down and rapidly replaced by new bone which allows for a pronounced disturbance in the normal architecture of the bone. The bone itself may be thickened in its actual measurements, but more radiolucent because of replacement of the more compact type of normal bone. Rickets is another example of this type of disturbance in the basic architectural pattern of bone due to the ossification which occurs mainly in the periosteal areas (Fig. 8.1).

## Changes in Contour and Size of Bone

The primary considerations involved in the change in contour and size of bone are generally categorized as follows:

1. Thickening of bone as in acromegaly and certain forms of osteoarthropathy
2. Increase in bone length as in arachnodactylia and Engelmann's disease
3. Decrease in the diameters of bone as in osteogenesis imperfecta and osteopsathyrosis
4. Shortening of bone length as in achondroplasia and hypoplasia
5. Irregular deformity of bone as in osteitis deformans, Paget's disease, chondrodysplasia and Ollier's disease
6. Traumatic or pathologic fractures
    a. Traumatic fractures of bone generally display a characteristic disruption of the normal contour, continuity or architectural organization of the structures which in most cases are easily recognized roentgenologically by reasonably careful survey of the films. However, compression type fractures—whether recent or healed—may be difficult to differentiate from some pathological processes on the basis of roentgen impressions alone
    b. Pathological fractures of bone may accompany an endless list of conditions in which bone destruction and/or osteoporotic processes are present. In the spinal column, pathological fractures are most frequently represented by partial or complete collapse of the vertebral bodies. Partial collapse is almost always related to the anterior or anterolateral aspect of the body because of the predominance of weight impressed on this area, and lack of support given to the posterior aspect by the articular processes (Fig. 8.2)

## Miscellaneous Considerations

### DISORDERS OF ALIGNMENT

Disorders of alignment of otherwise normal bone which impairs function of articulations are usually considered part of a routine roentgenologic survey. However, since that is the primary objective of spinographic interpretation procedure, this consideration will be covered in the preceding chapters.

## ALTERATIONS OF BONE DEVELOPMENT

Disorders of bone development wherein the maturation process is accelerated or retarded—aside from those discussed in Chapter 5 on spinal development—are another important area of study in roentgen diagnosis. Accelerated or retarded bone growth may be related to the following etiologies:

1. Nutritional factors
2. Endocrinopathies
3. Intrinsic bone diseases
4. Genotype variations

### Localization of Involvement

Localization of skeletal areas and parts of bone which may have a predilection for certain disease processes, or what is called "fields of most frequent involvement," also must be taken into consideration (Fig. 8.3, 8.4).

In the case of skeletal localization, for example, about 70% of all *osteosarcomas* are localized to the lower extremities, particularly the knee; about 30% of the *chondrosarcomas* are localized to the pelvis; about 50% of the *chondroblastomas* are localized to the knee; about 80% of the *chondromyxofibromas* are localized to the lower extremities; about 70% of the *giant cell tumors* are localized to the knee or distal radius (4).

In the case of predilection within a particular bone, the areas of most frequent involvement (particularly in the young) are those of most rapid growth, such as the epiphysis. Hereditary diseases may have a predilection for the epiphysis, metaphysis or diaphysis. Neoplastic disorders are frequently differentiated positionally by the type of tissue predominant in the area of involvement.

## PROCESS OF ROENTGEN FEATURE ANALYSIS

In summary, it should be recognized at this point that the spinographic evaluation

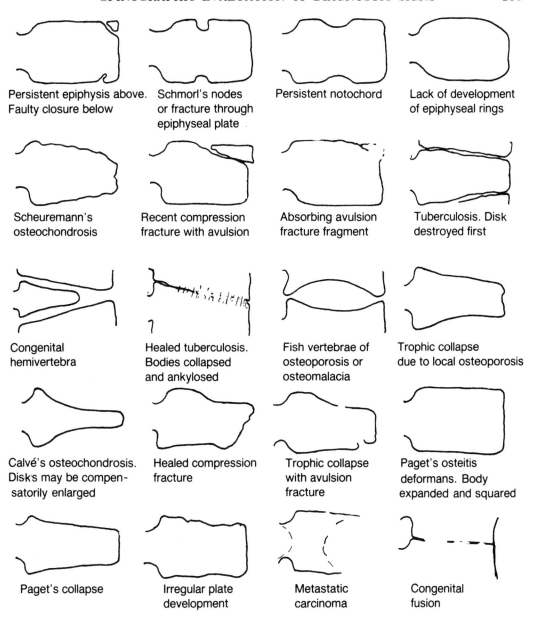

**Figure 8.2.** Differential diagnosis of skeletal disorders from vertebral body alterations in architecture, contour and size. (Adapted from unpublished work of Appa L. Anderson.)

of diagnositc signs is not directed toward an effort to memorize the classic roentgen appearance of the many disease conditions which may affect bone (many of which may present very similar roentgen impressions), but rather to a *process of roentgen feature analysis* effected by asking pertinent questions and then attempting to answer those questions based on one's knowledge of nor-

mal radiographic anatomy and the changes that may take place in response to disease processes—for example:

1. With respect to age, sex, etc., are the roentgen impressions of a particular bone normal in relation to tissue density, architecture, contour, size, and alignment to contiguous structures, or abnormal?
2. If abnormal with respect to those consid-

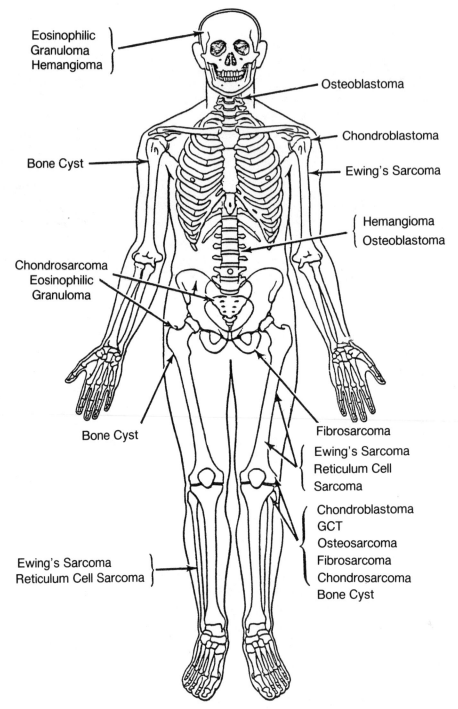

**Figure 8.3.** Localization of solitary lesions in the skeleton. [Adapted from Theros (4).]

erations, are the impressions that of pathology, trauma or abnormal development?

3. If pathological, is it localized to the cortical, medullary or periosteal areas?; more predominant in the epiphysis, diaphysis or metaphysis?; involve the articular surfaces?; extend into adjacent soft tissue?; etc.

4. What are the various conditions which

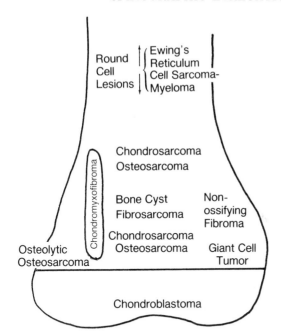

**Figure 8.4.** Localization of solitary lesions within a bone. [Adapted from Theros (4).]

may present such a roentgen appearance and what abnormal physical examination and laboratory findings (if any) are generally associated with those conditions?

In this manner, as stated by Greenfield (1), a list of differential diagnoses is prepared and a process of elimination is began whereby the list is narrowed down to the most likely possibilities. In some cases one may be left with one logical and definitive conclusion and in others several possibilities may remain. If several possibilities remain, further studies should be considered (either directly or by referral), keeping in mind that the roentgenological diagnosis of bone diseases is a very comprehensive skill which the general chiropractic practitioner can only hope to gain sufficient knowledge in to enable him or her to make wise and well considered decisions—including the decision to seek consultation, or refer, when indicated.

### References

1. Greenfield GB: *Radiology of Bone Diseases*. Philadelphia, Lippincott, 1969.
2. Teplick JG, Haskin ME: *Roentgenological Diagnosis*. Philadelphia, Saunders, 1971, vol 2.
3. Meschan I: *Roentgen Signs in Clinical Practice*. Philadelphia, Saunders, 1966, vol 1.
4. Theros EG: *Fundamental Patterns in the Diagnosis of Solitary Bone Lesions*. Washington, DC, American Registry of Pathology, Armed Forces Institute of Pathology.

# CHAPTER 9

# Spinographic Interpretation of Biomechanical Disorders

## INTERPRETIVE RATIONALE

To this point effort has been given to present chiropractic spinography interpretation procedure as a process not too unlike that of general radiographic diagnosis, the difference being mainly in terms of information sought—biomechanical as opposed to pathological considerations. However, it should be mentioned that two different concepts of interpretive rationale have been promoted within the chiropractic profession—the *traditional* rationale of static subluxation analysis and the *contemporary* rationale of biomechanical integrity interpretation. In order to clarify the objective of this chapter, a brief discussion of each concept is considered appropriate.

### Traditional Rationale of Static Subluxation Analysis

Spinographic x-ray procedure was introduced into chiropractic clinical procedure in 1910 by Bartlett Joshua (B.J.) Palmer as (according to him) a means of "scientifically proving the existence of chiropractic subluxations," which to that time were limited to palpatory examination procedures which he felt were highly inaccurate due to the developmental anomalies normally inherent to some degree in all spinal structures (1, 2). This claim, however, was quickly challenged by Daniel David (D.D.) Palmer who maintained that, in addition to the structural consideration of vertebral misalignment that B.J. was attempting to evaluate, the chiropractic concept of vertebral subluxation which he originally proposed in 1895 also included a neuropathic element which could not be visualized on spinographic x-ray films (3).

Although B.J. later attempted to qualify his claim for spinography by developing electronic instrumentation aimed at detecting and measuring the neurological component of the chiropractic subluxation, the concept (variations of paraspinal skin temperature as an index of spinal nerve root impingement) was based on a biologically implausible theory which the profession as a whole did not accept. However, his original claim that chiropractic subluxations in their entirety could be ascertained on spinographic x-ray films did persist to eventually spawn numerous *entrepreneurial systems* of analysis which attempted to evaluate static structural relationships of contiguous spinal components by measurement of lines drawn on the film images (4–8).

In most cases, it was inherent within the concept of such analysis procedures that vertebral misalignments of a certain magnitude resulted in concomitant nerve root impingement and, the more refined the system of spinographic analysis, the more exacting it was purported to be in determining the existence of a chiropractic subluxation in all its ramifications. In some cases, systems of spinographic analysis were developed which claimed to measure a vertebral subluxation within a parameter of one-half of 1°—a claim that the chiropractic profession in general rejects because it is felt that there is no conceivable way that such measurement procedures can so minutely differentiate between the *actual* vertebral misalignments which theoretically might be involved in a subluxation and the *apparent* misalignments which result from asymmetry of spinal structures and/or the illusion of asymmetries resulting from the effects of radiographic projectional distortion.

## Contemporary Rationale of Biomechanical Integrity Interpretation

As a technological procedure, chiropractic spinography is to be regarded as a noteworthy contribution of the chiropractic profession to health care science; when used in accordance with accepted contemporary knowledge of spinal biomechanics, it has the potential of providing clinically useful information which is not presently obtainable by any other means. However, as a result of the profession's efforts in recent years to more critically review its theories in relation to accepted, scientifically based knowledge, traditional chiropractic spinography analysis concepts have generally been found lacking in credibility for three primary reasons, which to some extent have already been touched upon in the preceding discussion:

1. The concept that spinographs can reveal the existence of a vertebral subluxation in all its ramifications (which in itself has not yet been scientifically substantiated) is presently without sufficient basis to justify *routine* clinical application
2. The use of spinographic analysis procedures based on the measurement of lines drawn on the film images (although sometimes helpful in arriving at a clinical decision) are inadequate when the information gained by such measurements is rotely used as a clinical decision in itself; i.e. when such information is taken at face value without integration into the total clinical picture of a particular patients' condition
3. The consideration of intervertebral relationships from a static concept of alignment or misalignment rather than the more realistic, presently accepted, functional concept of vertebral motor unit biomechanics—under no circumstances can the spinal column within a living body ever be considered static; even when in an immobilized state the vertebral motor units

of the spinal column do display their movement capacity in accordance with specific postural requirements under a given set of circumstances

Therefore, this presentation is an effort to provide a *new* approach to spinographic interpretation which is more consistent with contemporary knowledge of spinal biomechanics, more realistic in terms of what spinographic x-rays are actually capable of revealing, and more objective in evaluating the nature of the information gained in terms of the overall clinical picture of a particular patients' health problem. Unquestionably, accepting this new approach will require some reevaluation on the part of the proponents of traditional spinographic concepts, as well as their opponents.

## GEOMETRY OF X-RAY PROJECTION AND IMAGE FORMATION

In general radiographic diagnosis of bone disorders, emphasis was given to the evaluation of such factors as; alteration of bone density, architectural variations, changes in contour and size of structures, etc. At this point, in keeping with the statement made in Chapter 1 that "*spinographic views are to be considered diagnostic films with the added dimension of providing clinically significant information of a biomechanical nature,*" it is now necessary that the clinical skill which comprises the basis for that other dimension be added to our roentgenological diagnostic armamentarium—*the geometry of x-ray image formation and its relationship to the interpretive evaluation of biomechanical integrities of the pelvis and spinal column.*

The geometry of x-ray image formation has to do with an x-ray projectional phenomenon wherein three-dimensional body structures are projected to the flat, two-dimensional film surface in a magnified and distorted manner. Although opponents to spinography have used this as *an excuse* to justify their opposition, maintaining that it is an unsolvable dilemma, that is not the case—spinographic distortion can be interpretively dealt with to the extent that one may develop a biomechanical interpretive skill in much the same manner as one learns to interpret pathology by evaluating the films for evidence of certain tissue change characteristics. A good knowledge of pelvic and spinal anatomy and biomechanics, and a comprehensive understanding of the manner by which those three-dimensional structures project to the flat, two-dimensional film surface, is the key (9–12).

## An Exercise in Electromagnetic Beam Projection

As was learned in Chapter 2 on "X-Ray Physics and Radiologic Technology," x-rays are electromagnetic radiations which may be electronically produced in an x-ray

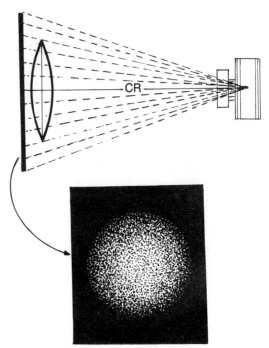

**Figure 9.2.** A disk-shaped object of equal density throughout, but tapered around its edge, is penetrated by the x-ray photons (minute particles of energy) in accordance with the object's varying thickness to expose the film with an image of the object. The thicker central area of the object absorbs more of the x-rays resulting in lesser exposure of the film (lighter) while the thinner object edges absorb less of the x-rays resulting in more exposure of the film. *CR*, central ray.

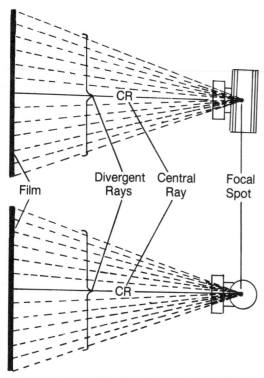

Film    Divergent   Central    Focal
       Rays       Ray      Spot

**Figure 9.1.** Side (*above*) and top (*below*) views of divergent projection of x-rays from focal spot of x-ray tube to the film. X-rays project outward in straight lines in all directions from the x-ray tube focal spot in a 360° pattern. The central beam of the cone of x-rays is the central ray (*CR*).

tube by bombarding its anode target surface with electrons. Arising from this *point-source*, the x-rays then project outward in straight lines in all directions: in the case of roentgenography, to the x-ray film surface (Fig. 9.1). If an object is placed in front of the film within the path of the x-rays, it will be penetrated to one extent or another to expose the film with an image of the object, the nature of the image depending upon the variable thickness of the object and the density of the material of which it is composed (Fig. 9.2).

This mechanism of x-ray image production in itself is easy enough to understand; however, when we begin to talk about the "geometric aspects" of image formation—

*projectional image magnification and distortion*—a "mental block" often arises in the mind of the viewer. In the case of students this mental block may be simply due to their inexperience in looking at radiographs/spinographs; in the case of the more experienced practitioner it may be due to their preconceived notions regarding the subject of spinography in general. Therefore, in an effort to get across a few basic physical principles on the subject by circumventing any mental blocks that may be present, we might initially forget about x-rays and use another form of electromagnetic radiation which projects in exactly the same manner; e.g. *visible light*.

## IMAGE MAGNIFICATION

In Figure 9.3 it is noted that the disk-shaped object used in the preceding experiment of x-ray image production has been again placed in front of the film, and a source of visible light has been positioned to take the place of the x-ray tube. It will also be noted that the plate placed in front of the light source, has a rectangular aperture (collimator) in its base to conform to the rectangular shape of the film, the rectangular aperture having no effect on the projection of light rays outward, in straight lines, in all directions, but only on the area of projected coverage.

Further observing this experiment, it is noted that the disk-shaped object is projected to the film surface in a magnified manner by the divergent beam of light rays so that the image of the object on the film is larger than the object itself. This projection (exactly the same as if x-rays were used) is primarily influenced by three geometric factors; (*a*) object size, (*b*) object-film distance, and (*c*) focal-film distance. These three physical factors of image magnification are further discussed as follows:

### Object Size

The larger the object, or the farther the extreme boundaries of the object from the central ray, the greater will be the magni-

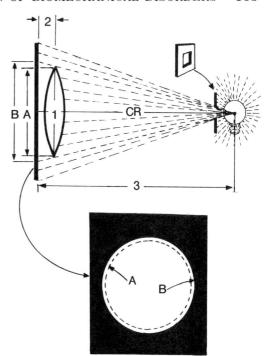

**Figure 9.3.** By replacing the x-ray tube with a visible light source which projects in the same manner as x-rays but is less penetrating, one is able to better study the effects of radiant energy magnification and its principal affecting factors. In this illustration it is noted that the image of the disk-shaped object is projected to the film in a magnified manner. *A* represents the actual size of the object and *B* represents the magnified size of the object as its image is projected to the film. The factors which influence this magnification are: *1*, size of the object or distance of its extreme borders from the central ray; *2*, distance of the object from the film (OFD, object-film distance); *3*, distance of the light (or x-ray) source from the film (FFD, focal-film distance). *CR*, central ray.

fication of the image. Conversely, the smaller the object or the closer its extreme boundaries to the central ray, the lesser the amount of magnification.

### Object-Film Distance

The farther the object from the film, the greater the magnification of the image. Conversely, the closer the object to the film, the lesser will be the magnification; i.e. the closer will be the size of the projected image to the actual size of the object.

## Focal-Film Distance

The shorter the focal-film distance, the greater the image magnification. Conversely, the longer the focal-film distance the lesser the image magnification.*

Uncomplicated (undistorted) magnification may be defined as "the equal enlargement of the image of an object in all directions relative to the actual size of the object," and is respondent to the *inverse square law* of radiant energies: i.e. the size of the projected image of an object is inversely proportional to the square of the focal-film distance (FFD) and directly proportional to the square of the object-film distance (OFD) (Fig. 9.4). The effect of the inverse square law on image magnification may be conceptually summarized as follows:

A. Focal-film distance: *increase* of FFD by 2 times equals *decrease* of image magnification by 4 times; *decrease* of FFD by 2 times equals *increase* of image magnification by 4 times.

B. Object-film distance: *increase* of OFD by 2 times equals *increase* of image magnification by 4 times; *decrease* of OFD by 2 times equals *decrease* of image magnification by 4 times.

As stated, image magnification responds to the three factors of: object dimensions (O), focal-film distance (D) and object-film distance (D). To find the true object dimension, the image dimension is multiplied by a number less than one (correction factor, CF). This correction factor may be obtained by means of the following equation (13) (Fig. 9.5).

$O$ = Object dimension (cm)
$I$ = Image dimension (cm)

---

* Although the longer the focal-film distance the closer will be the image size to the actual size of the object, there is theoretically no point at which the focal-film distance can be increased to completely eliminate magnification, since visible light and x-ray arise from a point-source and project *infinitely* outward in straight lines. Also, there is no practical way of "bending" visible light or x-rays to parallel line projection, as they apply to radiographic/spinographic procedure. However, the process of *laser*—light amplification by the stimulated emission of radiation—is able to conform visible light rays to parallel line.

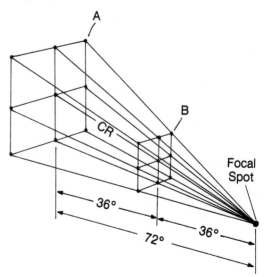

**Figure 9.4.** Schematic diagram representing the effects of the inverse square law on image magnification. In the case of visible light and x-rays, the distance not only affects object magnification but also the quantity of light or x-rays reaching the film. *CR*, central ray; (see text for *A* and *B* definitions).

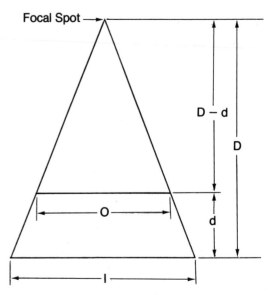

**Figure 9.5.** Schematic diagram of factors which comprise the geometric equation by which the inverse square law effects on magnification may be computed (see text for definitions).

$D$ = Focal-film distance (cm)
$d$ = Object-film distance (cm)

It is important to have all dimensions in the same units, then, by similar triangles,

$$\frac{O}{I} = \frac{D-d}{D} \text{ and } O = \frac{(D-d)}{(D)} I.$$

Therefore,

$$CF = \frac{D-d}{D}.$$

Ordinarily, one would not actually compute inverse square law magnification rates as a direct function of spinographic interpretation procedure. However, the ability to *conceptualize* the effect of this law on the spinographic film images is an important consideration.

## IMAGE DISTORTION

Distortion may be defined as "the unequal magnification of the image of an object as compared to the actual configuration of that object. Image distortion is dependent upon the basis factors of image magnification, and its nature is determined by the two considerations of (*a*) alignment of the object and central ray, and (*b*) alignment of the object and film.

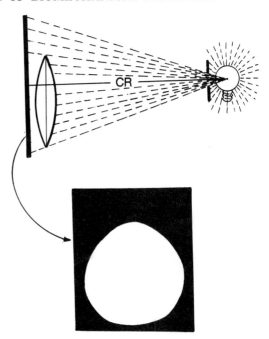

**Figure 9.6.** Example of distortion (unequal magnification) of the object image by lateral (or up-or-down) movement of the object out of alignment with the central ray (*CR*) of the light beam.

### Alignment of the Object and Central Ray

In the preceding examples of image magnification it will be noted that the central ray was aligned 90° degrees to the center of the object, thus the image was equally enlarged in all directions from its center. However, if the object and central ray are not so aligned, the image will be unequally magnified relative to its center. Either of two basic factors will essentially have the same distortional effect: (*a*) movement of the center of the object in any direction away from the central ray (Fig. 9.6), or (*b*) movement of the central ray in any direction away from the center of the object.

### Alignment of the Object and Film

In the preceding examples of image magnification (Fig. 9.3) it will be noted that the center of the object was not only aligned to the central ray, but was also in parallel alignment with the film. Thus, the image of the object was equally magnified in all directions from its epicenter. However, if the object and the film are not in parallel alignment to each other, the image of the object will be unequally magnified—distorted. Either of two principal factors will essentially have the same basic effect: (*a*) the object being out of parallel alignment with the film (Fig. 9.7), or (*b*) the film being out of parallel alignment with the object.

The foregoing examples of image magnification and distortion as an effect of visible light projection (exactly the same as if x-rays had been used), were on a two-dimensional basis; that is, the third dimension of *depth* was not considered. If, at this point, we replace the visible light source with an x-ray source, and replace the disk with a three-dimensional object (Fig. 9.8), we are able to see the combined effects of all of the aforedescribed factors of image magnification *and* distortion in a single image.

It will be at first noted that the film image of the three-dimensional object ap-

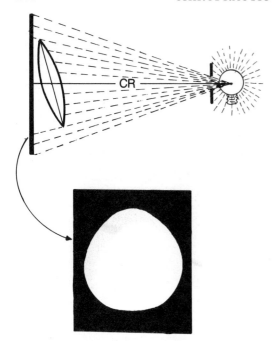

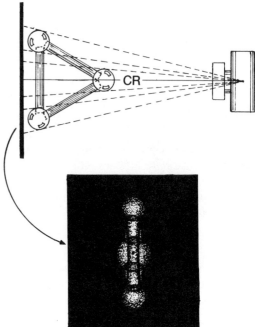

**Figure 9.7.** Example of distortion of the object image by altering its parallel relationship with the film. Although the object is centrally aligned to the central ray (*CR*) and film, that part farther from the film is magnified to a greater degree than that part closer to the film.

**Figure 9.8.** Example of combined magnification and distortion of a three-dimensional object being projected by a divergent pattern x-ray beam to the flat, two dimensional film surface. *CR*, central ray.

pears (and in fact is) two-dimensional—flat. However, if one first looks at the object itself and fixes an impression of its three-dimensional character in his/her "mind's eye" (as it is projected to the flat film by a point-source emission of x-rays from the x-ray tube) and then looks at the film image, it now begins to take on a visual impression of the three-dimensional character of the object it represents.

## SPINOGRAPHIC PROJECTION AND STRUCTURE RECOGNITION

Ordinarily, in general radiographic diagnosis procedure (and in most contemporary chiropractic spinograpy analysis concepts, as well) structure recognition is generally limited to simply identifying the film image structures. However, in this presentation, effort will not only be directed to recognizing film image structures, but also toward development of a visual skill of interpreting the manner by which those structures were

projected to the film in a magnified and distorted manner. The development of this skill is considered necessary as a requisite toward later efforts to expand that skill to the visual evaluation of biomechanical integrities of the pelvis and spinal column.

In the preceding experiment (Fig. 9.8) it was noted that if one first implants a picture in their "mind's eye" of the three-dimensional shape of the object and the manner by which it is being projected to the flat (two-dimensional) film surface, they are able to recreate the three-dimensional character of the object within the film image. Thus, two prerequisites to visualizing three-dimensions within a film image are evident:

1. One must have a good knowledge of the anatomy (architecture, shape and size) of the structure(s) being projected to the film,† and

---

† Later efforts will expand this prerequisite to include a good knowledge of normal and abnormal biomechanics of the pelvis and spinal column as well.

2. One must have a good knowledge of the physical principles by which the structure(s) are projected to the film by a point-source emission of x-rays from the x-ray tube.

## Anteroposterior Full Spine Projection

The anteroposterior full spine projection (posteroanterior view) is taken in one single exposure on a 14 × 36-in (35.6 × 91.4-cm) film, ideally at a 72-in (1.8-m) focal-film distance to best illustrate certain biomechanical considerations of the pelvic and upper cervical complexes. Note in Figure 9.9 that the patient has been positioned in his/her normal standing posture in close proximity to the film, the film has been vertically adjusted so as to allow an equal distance above the occiput and below the ischial tuberosities and the central ray is aligned 90° to the horizontal center of the film, which then passes approximately through the patient's sternal zyphoid process and 9th/10th thoracic vertebral bodies.

It will be further noted that the primary x-ray beam passes outward in ever-increasing divergent angles from the focal-spot of the x-ray tube, in a 180° pattern around the central ray, to project the various body structures—*in infinite frontal plane layers*—to the film. Thus, each infinite frontal plane layer of the three-dimensional body is projected in a magnified and inherently distorted manner to the flat, two-dimensional, film surface in accordance with the aforediscussed inverse square law factors of: (*a*) size of object or distance of a part from the central ray, (*b*) distance of a part from the film and (*c*) focal-film distance.

In essence, then, the spinographic view in Figure 9.9 is a two-dimensional representation of a three-dimensional body in which each infinite frontal plane layer has been individually magnified and distorted and then compressed (superimposed) onto the flat film surface. Insofar as the geographic center of the spinographic image is the *epicenter* point of the central ray, it is the only point on the film which is not magnified or distorted. Consequently, the film can be divided into four distinct projec-

tional zones separated by *dividing lines of horizontal and vertical projection*; individually designated as lower left quadrant (LLQ), lower right quadrant (LRQ), upper left quadrant (ULQ), and upper right quadrant (URQ).

The anteroposterior (AP) spinographic *projection* is a posteroanterior (PA) *view*, therefore, it is helpful in the visualization of film image structures to imagine one is standing behind the patient looking forward toward the source of the x rays—the x-ray tube focal spot. Insofar as in spinographic interpretation procedure the structures are compared on a bilateral basis from the pelvis upward, the lower left and lower right quadrants are viewed first (Fig. 9.10), followed by the upper left and upper right quadrants (Fig. 9.11). While orienting one's-self to the various pelvic and spinal structures, as they are projected to the film, it is also important to develop the habit of looking at the areas of various soft tissue structures (bladder, bowel, kidneys, spleen, liver, diaphragm, heart and great vessels, lungs, trachea, etc.) which may exhibit pathological impressions in need of further study.

## Lateral Full Spine Projection

The lateral full spine projection (left or right lateral view) is taken in two separate exposures on one 14 × 36-in (35.6 × 91.4-cm) film at a 60-in (1.5-m) focal-film distance to minimize distortion (which would be excessive if taken in a single exposure, even at a 72-in focal-film distance) and to consider the capacity of x-ray generator units usually used in chiropractic general practice—generally a maximum of 300 mA-125 kVp, single phase. However, if larger capacity equipment is used, increased focal-film distance is recommended.

Figure 9.12 indicates positioning of the patient for a right lateral projection (left lateral view) with the epicenters of the central ray passing approximately through top of the shoulder for the upper section and through the body of L3 for the lower sec-

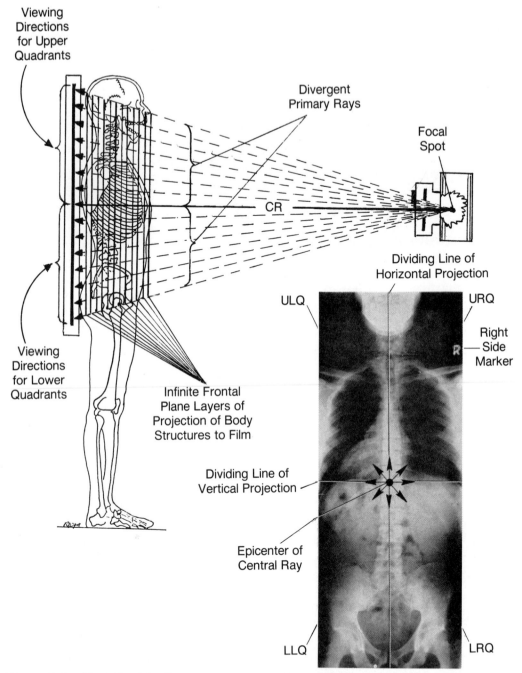

**Figure 9.9.** Example of the divergent pattern x-ray beam magnifying theoretical infinite coronal plane slices of a three-dimensional body, superimposing each individually magnified coronal plane layer onto the flat film surface. Interpreting biomechanical values on the film requires a very well-developed ability to visualize the manner by which the x-ray film images were projected to the film in a magnified and distorted manner. *CR*, central ray; *ULQ*, upper left quadrant; *URQ*, upper right quadrant; *LLQ*, lower left quadrant; *LRQ*, lower right quadrant.

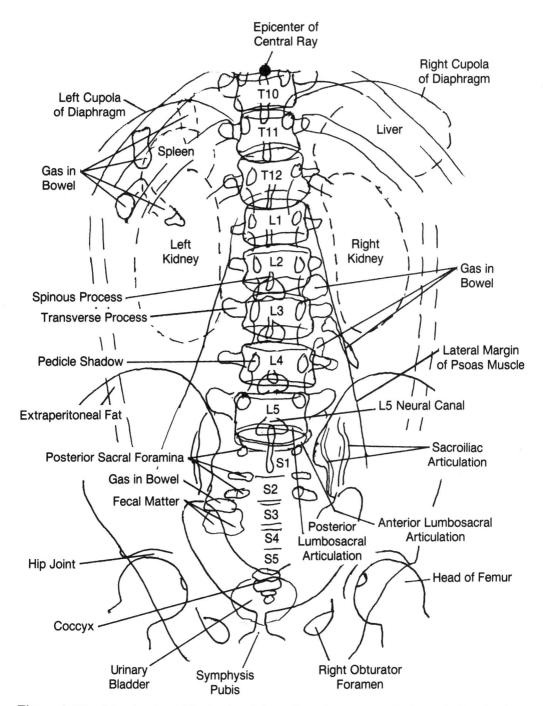

**Figure 9.10.**   Line drawing of the lumbopelvic section of an anteroposterior projection (postero-anterior view) of a full spine radiograph illustrating projected shapes and positions of various osseous and soft tissue structures of interest in spinographic interpretation.

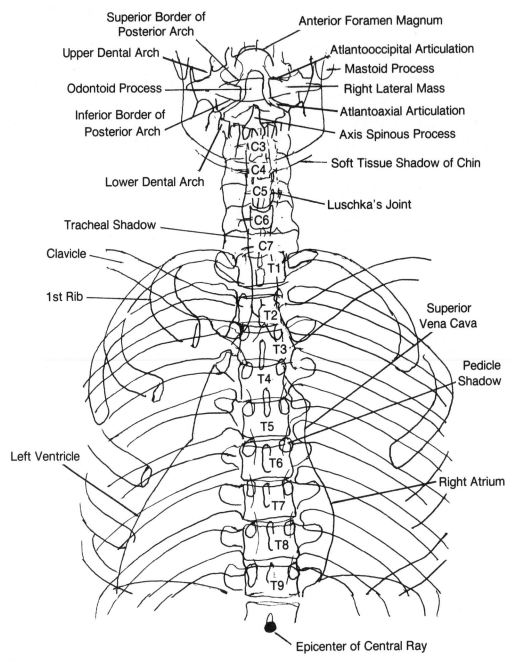

**Figure 9.11.** Line drawing of anteroposterior projection (posteroanterior view) of the upper section of a full spine radiograph.

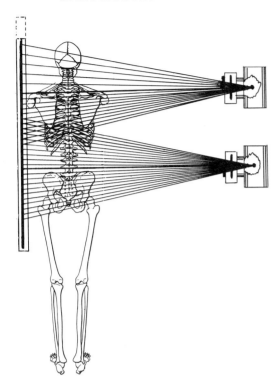

**Figure 9.12.** Left lateral view (right lateral projection) of a full spine radiograph taken in two separate exposures on a single 14 × 36-in film at a 60-in focal-film distance. Upper and lower sections are overlapped to insure projecting all spinal structures to the film.

tion. The lower section (Fig. 9.13) and upper section (Fig. 9.14) are individually viewed with reference to the epicenters of the central ray on each. Since bilateral comparisons are not made on the lateral view, as is the case with the posteroanterior view, separation of the film into quadrants is not applicable.

## SPINOGRAPHIC PROJECTION OF BIOMECHANICAL PATTERNS

At this point it should be firmly implanted in the mind's eye of the reader that x-rays emitting from the focal-spot of the x-ray tube project outward in ever-increasing divergent angles, in 360°, relative to the central ray. After *vectoring* with specific parts of the three-dimensional pelvis and spinal column, the divergent rays travel

onward to implant the images of those parts on the flat, two-dimensional, film in a magnified and *inherently distorted* manner. If the positions of the pelvis and spinal column in this situation are then biomechanically altered relative to the film, an *induced distortion* is superimposed over that which inherently existed as a natural consequence of three-dimensional radiographic projection. The process and significance of inherent and induced distortion are further explained as follows (11):

### Inherent Spinographic Distortion

Inherent spinographic distortion is that natural consequence of the three-dimensional structures of the pelvis and spinal column being projected to the flat, two-dimensional film surface via a point-source emission of x-rays from the x-ray tube. Inherent spinographic distortions are a normal occurrence in all roentgenographic images and the magnitude is determined by the three physical factors of focal-film distance, object-film distance and part-central ray distance.

### Induced Spinographic Distortion

Induced spinographic distortion is the consequence of inherently-distorted part images being further distorted by the effects of biomechanical deviations of the pelvis and spinal column, in whole or part. Induced spinographic distortion is a superimposition over the inherent distortion, such being equally affected by the physical factors of focal-film distance, object-film distance and part-central ray distance.

### Anteroposterior Projection

Figure 9.15 illustrates an experiment of the mechanism and effects of inherent and induced spinographic distortion on an anteroposterior full spine view. In this experiment, a life-size model of the pelvis and spinal column (in which manual effort was made to align all structural components) was positioned (first without rotation of the

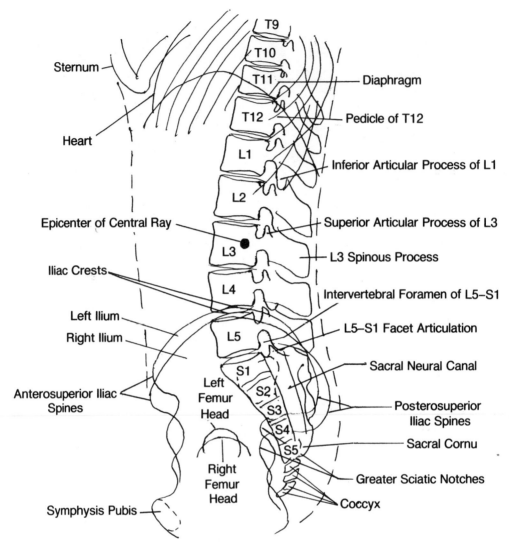

**Figure 9.13.** Left lateral view (right lateral projection) of lumbopelvic section of full spine radiograph.

pelvis and spinal column relative to the film) as for a standard AP full spine view taken at a 72-in focal-film distance. A series of actual exposures were then made of the model, in the neutral position and at 6°, 12° and 18° of left anterior rotation around a central vertical axis of the pelvis and spinal column.

It will be noted in the *neutral view* that the pelvis is bilaterally symmetrical, while the spinal column illustrates a moderate left lower lumbar curvature, a slight right thoracolumbar curvature, and a relatively straight thoracocervical spine. As the pelvis and spinal column are then rotated anterior on the left and posterior on the right, the pelvis and spinal column begin to take on a change in configuration due to the gradual introduction of the *normal anteroposterior spinal curves* into the anteroposterior projection—at 6° anterior rotation on the left, the left lumbar and right thoracolumbar curvatures are cancelled out and the thoracocervical spine begins to show an illusion of a right lateral bending; at 12° and 18° anterior rotation on the left, the pelvis be-

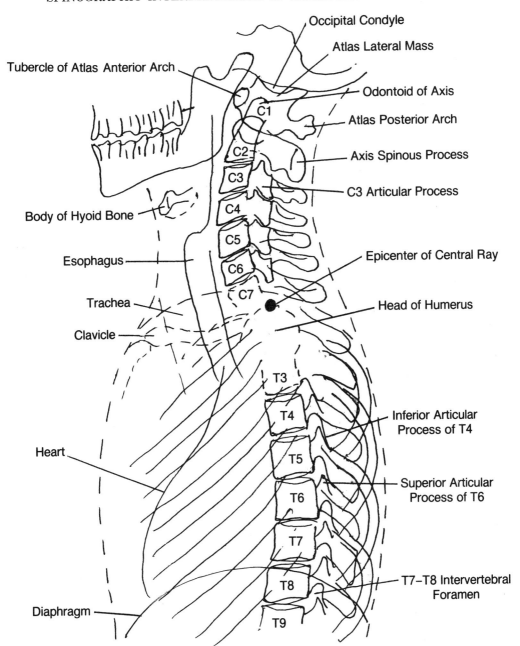

**Figure 9.14.**   Left lateral view (right lateral projection) of thoracocervical section of full spine radiograph.

gins to show increasing asymmetry and the spinal curvatures, slightly evident on the neutral view, begin to show what appears to be an increasing amount of lateral bending in the opposite direction.

On the surface, the phenomenon of spinographic projection, resulting in the af-

fecting of inherent and induced distortion, may, in fact, seem to constitute an insolvable dilemma. However, in principal at least, that is not the case—the mechanism of spinographic projection is a function of known physical laws and the quantitative factors of inherent and induced distortion

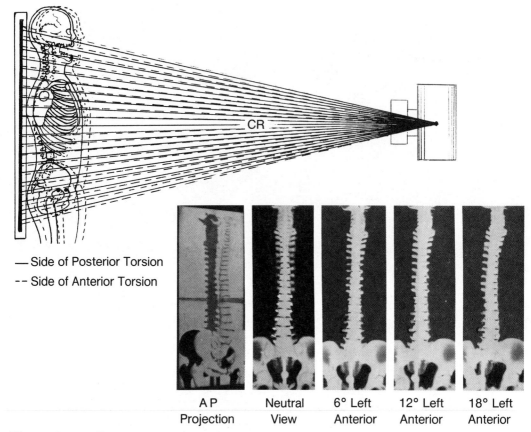

— Side of Posterior Torsion
-- Side of Anterior Torsion

| A P Projection | Neutral View | 6° Left Anterior | 12° Left Anterior | 18° Left Anterior |

**Figure 9.15.** Experiment illustrating standard 72-in anteroposterior full spine projection to a model pelvis and spinal column and the affects of inherent-induced distortion with rotation of the model at specific degrees of central axis rotation. See text for discussion of specific consideration of experiment.

are geometrically calculatable by virtue of a *projection summation angle principle* (11).

In Figure 9.16 it will be noted that a scaled, theoretical projection-plotting grid is placed in the positioning field of an anteroposterior full spine projection. Example divergent-beam x-rays are projected to the subject's femur heads and occipital condyles, and onward to the point where the images of those structures are projected to the film (*A* = occipital condyles; *B* = femur heads). In the illustrated example of an average 5 ft, 8-in (172.7-cm) subject, the projection summation angles of: *1* = object-film distance, *2* = object-central ray distance and *3* = focal-film distance) to the femur heads is approximately 9° and to the occipital condyles 12°, resulting in about 1¼ in of inherent film distortion from the

central ray to each point of measurement—about 2½ in of total vertical distortion from the femur heads to the occipital condyles.

Because there is currently no method by which the actual component parts of the pelvis and spinal column can be measured *in vivo*, no actual computations of inherent and/or induced distortion in each individual are possible. However, by conceptual application of the *projection summation angle principle*, sufficiently accurate estimates are possible to enable reasonably accurate judgments of projected biomechanical patterns.

With respect to this projection summation angle, it should be remembered from the previous discussion of Figure 9.9 that the projection of x-rays from the focal spot of the x-ray tube is in a 360° pattern around

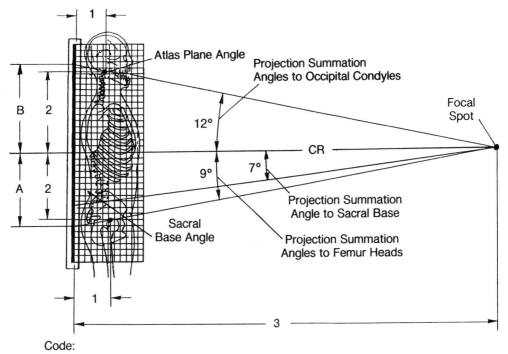

Code:
1. Object-Film Distance
2. Object-Central Ray Distance
3. Focal-Film Distance

A. Occipital Condyle Projection to Film
B. Femur Head Projection to Film
(Subject Height = ~5 ft 8 in

Scale: 1/16 in = 1 in

**Figure 9.16.** Projection-summation angle principle illustrating manner by which spinal and pelvic structures are projected to the film in a predictable magnitude making it possible to visualize biomechanical relationships of structures as they are projected to the film. *CR*, central ray.

the central ray. Therefore, the projection summation angles correspondingly apply— as the distance of a particular divergent ray spreads outward from the central ray, the projection summation angle increases correspondingly.

## PROJECTION OF PELVIC BIOMECHANICAL PATTERNS

The biomechanical patterns that may relate to normal and/or abnormal structural deviations of the pelvis (as discussed in the Chapter 6 on the Postural Complex of the Human Body) are basically confined to those which involve the pelvis as a total unit (lateral shifting, rotation and anteroposterior rocking on the femur heads) and those which involve interpelvic—*sacroiliac subluxation-inducing*—deviations (opposed anteroposterior deviations of the innomi-

nate bones, primary deviation of the sacrum relative to aligned innominate bones, and combined sacrum and innominate bone disrelationships). Each of these result in characteristic spinographically projected patterns as a result of alterations in the respective projection summation angles.

### Lateral Pelvic Shift

As was previously discussed, lateral shift of the pelvis as a unit on the femur heads, when normally positioned directly over the heels does not result in any significant sagittal plane pelvic unleveling, other than what may be present due to actual shortening of an extremity. Consequently, insofar as the pelvis is generally centered to the center of the film in standard full spine positioning, no change in biomechanical pattern from the normal would be anticipated.

Pelvic Rotation

Rotation of the pelvis as a unit on the femur heads is that biomechanical consideration referred to as a *Left Anterior Pelvis* (LAP) on *Right Anterior Pelvis* (LAP). Such rotation of the pelvis as a unit on the femur heads may or may not be considered a biomechanical irregularity depending upon its assignment to one or more of the following structural classifications‡:

1. Rotation of the entire pelvis as a unit on the femur heads as a consequence of complete torsion of the body during positioning
2. Rotation of the entire pelvis as a unit on the femur heads independent of (or underneath) the spine above
3. Rotation of the entire pelvis as a unit on the femur heads as a consequence of opposing anteroposterior innominate disrelationship:
   a. With concomitant rotation of the entire body above, or
   b. Independent of (or underneath) the spine above

Figure 9.17 depicts the representative projection summation angles to various pelvic structures (crest of ilia, sacral promontory, femur heads and symphysis pubis) in the neutral and left anterior rotation positions. Because of the increase of projection summation angles to the left innominate (which is farther from the film) as compared to the right innominate, a typical spinographically projected biomechanical pattern is evident. The uncomplicated (without interpelvic innominate or sacral misalignments) spinographic pattern of a left anterior pelvis (LAP) would then be represented by the following classic findings:

1. The left innominate bone will appear narrower than the right, including the sacroiliac articulation overlap
2. The apex of the sacrum will appear diagonally deviated toward the side of the anterior innominate and the symphysis pubis deviated away from the anterior innominate
3. The pelvic outlet will be diagonally deviated away from the side of the anterior innominate
4. All structures on the left will be projected lower than the right, namely:
   a. The left iliac crest will be projected lower, with the left ischeal tuberosity additionally lower, resulting in an increase of vertical measurement of the left innominate as compared to the right
   b. The left femur head will be projected lower, resulting what is sometimes referred to as a "projectional leg deficiency"
   c. The sacral base will be projected lower on the side of the LAP, assuming no complication from independent, primary sacral deviation within the ilia of the innominate bones.

In this illustration note that the lumbar spine appears to be in a state of right posterior rotation and right compensated scoliosis. However, this is actually representative of a left anterior pelvis resulting from *left anterior torsion of the entire body in spinographic positioning*, with the lumbar spine impressions being an illusion created by the normal anterior lordotic lumbar curve being projected into the anteroposterior view. If the sacral base were actually low on the left, as it is projected, the lumbar spine would tend to compensate to the left rather than the right; e.g. toward the side of the low sacral base§.

Again, the objective of this exercise in "contemporary spinographic interpretation" procedure (as opposed to "traditional spinographic analysis" procedure) is to evaluate *projected structural patterns* in terms of biomechanical probabilities. Although measured analysis procedure can

‡ Biomechanical significance would be presupposed in those cases where pelvic rotation occurred independent of the spine above, but not in those cases where the rotation was a result of complete body torsion; classification three excepted on the basis of the opposed anteroposterior innominate disrelation which is a separate consideration from LAP-RAP pelvic subluxation classifications. In all cases, the spinographic projectional pattern would be identical or similar and would require specific interpretive evaluation of the individual biomechanical patterns for differentiation.

§ For confirmation, compare this illustration with the pelvis in Figure 9.15 in which the entire spine was purposefully rotated in positioning—anterior on the left.

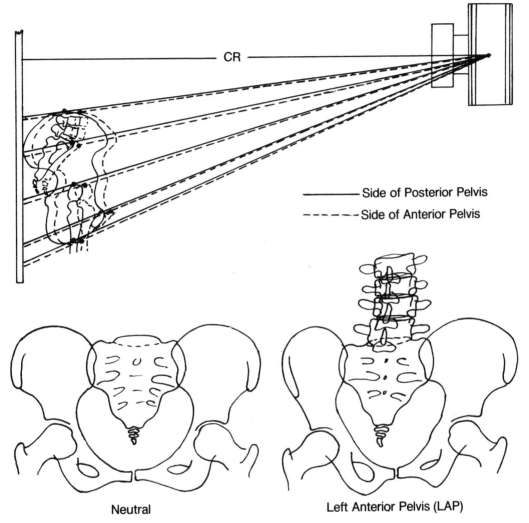

**Figure 9.17.** Projectional characteristics of a left anterior pelvis (LAP) as compared to a nonrotated pelvis. *CR*, central ray.

assist in this interpretive effort, the final diagnostic judgement must rest on one's knowledge of pelvic and spinal biomechanics and the manner by which that biomechanics projects to the film.

### Pelvic Flexion and Extension

Pelvic flexion (anterior rocking) and extension (posterior rocking) on a bilateral femur head pivot is a normal mechanism of sagittal plane postural accommodation to body weight distribution to the anterior or posterior, as that pelvic action influences (or is influenced by) the magnitude of the anterior and posterior spinal curves. Clinically, pelvic flexion and extension is not significant in itself unless it is of a magnitude which may result in lumbosacral and sacroiliac articulation stresses, and then it is more inclined to be an *effect* of postural balance requirements than it is to be a biomechanical *cause* in itself. Spinographically, the observation of pelvic flexion and extension is almost entirely an exercise in visualizing the third dimension of depth on the anteroposterior projection (i.e. the posteroanterior view).

In most anteroposterior projection evaluations, however, contour comparisons are

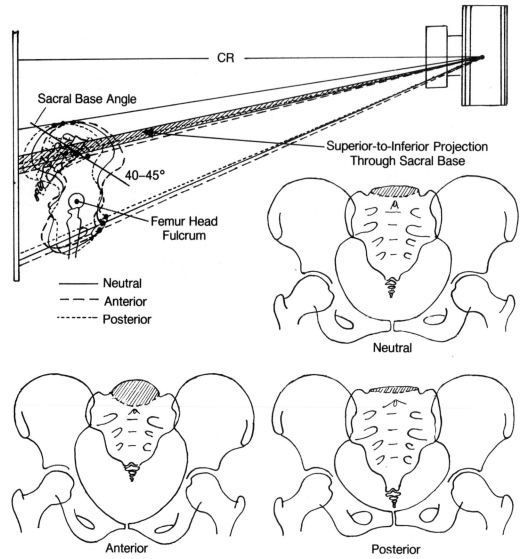

**Figure 9.18.** Projectional characteristics of an *anterior* (flexion) or *posterior* (extension) pelvis as compared to what may be regarded normal. Note how base of the sacrum increases long axis to divergent rays in anterior flexion and decreases long axis to divergent rays in posterior extension, and provides increase of pelvic outlet in flexion similar to what is sometimes called an "obstetric view." *CR*, central ray.

made of like structures on a bilateral basis (in opposite horizontal film quadrants). In the case of uncomplicated (without concomitant pelvic rotation or interpelvic deviations) pelvic flexion and extension is an exercise in evaluating equal bilateral projection summation angles as they are influenced by sagittal plane anteroposterior rocking of the pelvis as a unit on the femur heads.

Figure 9.18 depicts the representative projection summation angles to various pelvic structures (crests of the ilium, anterior and posterior borders of the sacral base, superior and inferior borders of the pubic bodies) and spatial distances in between as they would project to the neutral, anterior and posterior pelvic configurations.

As compared to the neutral view, the configuration of an uncomplicated anteriorly rocked (flexion) pelvis would be characteristically illustrated by:

1. Increase in vertical dimensions of the pelvic outlet, along with corresponding increase in the vertical measurements of the innominate bones
2. Decrease in vertical dimensions of the sacrum, with increase in depiction of the sacral base
3. Decrease in vertical dimensions of the pubic bodies

As compared to the neutral view, the configuration of an uncomplicated posteriorly rocked (extension) pelvis would be characteristically illustrated by:

1. Decrease in vertical dimensions of the pelvic outlet, along with corresponding decrease in the vertical measurement of the innominate bones
2. Increase in vertical dimensions of the sacrum, with decrease in depiction of the sacral base
3. Increase in vertical dimensions of the pubic bodies

In visualizing the anteroposterior projection of the pelvis on a full spine view, a number of qualifying factors must be taken into consideration aside from the possible complication of impressions by pelvic rotation and/or interpelvic deviations. The most significant factor is that of patient gender, insofar as there are distinct differences in the comparative configurations of the male and female pelvises (Fig. 9.19). Another factor is that of focal-film distance insofar as longer focal-film distances (than the 72 in recommended in this presentation) tend to simulate what might appear to be a posteriorly rocked pelvis.

As an interesting postscript to our earlier reference to visualization of the third dimension of depth on the anteroposterior projection (PA view), the appearance of what is called a "bow sign" is indicative of a possible spondylolisthesis condition of L5 on the sacrum which may be confirmed on the lateral view (Fig. 9.20). The appearance of an L5/sacral base bow sign is particularly significant to this discussion in that it may be simulated by an anteriorly rocked pelvis which tends to face the articular base of the

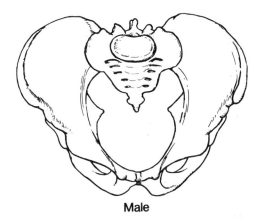

Male

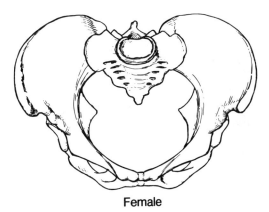

Female

**Figure 9.19.** Differences of male and female pelves which must be considered when evaluating possible flexion or extension on the pelvis on the anteroposterior full spine projection. (Male-female pelvic illustrations by courtesy of Williams & Wilkins *Medical Art: Graphics for Use* by Diane Abeloff.)

sacrum more in line with the divergent rays.

Innominate Cleave

Innominate cleave (a term coined for this presentation) may be described as "a normal interpelvic biomechanical action in which the bilaterally opposed ilia of the innominate bones move in an anterolateral/posteromedial direction, relative to each other and to the sacrum, on a point of pivot located at the symphysis pubis articulation. Innominate cleave is a normal, synchronous intrapelvic innominate action in locomotion and in postural accommo-

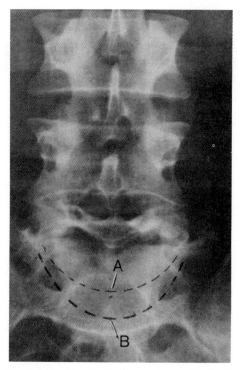 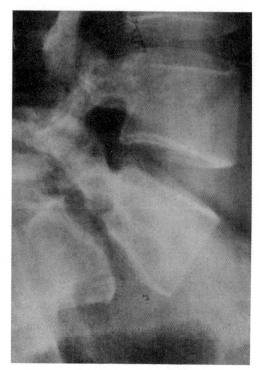

**Figure 9.20.** Indication of spondylolisthesis as may be suspected by "bow sign" impression on anteroposterior full spine view. *Left, A* = normal; *B* = abnormal. *Right,* lateral view of same patient. (Illustration from *U.S. Military X-Ray Manual.*)

dation to standing on an unlevel surface or in compensation to a scoliotic spinal curvature. When such bilaterally opposed innominate movement is carried to an extreme (perhaps beyond 2° at each sacroiliac articulation), bilateral or unilateral sacroiliac subluxation may be suspect (Fig. 9.21).

With respect to this normal and sacroiliac subluxation-inducing action of the innominate bones, four commonly accepted misnomers associated with certain traditional systems of spinographic analysis require identification in order to emphasize the uniqueness of the preceding explanation of intrapelvic biomechanics:

1. The traditional concept of the ilia of the bilaterally opposed innominate bones moving anterosuperior/posteroinferior (AS/PI) is insufficiently descriptive insofar as when an innominate ilia moves anteriorly and superiorly it correspondingly moves laterally relative to the sacrum (anterolateral-superior) and, conversely, when the opposite innominate ilia moves posteriorly and inferiorly it correspondingly moves medially relative to the sacrum (posteromedial-inferior)

2. The proposition that the innominate bones can "flare" internally or externally (IN/EX) as an independent movement is an implausible concept insofar as the spinographic appearance of such innominate flaring is a concomitant action of anterolateral/posteromedial movement of the ilia relative to the sacrum and/or the projectional effect of LAP/RAP pelvic torsion

3. The idea that the opposed innominate bones move anterior and posterior on a femur head pivot (as a normal or subluxation-inducing action) is incorrect insofar as the ligamentous restriction of the symphysis pubis would (unless traumatically or pathologically loosened) disallow this action

4. The designation of "innominate subluxation" is inappropriate insofar as bones in themselves do not subluxate, but rather the articulations between bones do—in the case of the above-discussed movement of the opposed innominate bones on a symphysis pubis pivot, the associated orthodysarthria is a *sacroiliac* subluxation.

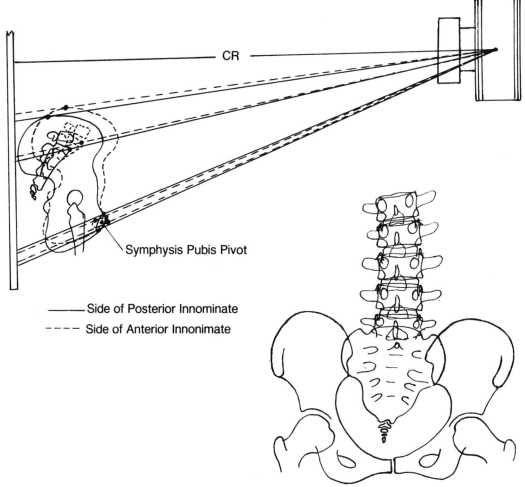

CR

Symphysis Pubis Pivot

———— Side of Posterior Innominate

– – – – Side of Anterior Innonimate

**Figure 9.21.**    Projectional characteristics of innominate cleavage on a symphysis pubis point of pivot: *right*, posteromedial innominate; *left*, anterolateral innominate; *CR*, central ray.

Thus, the following spinographic evaluation of intrapelvic biomechanics as was depicted in Figure 9.21 is based on the proposed concept of *innominate cleavage*; e.g. "movement of the bilaterally opposed ilia of the innominate bones in an anterolateral/posteromedial direction, relative to each other and to the sacrum, on a point of pivot at the symphysis pubis articulation":

1. The cleaving action of the two opposed innominate bones on a symphysis pubis pivot will result in:
   a. The posteriorly disposed innominate ilium moving medially (toward the center of the sacrum) and the anteriorly disposed innominate ilium moving laterally (away from the center of the sacrum)
   b. The pelvic rim projecting a shorter radius on the side of the posteromedially disposed ilium and a greater radius on the side of the anteromedially disposed ilium
   c. An increase in the vertical dimensions (wider) of the pubic body on the side of the posteromedially disposed ilium and a decrease in vertical dimensions (narrower) on the side of the anterolaterally disposed ilium.
2. Unless complicated by independent movement, the sacrum will tend to move inferiorly with the inferiorly disposed posteromedial ilium, resulting in:
   a. The sacral base being structurally low as well as being projected additionally lower on the side of the posteromedial ilium
   b. The sacroiliac articulation showing

greater overlap on the side of the posteromedial ilium as compared to the
side of anterolateral ilium.

c. The sacral base being diagonally deviated toward the side of the anteromedially disposed ilium and way from
the side of the posteromedially disposed
ilium.

3. If the lumbar spine vertebral motor units
are capable of normal functional response
(i.e. not in a state of subluxation fixation)
to the sacral unleveling, the lumbar spine
will assume a *normal* functional scoliosis,
convexing and rotating posteriorly on the
side of the low (and incidently, anteroin-
feriorly rotated) sacral base.

The foregoing description of innominate
cleavage represents the characteristic
impressions of what is sometimes called a
"basic pelvic distortion pattern" (Fig. 9.22)
and provides a good study in the visualization of pelvic biomechanics as it is spinographically projected to the film. Also, this
basic pelvic distortion pattern provides a
good study in the contemporary concept of
spinographic interpretation of biomechanical integrities, as opposed to the traditional static concept of alignment versus
misalignment—the object being to ascertain whether or not the component parts of
the pelvis and spinal column are capable of
functioning in accordance with the demands of human bipedal posture and locomotion.

In this regard, the affecting of a basic
distortion pattern of the pelvis—up to
that magnitude allowed by the symphyseal
and sacroiliac articulations—in response to
balance control requirements of the body is
a biomechanically diagnostic sign of functional integrity. However, beyond that
magnitude allowed by the articulations, a
sacroiliac subluxation *secondary* to the pos-
teromedial/anterolateral disrelationship
may be suspect.

Sacral Flexion, Extension and Rotation

Flexion, extension and rotation of the
sacrum within the bilaterally opposed ilia
of the innominate bones are generally concomitant, synchronous movements designed to serve as a *postural control link*
between the pelvis as a unit below and the

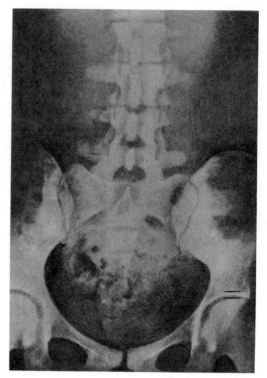

**Figure 9.22.** Spinographic impression of a
"basic pelvic distortion" pattern in the case of a
right posteromedial/left anterolateral innominate cleavage on a symphysis pubis point of
pivot. Note: (*a*) widening of the right pubic body
as compared to the left, (*b*) decrease in contour
of the right pelvic outlet as compared to the left,
(*c*) lowering of sacral base on the right, (*d*)
compensatory right functional scoliosis to the
side of the lowered sacral base.

spine as a unit above. While the sacrum
may move *in sympathy* to its innominate
support, as discussed, it can also move to a
certain degree independent of the bilaterally opposed ilia—the primary movement
being rotation around a 35–40° inclined
vertical axis with flexion and extension
being secondary movements designed to
regulate the magnitude of rotation effect
(in a universal-joint type of action) upon
the fifth lumbar vertebra (11, 14, 15).

In Figure 9.23 the flexion, extension and
rotation movement characteristics of the
sacrum within the ilia are schematically
illustrated, along with the manner by which
these biomechanical actions are projected
to the film. The spinographic line drawing
then illustrates the sacrum rotated ante-

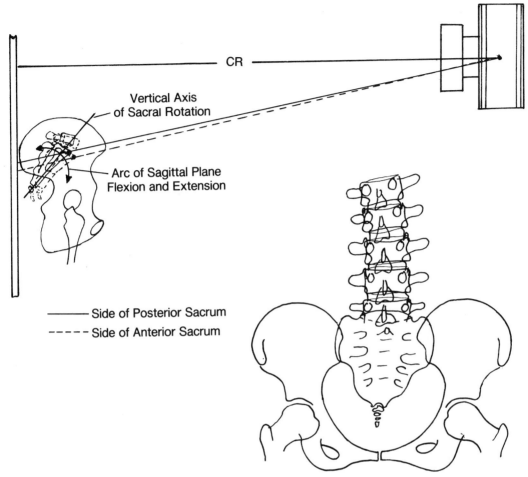

**Figure 9.23.** Projectional characteristics of a right anteroinferior-left posterosuperior rotation of the sacrum within the innominate ilia which, along with the anterior flexion-posterior extension action of the sacrum, initiates a variable "universal joint" action to control magnitude of lumbar curvature compensation. *CR*, central ray.

riorly and inferiorly within the ilia of the bilaterally aligned innominate bones—the anteroinferior rotation being the predominant spinographically identifiable movement insofar as the illustrated projection summation angles to the sacrum would not clearly indicate flexion or extension, or the lesser possibility of lateral sacral tilt as a normal movement consideration.

Thus, as the sacrum rotates anteriorly and inferiorly on the right (Fig. 9.24) (which may occur as an independent action of the sacrum within the ilia or in sympathy to innominate cleavage) the lumbar spine initially is deviated off balance to the right but (if the lumbar vertebral motor units are

normally functional) is corrected by the proprioceptively initiated pull of the paraspinal muscles affecting a compensatory scoliosis which in turn is mechanically integrated with sacral flexion, extension and rotation (see Chapter 6, Figures 6.22–6.25 and accompanying discussion for review of this concept of integration of spinal function).

Although a certain degree of sacral flexion, extension and rotation within the ilia is a normal biomechanical action, excessive movement in these directions can result in sacroiliac articulation subluxation by the resulting *jamming* effect. As previously stated, the probable amount of normal

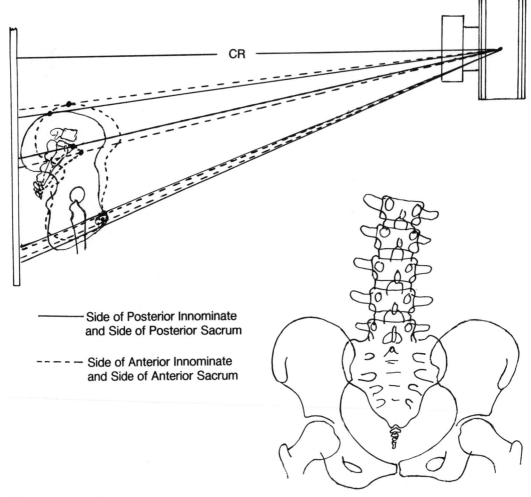

—— Side of Posterior Innominate
and Side of Posterior Sacrum

- - - - Side of Anterior Innominate
and Side of Anterior Sacrum

**Figure 9.24.** Projectional characteristics of a combined "primary" subluxation of the sacrum (low on the left) in the presence of a "secondary" sacroiliac subluxation on the right due to a right posteromedial innominate on a symphysis pubis point of pivot. *CR,* central ray.

movement of the sacroiliac articulation is somewhere around 2°, and beyond that point a *primary* subluxation of the sacrum relative to the ilia may be suspect.

In summary, the movement of the sacrum beyond the limits of its articulation with the ilia has been designated as a "primary sacroiliac subluxation" and movement of the ilia beyond their normal limits with the sacrum has been designated as a "secondary sacroiliac subluxation." Conceivably, also, both types of sacroiliac subluxations may occur simultaneously; e.g. (Fig. 9.24), the sacrum might undergo a *primary* sacroiliac subluxation on one side

(perhaps due to a universal joint type torsion from a scoliotic condition of the spine above) while at the same time undergo a *secondary* sacroiliac subluxation on the other side due to posteromedial cleavage of the innominate bone (perhaps as a result of an iliopsoas muscle dystonia).

## PROJECTION OF SPINAL BIOMECHANICAL PATTERNS

As maintained throughout this presentation of contemporary (as opposed to traditional) spinographic interpretation, effort is directed to ascertaining *losses of normal* biomechanical integrities as departures from the normal, rather than to the arbitrary assumption that a subluxation does or does not exist on the basis of whether or not a vertebra is in proper alignment with another vertebra, above and/or below. This is an important distinction that bears repetition: "in contemporary spinographic interpretation we are not so concerned with whether or not a vertebra is in proper alignment with the one above or the one below or both, but rather we are concerned with the question of whether or not the vertebral motor units of the spinal column (individually or collectively) are responding normally to postural requirements under a given set of circumstance in a particular case" (Fig. 9.25).

Contrary to the implied concept of traditional spinographic analysis that "spinal subluxations are absolute conditions which may be definitively ascertained by spinographic analysis procedures," the arriving at a decision of a biomechnical impropriety AND ITS CLINICAL SIGNIFICANCE is a matter of *professional judgment* based on one's knowledge of spinal biomechanics and the manner by which that biomechanics projects to the x-ray film. Paraphrasing Greenfield (see "Overview of Roentgen Diagnosis" in Chapter 8), "The basic approach should be simple. The roentgen pattern should be accurately and objectively analyzed with respect to certain distinct, independent features ..." (16). With respect to the biomechanical considerations of the spinal column, the distinct, independent features relate to three primary classifications of abnormal spinal function referred to in Chapter 7 as "orthodysarthric lesions." These are:

**Type A:** the condition of a vertebral motor unit wherein a spinal structure is unable to *move from* its normal resting position in relation to its supporting structure below ...

**Type B:** the condition of a vertebral motor unit wherein a spinal structure is unable to *move through* its normal ranges of movement ...

**Type C:** the condition of a vertebral motor unit wherein a spinal structure is unable to *return to* its normal resting position after movement ...

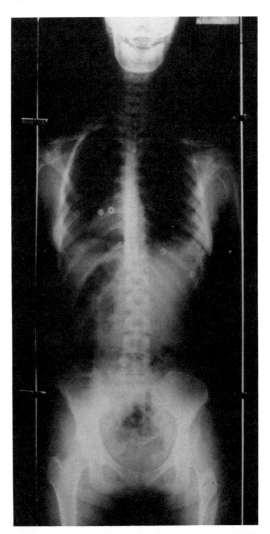

**Figure 9.25.** Example of spontaneous initiation of spinal vertebral motor unit action, under integrated neuromuscular control, to unleveling of the pelvis. Example is a case where patient inadvertently flexed right knee half-way through exposure, lowering the pelvis on the right and immediately causing a right thoracolumbar/left thoracocervical compensatory (functional) scoliosis. An unusual and extraordinary example of integrated vertebral motor unit function as a unitized action throughout the entire spinal column which further emphasizes that the spine is in fact a complete "organ structure" in which a subluxation in one part may affect the entire spinal column.

As a practical exercise in the application of this functional concept of spinographic interpretation, it will be noted in Figure 9.26A that the spine as a whole exhibits a mild (as opposed to moderate or severe)

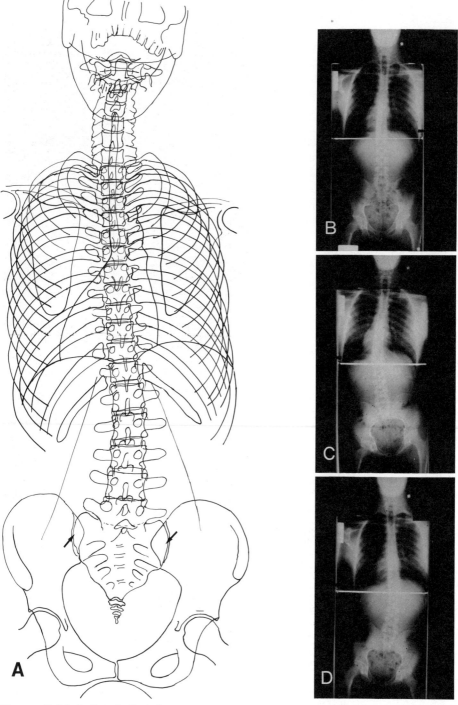

**Figure 9.26** *A–D. A,* line drawing of an actual AP full spine radiograph indicating normal function of the vertebral motor units in assuming a compensated functional scoliosis as a result of a lowering of the sacral base on the right and a raising on the left. *B,* anteroposterior full spine view of a patient with all vertebrae in apparent good alignment although exhibiting a very slight total left curvature. *C,* same patient, where activation of the vertebral motor units are forced into controlled neuromuscular response by placing a block under the right foot (technique of Chamberlain). *D,* same patient, where inactivation of the vertebral motor units are forced into controlled neuromuscular response by placing a block under the left foot (see pelvic response of this same patient where technique of Chamberlain illustrated resistance of symphysis pubis to vertical shearing).

right thoracolumbar/left thoracocervical functional (compensated, nonstructural) scoliosis as a result of a right anteroinferior/left posterosuperior sacral deviation due to a right posteromedial/left anterolateral innominate cleavage. Insofar as a *functional* spinal scoliosis is not an abnormal condition in itself, but rather is a normal response of the vertebral motor units to an unleveling of its postural base at some point below, the *provisional diagnosis* in this case (depending upon lateral view observations and correlation with other examination findings) would be that, although sacroiliac subluxation(s) are probably present, no spinal vertebral motor unit subluxations are suspected because of the following:

1. The involved vertebrae were obviously able to *move from* their normal resting positions
2. The involved vertebrae (barring other findings to the contrary) are probably able to *move through* their normal ranges of motion
3. The involved vertebrae (barring other findings to the contrary) are probably able to *return to* their normal resting positions after their prior movement into a functional scoliotic state; e.g. when the sacral base unleveling condition is corrected.

With respect to this example, two observations are of some importance—*spinographic analysis* implications and *clinical significance* implications:

## Spinographic Analysis Implications

Although certain traditional spinographic analysis procedures (5) would arbitrarily designate any vertebra that is in a state of "wedging" above a level vertebra as a "subluxation," such a diagnosis in this case would be fallacious insofar as the four vertebrae in the transitional scoliotic areas would erroneously meet that classification.

Although certain traditional spinographic analysis procedures (4–8) would tend to be arbitrarily definite (as opposed to the herein used professional judgement criterion) in designating the existence and magnitude of spinal subluxations, such definitive conclusions are not based on any presently accepted scientific support.

## Clinical Significance Implications

Because a functional scoliosis is a normal response of vertebral motor units to compensatory demands of a postural unleveling at some point below, this does not mean that such a condition is not without a negative clinical significance—a functional scoliosis imposes microtrauma stresses to the vertebral motor units which if not alleviated may result in clinically significant interarticular pathologies at a later stage.

Because a particular case may not present findings indicative of an A, B or C type orthodysarthric lesion, this does not mean that one may not be present which may require other means of detection: i.e. functional radiographic studies,¶ motion palpation, etc.

Continuing our practical exercise in the application of the "functional concept" of spinographic interpretation, it will be noted in Figure 9.27 that the patient exhibits various forms of normal and abnormal vertebral motor unit responses to an unleveling of the spinal column base—subluxation of the sacrum relative to the ilia due to a left posteromedial/right anterolateral innominate cleavage at a symphysis pubis pivot. In addition to the presence of sacroiliac subluxation, the following diagnostic findings are either evident or suspected:

---

¶ Although considerable effort has been given to the evaluation of potential spinal motion by the use of static and cineroentgenographic stress films, (17–58) these procedures do not necessarily provide adequate information on which to assess *normal* vertebral motor unit movement capability. Although such stress studies may force movement in spinal articulations which are in *fixed* states of subluxation, they do not necessarily demonstrate orthodysarthrias due to inefficient neuromuscular activation of the vertebral motor units. Ideally, the best manner of radiographically demonstrating such propriety of the vertebral motor units would be to take postural films under conditions which activate neuromuscular control of the vertebral motor units, as in the experimental studies depicted in Figure 9.26 *B–D*. However, at the present time, insufficient data is available to justify patient radiation exposure to such studies on a routine clinical basis. On the other hand, the newer procedures using *Nuclear Magnetic Resonance*—NMR—may eventually be capable of providing such information without the usual x-radiation hazards to patients (59–70).

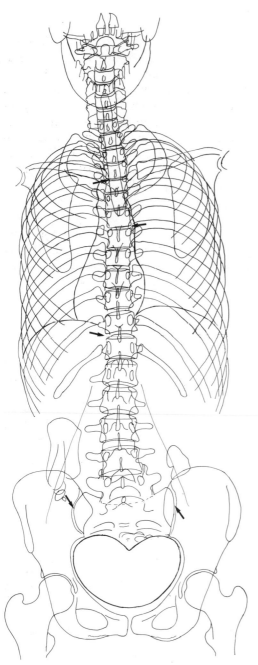

**Figure 9.27.** Line drawing of actual AP full spine radiograph illustrating various normal and abnormal vertebral motor unit impressions (see text for discussion).

1. The lumbar vertebral motor units appear to be normally functional insofar as the lumbar spine has assumed an expected left functional scoliosis in compensation to the lowered sacral base on the left
2. T11 vertebra appears to be in a left lateral

flexion subluxation on T12 insofar as it deviated abruptly out of continuity to the functional scoliosis from T12 downward
3. T11 upward to T7 appear to have resumed normal movement action (left functional scoliosis) in compensation to the subluxation of T11 on T12
4. T6 upward to T4 appear to be functional, while T3 has assumed a left lateral flexion subluxation on T4
5. The thoracocervical spine from T3 upward to the occiput appears to be in a normally functional state in compensation to the left lateral flexion subluxation of T3 on T4

While Figures 9.26 and 9.27 were examples of sacroiliac subluxations *secondary* to innominate cleavage, Figure 9.28 is an example of combined *primary* subluxation of the sacrum (low on the right) and *secondary* subluxation (high on the left) due to a posteromedial innominate cleavage to the side (left) opposite the side of low sacral base. Additionally, in this example, the diagnostic findings may be noted or suspected:

1. Because of the increased depth of the lumbosacral *bow line*, a spondylolisthesis condition is suspected which will require a lateral view for confirmation
2. A congenital fusion of L4 on L5 is evident, with both segments deviating as a unit to the side of the lowered sacral base
3. Fixation subluxations of L3 on L4 and L2 on L3 (in normal juxtaposition alignment) are evident due to the fact that they did not assume expected compensatory action to the right lateral deviation of L4 and L5
4. A left lateral *hypermobile* subluxation of L1 on L2 is noted insofar as it compensated abruptly to the fixations below
5. Compensatory action of the vertebral motor units from T12 to C7 appears normal
6. There is evidence of a healed compression fracture of C6 which reverses compensation of C5 to C2
7. There is a suggestion of fixation subluxations of atlas on axis and the occiput on atlas due to the absence of compensatory action which would have been expected as a neuromuscular (vestibular/proprioceptive-controlled) effort to level the head to gravity

## PROJECTION OF UPPER CERVICAL BIOMECHANICAL PATTERNS

The upper cervical complex (atlas and axis) is designed to function somewhat pas-

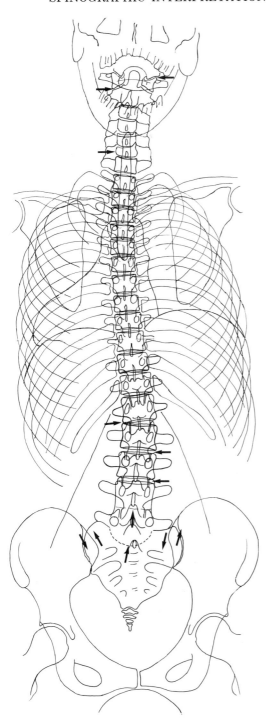

**Figure 9.28.** Line drawing of actual AP full spine radiograph illustrating various normal and abnormal vertebral motor unit impressions (see text for discussion).

sively as a postural balance mechanism for the head, as opposed to the pelvis which is designed to function more actively as a

mechanism of bipedal locomotion. Whereas in traditional spinographic analysis procedure effort is directly mainly to arriving at minutely measured misalignments of the upper cervical structures with the supposition that such misalignments represent subluxations, concern here (as was the case of pelvis and spinal column as a whole) is directed to evaluating the functional efficiency of these structures in fulfilling their objectives—supporting the head while at the same time allowing it to seek a gravitational balance in accordance with the dictates of the vestibular apparatuses of the inner ear.

In fulfilling their objectives, the atlas and axis are designed to allow for movement of the head on the three axes, or freedoms, of movement—lateral flexion around a sagittal axis, rotation on a vertical axis and flexion/extension on a transverse axis. Lateral flexion and rotation movements are most discernible on the anteroposterior projection (PA view) and flexion/extension movements are most discernible on the left lateral projection (right lateral view) or the right lateral projection (left lateral view). However, as was the case of the lumbosacral area wherein impressions of sagittal plane movements (as in the bow sign of spondylolisthesis) were sometimes discernible on the anteroposterior projection, similar impressions of atlas flexion and extention may be equally discernible in this manner.

In Figure 9.29 the projection of the divergent rays through the open mouth on the anteroposterior projection provides for posteroanterior visualization of the atlas, occiput and axis in a superior-to-inferior direction. Thus, movements of these structures relative to each other requires exercise of our previously acquired skill at three-dimensional visualization.

### Lateral Flexion and Rotation

Lateral flexion and rotation of the occipitocervical junction are concomitant movements, quite similar to that of the lower lumbar spine, even to the possible affecting of a variable universal joint type action to

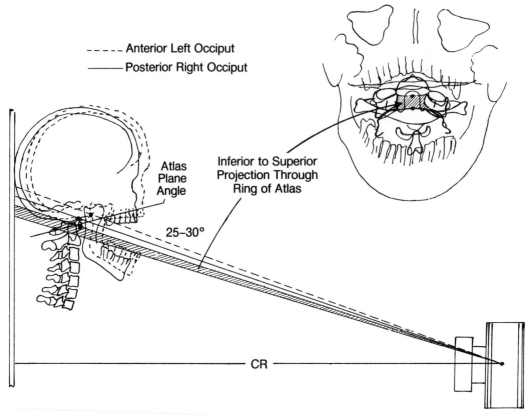

**Figure 9.29.** Projectional characteristics of the upper cervical complex on the anteroposterior full spine projection. Note that anterior rotation of the occiput on the atlas projects the occiput higher on the side of anterior occiput rotation. Also note that because of the inferior-to-superior projection of x-rays through the atlas ring and foramen magnum, the posterior-to-anterior viewing position is downward through the atlas ring.

increase or decrease the magnitude of compensatory action of the upper cervical area in balancing the head to gravity—increased rotation and lateral flexion of the head occurring concomitant with increased extension of atlas on axis and decreased rotation and lateral flexion of the head occurring concomitant with decreased extension (tending toward flexion) of the atlas on axis.

Projectionally, it will be noted in Figure 9.29 that because the divergent rays project upward to the occiput and to the film, rotation of the head results in it being projected upward on the side of anteriority, which will generally occur on the side opposite to the direction of head lateral flexion. Consequently, functional propriety of the upper cervical complex will be demon-strated if the head rotates anterior and flexes laterally (tilts toward) the side of a cervical spine scoliotic convexity. Failure of such action to occur would, of course, indicate a possible biomechanical orthodysarthria of the upper cervical articulations—particularly atlas on axis since most of the related compensatory movement of the head on the upper cervical area occurs at that articulation. The possibility of such a biomechanical impropriety was noted in Figure 9.28.

Flexion and Extension

As mentioned above, it is also possible to detect sagittal plane flexion and extension of the occiput, atlas and axis on the antero-posterior projection—a biomechanical activity which is most observable on the lateral view. This is accomplished by two principal observations: the relative distance of the atlas posterior arch to the axis spinous process and/or to the base of the occiput and the plane angle of the atlas as it relates to the incident divergent x-rays.

In the first of these considerations, the superior and inferior borders of the atlas posterior arch are normally equidistant to the axis spinous process and base of the occiput, and increase or decrease of these distance relationships would suggest possible increased flexion or extension of the head—increase in flexion, decrease in extension. If either of these distance relationships increases or decreases independently, hypermobile and/or fixation orthodysarthrias may be suspect.

In the second of these considerations, the normal mean plane angle of the atlas (relative to a horizontal) of about 15° vectors with the inferiorly to superiorly projected incident ray (of about 12°) at an interrelated angle of about 27° degrees, which in effect provides a superior to inferior PA view downward through the atlas ring. Thus, an increase in vertical dimension of the atlas ring would suggest extension of the head and a decrease would suggest flexion of the head.

These impressions, of course, would only be suggestive and confirmation would require lateral view evaluation to form a more conclusive diagnostic judgement of biomechanical impropriety.

## Lateral Projection

As was previously discussed in the chapter on spinographic technology, the lateral full spine projection is customarily taken in two separate exposures, at 60-in focal-film distances, while the patient is immobilized in what is referred to as "his/her normal standing posture."

While a single exposure at 72 in (as with the AP projection) may initially seem more advisable, this is generally contraindicated due to the unacceptable amount of radiographic distortion occurring at the upper

and lower extremes of the film and by the excessive power loads impressed on the x-ray tubes of standard single-phase x-ray machines used in many private practice settings. Three-phase x-ray generator spinography units have been developed which allow for anteroposterior and lateral full spine views taken at up to 108-in (27.4 m) focal-film distance have been developed (71), but the cost of such units (in excess of $125,000) make them cost prohibitive for most general chiropractic practice applications.

As was the case with the PA full spine view, projection of the three-dimensional components of the spine and pelvis to the flat, two-dimensional film can be geometrically plotted with the projection-summation angle principle. In Figure 9.30 it is noted that the patient is positioned for a left lateral view (right lateral projection) and the hypothetical scaled projection plotting field allows for rather precise measurements of the image distortion patterns as they are projected to the film.

For the thoracocervical section the central ray is aligned 90° to the film (parallel with the floor), passing across the acromial process of the shoulder and approximately through the second-third thoracic vertebrae. The collimated field for this thoracocervical section will include the base of the occiput to about the 11th thoracic vertebra, while the collimated field for the lumbopelvic section will include the ninth thoracic vertebra (overlapping at about the tenth) to the symphysis pubis articulation—the symphysis pubis articulation being required on the film to allow for certain measurements of sacroinnominate biomechanical relationships (see Chapter 4 on positioning for explanation of tube and film shift between exposures for the lateral projection exposure).

Although the lower thoracic overlap between exposures (to ensure projecting all thoracic vertebrae to the film) may appear to be offset, this is only a projectional impression which can be visually dealt with by accepting the fact that, since the patient did not move during the two exposures, the

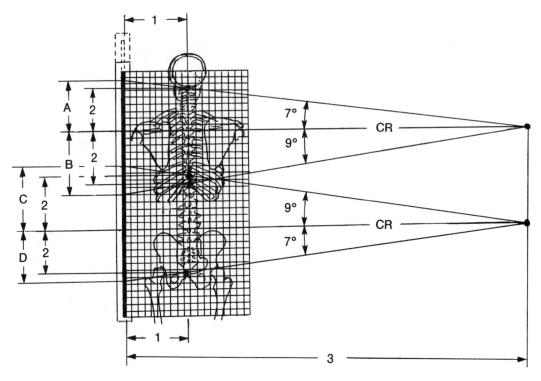

Code:
1. Object-Film Distance
2. Object-Central Ray Distance
3. Focal-Film Distance

A. Occipital Condyle Projection to Film
B. T10 Projection to Film
C. T9 Projection to Film
D. Symphysis Pubis Projection to Film      Scale: 1/16 in = 1 in

**Figure 9.30.** Projection summation angle plotting chart for a two-exposure left lateral full spine view as is customarily used in many systems of spinographic analysis (see text for discusson). *CR*, central ray.

lowest vertebra in the thoracocervical section and the upper vertebra in the lumbopelvic section were actually in approximately correct relationship, assuming they were not offset by sagittal plane subluxation.

Ideally, however, it would be more desirable to take the lateral full spine view in a single exposure if the technical limitations relative to required equipment cost could be minimized to practical limits for general chiropractic practice use. Although at the time of this writing the author did not have an opportunity to evaluate the *Gilardoni Total Body Radiography* (GTBR) homographic filtration system (see Chapter 4 for details), the information provided by the manufacturer indicates that this system may well be worth considering.

## PROJECTION OF LATERAL SPINE BIOMECHANICAL PATTERNS

Although not necessarily of greater or lesser importance, information-wise, interpretation of the lateral full spine view is considerably less complicated than the anteroposterior projection view. Whereas the lateral view mainly concerns evaluation of biomechanical integrities on only one movement plane (sagittal), the evaluation of the posterior view concerns primary evaluation of two planes (coronal and transverse), with some additional consideration of movements on the third (sagittal) plane.

In evaluating the lateral full spine view for possible biomechanical irregularities, it is significant to recall that it consists of four *normal* sagittal plane curves (two anterior in the cervical and lumbar sections and two posterior in the thoracic and sacral sections) which are composed of 26 movable units (24 vertebrae plus the sacrum and coccyx). While traditional spinographic analysis procedures often measure the depth of these normal sagittal plane curves with the idea that increases or decreases from "normal" are in some manner representative of individual or sectional subluxations, these judgements are more often than not only conjectural insofar as no normals for the depth of these curves on a particular person have ever been established—*average*, perhaps, but not *normal*.

Therefore, our objective at this point is not to be overly concerned with the depth of the normal sagittal plane curves, but rather to assess whether or not the depth (and contour) of these curves indicate proper functional integrity of the spinal components of which the curves are composed. For example, in the case of a functional scoliosis of the spine due to an unleveling of the pelvis, we may make a reasonable assumption that the vertebral motor unit within the scoliosis are simply functioning in a normal fashion to attempt to rebalance the body to a state of postural equilibrium. By the same token, if the normal sagittal plane curves of an obese person are increased beyond what might be considered average, this would likewise tend to indicate that the vertebral motor unit were simply responding normally in an attempt to rebalance the body to a state of postural equilibrium on the sagittal plane. It also then follows that a vertebra that did not respond in such a manner might be considered in a subluxated state.

To illustrate this concept of contemporary spinographic interpretation of functional adequacy of the vertebral motor units, we might note in Figure 9.31 that the spinal curves are relatively normal (e.g. average) for the 180-lb (81.8-kg), 5 ft 10-in (17.8 m) male represented by this left lateral spinographic view. Basically, two visual observations are made relative to the biomechanical relationship-functional re-

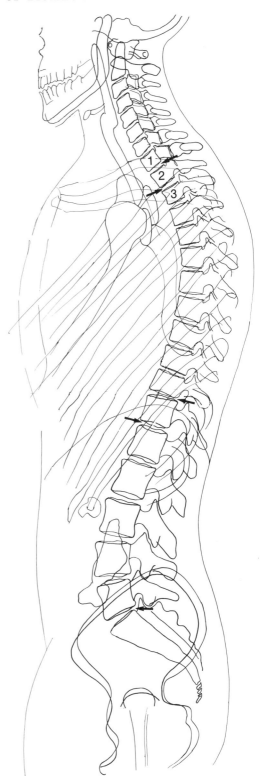

**Figure 9.31.** Line drawing of an actual left lateral full spine view illustrating various considerations of normal and abnormal vertebral motor unit actions.

sponse of the vertebrae: the aligned contour of the posterior aspect of the vertebral bodies from the sacrum to the atlas (commonly called "George's line") and the wedging (or nonwedging) of intervertebral spaces.

Thus, the following might be suggested at the points indicated by arrows starting at the lumbosacral junction:

1. There is a noticeable lack of alignment between the sacral base and L5 body— sacrum is anterior to L5 or L5 is posterior to the sacrum. Because L5 is in relatively good alignment to L4, we would tend to believe that the sacrum is abnormally anterior to L5; e.g. possible bilateral sacroiliac articulation subluxations.

2. Normally, when the patient's arms are raised in positioning for the lateral view, there is a tendency for them to arch the lower back to maintain standing balance, which normally (if the lumbar spine vertebral motor units are functional) results in some degree of posterior shifting of the upper lumbar vertebra on the one below, particularly from L2 to the sacral base. In this case, such posterior shifting of the lumbar vertebrae has occurred indicating the vertebral motor units are normally functional. However, since L5 has shifted posteriorly relative to the sacrum to an excessive amount, we have some confirmation that the sacrum has subluxated anteriorly to L5 rather than L5 subluxating posteriorly to the sacrum.

3. There is an impression that T12 (by virtue of its slight anterior intervertebral space wedging, or lack of any wedging, may be in a state of fixation subluxation relative to L1. This is somewhat confirmed by the fact that T11 has over-compensated by excessive wedging to the posterior; e.g. has assumed a hypermobile state.

4. All vertebrae from T11 up to T3 appear to be in a relatively normally aligned posterior curve expected for that region under the circumstances.

5. T2 appears to be in a state of anterior flexion subluxation on T3. Additionally, since L1 would have been expected to initiate the start of the normal anterior cervical curve, it may be in a state of fixation subluxation on L2 because it does not illustrate a slight posterior wedging of the intervertebral articulation.

6. No significant abnormalities in alignment are noted from T1 to the occiput, therefore no subluxations are suggested unless other examination findings indicate otherwise.

## References

1. Remier PA: *Modern X-Ray Practice and Chiropractic Spinography.* Davenport, Iowa, Palmer School of Chiropractic, 1957, pp 1–25.
2. Palmer BJ: *A Textbook on the Palmer Technique of Chiropractic.* Davenport, Iowa, Palmer School of Chiropractic, 1920.
3. Palmer DD: *The Science, Art and Philosophy of Chiropractic.* Portland, Oreg, Portland Printing House, 1910, p 1.
4. Logan HB: *Textbook of Logan Basic Methods.* St. Louis, Mo, L.B.M., 1950.
5. Herbst RW: *Gonstead Chiropractic Science and Art.* Mt. Horeb, Wisc, Sci-Chi Publications, 1968.
6. Grostic JD: Origins of the Grostic procedure. *Int Rev Chiropractic,* March:33–35, 1978.
7. Mears DB: *The Mears Technique: a Biomechanical Study of Occipitocervical Spine Displacement and Correction.* St. Albans, Vermont, DB Mears, 1976.
8. Pettibon BR: Pettibon method: cervical x-ray analysis and instrument adjusting. Tacoma, Wash, Pettibon & Associates, 1968.
9. Hildebrandt RW: *X-Ray Projection and Image Formation.* Davenport, Iowa; Palmer College of Chiropractic, 1964.
10. Hildebrandt RW: *Synopsis of Chiropractic Postural Roentgenology.* Lombard, Ill, National College of Chiropractic, 1974.
11. Hildebrandt RW: *Chiropractic Spinography; A Manual of Technology and Interpretation,* ed 1. Des Plaines, Ill, Hilmak Publication, 1977.
12. Hildebrandt RW: Clinical basis of chiropractic postural roentgenology. *J Clin Chiropractic,* 1974.
13. Lusted LB, Keats TE: *Atlas of Roentgenographic Measurement,* ed 4. Chicago, Yearbook Medical Publishers, 1978.
14. Illi F: *The Vertebral Column: the Lifeline of the Body.* Chicago, National College of Chiropractic, 1951.
15. Janse J: *The Work of Illi.* Chicago, National College of Chiropractic, 1954.
16. Greenfield GB: Radiology of Bone Diseases. Philadelphia, Lippincott, 1969.
17. Bronfort G, Jochumsen OH: The functional radiographic examination of patients with low-back pain: a study of different forms of variations. *J Manipulative Physiol Ther* 7:89–97, 1984.
18. Allbrook D: Movements of the lumbar spinal column. *J Bone Joint Surg* 39B:339–345, 1957.
19. Bakke SM: Rontgenolgische beobachtungen uber die bewegungen der wirbelsaule. *Acta Radiol (Suppl)* vol 13, 1931.
20. Benson RH, Schultz AB, Dewald RL: Roentgenographic evaluation of vertebral rotation. *J Bone Joint Surg* 58A:1125–1129, 1976.
21. Brown RH, Burstein AH, Nash CL, Schock CC: Spinal analysis using a three-dimensional radiographic technique. *J Biomech* 9:355–365, 1976.
22. Cassidy JD: Roentgenological examination of the functional mechanics of the lumbar spine in lateral flexion. *J Clin Chiropractic* 20:13–16, 1976.
23. Dimmet J, Fischer LP, Gonon G, Carret JP: Radiographic studies of the lateral flexion in the lumbar spine. *J Biomech* 11:143–150, 1978.
24. Duncan W, Hoen TJ: A new approach to the diagnosis of herniation of the intervertebral disk.

*Surg Gynecol Obstet* 75:257–267, 1942.

25. Frohning EC, Fromann B: Motion of the lumbar spine after laminectomy and spine fusion. *J Bone Joint Surg* 50A:897–918, 1968.

26. Frymoyer JW, Frymoyer NN, Wilder DG, Pope MH: The mechanical and kinematic analysis of the lumbar spine in normal living subjects in vivo. *J Biomech* 12:165–172, 1979.

27. Gianturco CA: A roentgen analysis of the motion of the lower lumbar vertebrae in normal individuals and in patients with low back pain. *Am J Roentgenol* 52:261–268, 1944.

28. Gregersen GG, Lucas DB: An in vitro study of the axial rotation of the human thoraco-lumbar spine. *J Bone Joint Surg* 49A:247–262, 1967.

29. Grice AS: Radiographic, biomechanical and clinical factors in lumbar lateral flexion, part 1. *J Manipulative Physiol Ther* 2:26–34, 1979.

30. Hanley IN, Matteri RE, Frymoyer JW: Accurate roentgenographic determination of lumbar flexion-extension. *Clin Orthop* 115:145–148, 1976.

31. Hasner E, Schalimtzek, Snorrason E: Roentgenological examination of the function of the lumbar spine. *Acta Radiol* 37:141–149, 1952.

32. Higley HG, Goodrich T: *Report of a Study of Spinal Mechanics L3, L4, L5.* Project sponsored by the Foundation for Chiropractic Education and Research, 1916 Wilson Blvd., Arlington, Va, March, 1968.

33. Howe JW: Preliminary observations from cineroentgenological studies of the spinal column. *J Am Chirop Assoc* 4:65–70, 1970.

34. Jirout J: Studies in the dynamics of the spine. *Acta Radiol* 46:55–60, 1956.

35. Jirout J: The normal mobility of the lumbosacral spine. *Acta Radiol* 47:345–348, 1957.

36. Keegan JJ: Alterations of the lumbar curve related to posture and seating. *J Bone Joint Surg* 35A:589–603, 1953.

37. Knutsson F: The instability associated with disc degeneration in the lumbar spine. *Acta Radiol* 25:593–609, 1944.

38. Matteri RE, Pope MH, Frymoyer JN: A biplane radiographic method of determining vertebral rotation in postmortem specimens. *Chirugia Orthop* 116:95–98, 1976.

39. Mensor MC, Duvall G: Absence of motion at the fourth and fifth lumbar interspaces in patients with and without low back pain. *J Bone Joint Surg* 41A:1047–1054, 1959.

40. Miles M, Sullivan NE: Lateral bending at the lumbar and lumbosacral joints. *Anat Rec* 139:387–393, 1961.

41. Morgan F, King T: Primary instability of lumbar vertebrae as a common cause of low back pain. *J Bone Joint Surg* 39B:6–22, 1957.

42. Nachemson AI, Schultz AB, Berkson MH: Mechanical properties of human spine motion segments: inluences of age, sex, level, and degeneration. *Spine* 4:1–8, 1979.

43. Pennal GF, Garson SC, McDonald G, Dale G, Garside H: Motion studies of the lumbar spine. *J Bone Joint Surg* 54B:442–452, 1972.

44. Pope MH, Wilder DG, Matteri RE, Frymoyer JN: Experimental measurements of vertebral motion under load. *Orthop Clin North Am* 8:155–167, 1977.

45. Sandoz RW: Technique and interpretation of functional radiography of the lumbar spine. *Ann Swiss Chiropractic Assoc* 3:66–110, 1965.

46. Schalimtzek M: *Roentgenological Examination of the Lumbar Spine.* Universitetsforlaget, Aavhus, Denmark, 1958.

47. Schram SB, Hosek RS: Error limitations in x-ray kiniematics of the spine. *J Manipulative Physiol Ther* 5:5–10, 1982.

48. Stokes IAF, Medlicott PA, Wilder DG: Measurement of movement in painful intervertebral joints. *Med Biol Eng Comput* 18:694–700, 1980.

49. Stokes IAF: *Computational Technique for Optimizing Accuracy of Radiographic Measurements of Intervertebral Joint Motion.* Proceedings of the Ninth North-East Conference on Bioengineering; Welkowitz W (ed). New York, Pergamon Press, March, 1981.

50. Stokes IAF, Wilder DG, Frymoyer JW, Pope MH: Assessment of patients with low back pain by biplaner radiographic measurement of intervertebral motion. *Spine* 6:233–240, 1981.

51. Suh CH: The fundamentals of computer-aided x-ray analysis of the spine. *J Biomech* 7:161–169, 1974.

52. Tanz SS: To and fro motion range at the fourth and fifth lumbar interspaces. *J Mount Sinai Hosp* 16:303–307, 1950.

53. Tanz SS: Motion of the lumbar spine. *AJR* 69:399–412, 1953.

54. Weitz EM: The lateral bending sign. *Spine* 6:388–397, 1981.

55. White AA, Panjabi MM: The basic kinematics of the human spine. *Spine* 3:12–20, 1978.

56. Wiles P: Movements of the lumbar vertebrae during flexion and extension. *Proc R Soc Med* 28:647–651, 1935.

57. Triano J: *Accurate Determination of Motion from Plane Films.* Abstract presented to the American Biomechanics Society Conference, Tuscon, Ariz, Oct 3–5, 1984.

58. Meeker WC: The role of functional radiographs of the lumbar spine. In Coyle BA (ed): *Proceedings Conference on Current Topics in Chiropractic-Review of the Literature.* Palmer College of Chiropractic-West, May 19–20, 1984.

59. Coyle BA: Nuclear magnetic resonance: a review of principles and applications in medicine and chiropractic. *J Manipulative Physiol Ther* 6:139–142, 1983.

60. Coyle BA: Leaping ahead: nuclear magnetic resonance imaging could revolutionize chiropractic if FCs pain access to the new technology. *Int Rev Chiropractic* May/June:25–28, 1984.

61. Coyle BA: In vivo studies using NMR. In Coyle BA (ed): *Proceedings Conference on Current Topics in Chiropractic—Review of the Literature.* Palmer College of Chiropractic-West, May 19–20, 1984.

62. Geard CR, Osmak RS, Hall EJ, et al: Magnetic resonance and ionizing radiation: a comparative evaluation in vitro of oncogenic and genotoxic potential. *Radiology* 152:199–202, 1984.

63. Howe JW, Tong VYW: Sophisticated diagnostic imaging: boom or bust for chiropractic? *Articulations* March:17–21, 1984.

64. Modic MT, Weinstein MA, Pavlicek W, et al:

Magnetic resonance imaging of the cervical spine: technical and clinical observations. *Am J Radiol* 141:1129–1136, 1983.

65. Modic MT, Pavlicek W, Weinstein MA, et al: Magnetic resonance imaging of intervertebral disk disease: clinical and pulse sequence considerations. *Radiology* 152:103–111, 1984.

66. Murphy WA: How does magnetic resonance compare with computed tomography? *Radiology* 152:235–236, 1984.

67. Gerard G, Rossi DR: Nuclear magnetic resonance imaging of the brain. *Hosp Pract* July:143–156, 1984.

68. Runge VM, Foster MA, Clanton JA, et al: Contrast enhancement of magnetic resonance images by chromium EDTA: an experimental study. *Radiology* 152:123–126, 1984.

69. Schultz CL, Alfidi RJ, Nelson AD, et al: The effect of motion on two-dimensional fourier transformation magnetic resonance images. *Radiology* 152:117–121, 1984.

70. NMR uncovers body's secrets. *Hinsdale Hosp Pacesetter*, 2:8, 1984.

71. Siemans Spinal Radiography Equipment; Erlangen, Germany. Aktiengesellschaft, S 40/662 d.e.

# CHAPTER 10

# Spinographic Measurement Procedures

## PRINCIPLES AND PROCEDURES OF SPINOGRAPHIC MEASUREMENT

As stated in Chapter 1 relative to the "Fundamentals of Spinographic Interpretation," following a survey of the films for indications of pathology, trauma and abnormal development which may constitute disease conditions in themselves and/or may qualify biomechanical factors, a visual examination is made for evidence of biomechanical irregularities which may constitute orthodysarthric subluxations. Following this, various measurement procedures may or may not be employed in a particular case depending upon the following general considerations:

1. To arrive at a judgement of the presence and character of a structural problem in borderline cases where visual impressions may be inconclusive
2. To assist in arriving at a decision of need for, and type of, treatment procedures which may be indicated
3. To make comparative evaluations on subsequent studies for an estimate of corrective progress following a course of treatments, and/or
4. To collect data on normal and abnormal biomechanical values for clinical research purposes

From a more specific clinical aspect spinal, pelvic and/or other measurements may be made for either a *general diagnostic* or *chiropractic analytical* purpose, briefly differentiated as follows:

## General Diagnostic Measurements

General diagnostic measurements are those made to arrive at a judgement of the presence of a suspected structure-altering condition and/or to determine the magnitude of a structural alteration known to exist on the basis of the preceding visual evaluation. These conditions usually involve a single measurement and may be biomechanical, developmental or pathological in nature. For illustrative purposes, the following examples are given:

1. Measurement of the axial angle of the femoral neck and shaft to ascertain bilateral inequality which may be responsible for a structural leg deficiency
2. Measurement of the acetabular angle of the growing hip to detect possible anomalous development
3. Measurement of spondylolisthesis
4. Measurement of spinal curvatures—scolioses, kyphoses and/or lordoses
5. Measurement of the spinal canal to ascertain possible stenosis
6. Measurement of the atlantodental interval (ADI) to determine possible pathologic or traumatic anterior subluxation of the atlas relative to axis
7. Measurements of the base of the skull to determine possible abnormal basilar invagination condition
8. Measurement of the heart to determine possible irregularities, such as ventricular hypertrophy
9. Measurement of the size of a mass or growth in the body to monitor future growth

## Chiropractic Analytical Measurements

Chiropractic analytical measurements are generally confined to the evaluation of biomechanical patterns of the pelvis and spinal column to ascertain the possible existence of subluxations, their magnitude and manipulative correction requirements. Such measurements may be singular in an effort to more precisely define biomechanical irregularities determined to be present on the basis of visual observations, or they may be multiple and organized into a "systematic" approach whereby most (if not all) articular relationships are measured to gather information leading to a decision regarding the existence and character of pelvic or spinal subluxations.

As previously mentioned in other parts of this text, some such spinographic measurement *systems* have been used in manners which arbitrarily assume certain subluxation factors which cannot be ascertained on the basis of spinographic measurements alone. Also, erroneous judgements regarding subluxation which cannot be made at all on the basis of current scientific or clinical knowledge of the subject are often proposed. With these ideas in mind, it is emphasized that this present effort is not so directed, but rather uses the word *analysis* in terms of its general clinical meaning; i.e. to collect informational data (as by clinical laboratory analysis) to assist in making diagnostic judgements of the possible existence of biomechanical irregularities and, if present, their particular configurations which may be helpful in determining corrective effort (if any) which may be indicated.

### Measurement Procedures and Equipment

With the foregoing objectives in mind (both general diagnostic and chiropractic analytical), the measurement procedures described may include methods used within the health care professions at large, procedures incorporated into various chiropractic spinography analysis systems, or concepts which may be peculiar to this presentation.

Insofar as measurements will be made, it naturally follows that certain measuring equipment will be required; such as, a millimetric ruler for linear measurements, a protractor for angular measurements, special film making pencils (Dixon Black No. 2225 is recommended), etc. Additionally, the following two specialized spinographic measuring instruments are recommended:

### SPINOGRAPHIC PARALLEL RULER

The Gonstead Spinographic Parallel ruler is a device comprised of a heavy duty, 10 or 12-in long plastic rule (marked off in both inches and millimeters, and sometimes including a protractor) with metal rollers on each end of a finger grip mounted on the trailing edge of the ruler (Fig. 10.1). In film marking and measuring procedure a parallel ruler is a helpful device in that its finger grip allows for easy maneuvering control on the flat film surface and its rollers allow for quick drawing of parallel lines at some distance to each other.

### SPINOGRAPHIC PROTRACTORULE

The Hilmark Spinographic Protractorule is an instrument which allows for rapid and accurate measurement of angles on postural spinographic films, placed on an upright viewing illuminator, without drawing any of the customary lines on the film that are generally required. Virtually all angles generally measured on the posteroanterior (PA) [or anteroposterior (AP)] and lateral views may be quickly and easily measured with the Protractorule, including some angles that may be difficult to measure because their reference lines extend off the border of the film (Fig. 10.2).

### Spinographic Measurement Qualifications

Spinographic measurement procedures may be qualified in terms of biomechanical significance as they do or do not actually represent the patient's postural pattern at the time the films were taken and in terms of the technical accuracy of the actual measurements themselves.

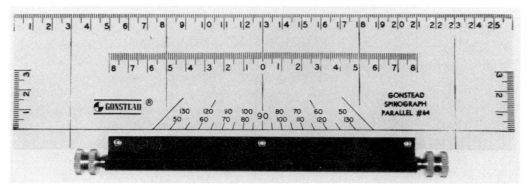

**Figure 10.1.** Gonstead Spinographic Parallel (Courtesy of the Gonstead Chiropractic Clinic, Mt. Horeb, WI.)

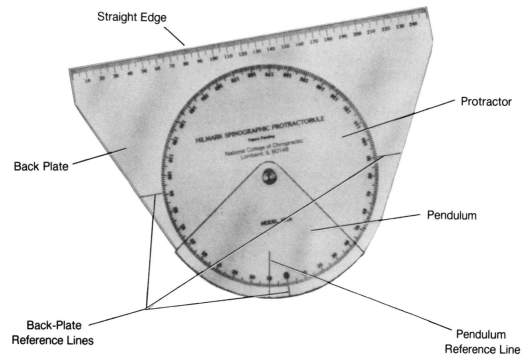

**Figure 10.2.** Hilmark Spinographic Protractorule (Courtesy of the National College of Chiropractic, Lombard, Ill.

## BIOMECHANICAL SIGNIFICANCE

Biomechanical significance of the postural full spine films in terms of how they actually represent the patient's postural pattern at the time the films were taken is primarily *controlled by* the positioning of the patients, themselves, (in that attitude they naturally assume at the time of the procedure) and secondarily *influenced by* the following:

1. Alignment of the x-ray tube and Bucky grid unit
2. Levelness of the floor on which the patient is standing
3. Alignment of the film in the cassette and the cassette in the Bucky-grid unit—although the patient may be in his/her nat-

urally assumed posture, on a level floor, in front of a gravitationally aligned Bucky-grid unit and x-ray tube, if the film and cassette are not equally well aligned, one starts out with a measurement accuracy qualification built into the film image itself.

## MEASUREMENT ACCURACY

Accuracy of the actual measurements as representing measurements within the body of the patient, are also secondarily *influenced by* the following:

1. Alignment of the upright illuminator to a gravitational plumb, as well as the film in the illuminator, to a degree comparable to that of the spinographic x-ray equipment
2. Care exercised in drawing the lines on the film and making the measurements

It is, of course, recognized that accuracy of all these controlling and influencing factors is more or less impossible to achieve to an absolute degree. However, insofar as a variance of 1 mm or 1° in each consideration could result in an error factor between the film measurements and the patient of several (4, 5 or more) units, all possible effort should be given to each consideration individually in order to reduce the error factor as much as possible.

## POSTEROANTERIOR FULL SPINE VIEW MEASUREMENTS

Posteroanterior full spine view measurements, as was the case with visual examinations, are primarily concerned with bilateral structural evaluation of the pelvis and spinal column on the transverse and sagittal body planes. Because in the standing postural state each pelvic or spinal component above is dependent upon its biomechanical support from the component immediately below, initial evaluation concerns a determination of bilateral leg length equality or inequality.

While considerable general information has been published on the etiology, (1) effects, (2–29) and detection or measurement (30–41) of leg length inequalities, few controlled studies have been conducted which

attempt to statistically establish quantitative values and correlate them with observed effects. One notable exception is a study conducted by Rush and Steiner (42, 43) in which they radiographically evaluated comparative leg lengths of 1000 cases presenting with low back pain (LBP) and 100 asymptomatic controls using a specially designed positioning device. They summarized their findings as follows:

"Observations have been presented on a series of 1000 lumbosacral spines examined in the X-Ray Department of the Regional Station Hospital of Fort Leonard Wood, Missouri. The technique of examination is described and is unique in that it utilizes a new stabilization device which necessitates that all lumbosacral spines be examined in the standing position. By this method it is possible to accurately measure differences in lower extremity lengths as manifested by differences in the heights of the femoral heads.

"The 1000 cases were reviewed, both for the purpose of measuring differences in lower extremity lengths, and also from the standpoint of roentgenological pathology. Of the 1000 cases 230, or 23%, were found to have legs of equal length while the remaining 770, or 77%, had lower extremities of unequal length. The average shortening of the right lower extremity was 7.47 mm, while the shortening of the left lower extremity was 6.50 mm (42) (Table 10.1).

"The cases were reviewed for roentgenological pathology and it was found that of the 1000 cases, 293, or 29.30%, had evidence of roentgenological pathology. Of this number, 63, or 27.39%, were of the 230 cases of equal leg lengths, while 230, or 29.87 percent, were of the remaining 770 cases of unequal leg lengths (42) (Table 10.2).

"A consistent observation which has been made is that in those cases with a shortened leg there is a corresponding tilt of the pelvis and a compensatory scoliosis of the lumbar spine. While the existence of roentgenological pathology does not seem to be correlated in any way with difference of leg lengths, it was found that in most cases with a difference in leg lengths in excess of 5 mm, and there were 375 such cases, only 93, or 24.80%, had any roentgenological pathology while the remaining 282, or 75.20%, had no roentgenological pathology other than the shortened leg with the corresponding tilt of the pelvis and the compensatory scoliosis of the lumbar spine. Since all of these had low back complaint it is possible that the remaining 75.20% had

Table 10.1.
Measurements of lower extremity lengths (1000 cases)[a]

| Lower extremity lengths | Millimeter difference | Total millimeter differences | Number of cases | Average millimeter difference |
|---|---|---|---|---|
| Equal Total | None | None | 230 | None |
| Right shorter than left | 0–5 | 665 | 199 | 3.34 |
| | 6–10 | 963 | 119 | 8.09 |
| | 11–20 | 1128 | 78 | 14.46 |
| | 21 over | 278 | 10 | 27.80 |
| Subtotal | | 3034 | 406 | 7.47 |
| Left shorter than right | 0–5 | 604 | 196 | 3.08 |
| | 6–10 | 836 | 106 | 7.88 |
| | 11–20 | 739 | 55 | 13.43 |
| | 21 over | 188 | 7 | 26.86 |
| Subtotal | | 2367 | 364 | 6.50 |
| Total cases | | | 1000 | |

[a] From Rush and Steiner (42).

complaint in association with the changes seen due to a shortened extremity (42) (Table 10.3).

"A similar analysis was done on 100 general duty soldiers who were selected as individuals who had no physical complaints. The analysis showed that a slightly greater percentage had legs of equal length and the average amount of difference of lower extremity lengths was definitely less than in the series of 1000 cases with low back complaint (Table 10.4). Furthermore, the amount showing any evidence of roentgenological pathology was small, being 8, or 8%, as compared with 293, or 29.30%, for the series of 1000 cases. Finally, among the 100 general duty soldiers with lower extremity differences in excess of 5 mm, only 1 showed any evidence of roentgenological pathology." (42).

It might be noted in this study that Rush and Steiner "suggest" 5 mm as the point at which a femoral head deficiency becomes clinically significant, while in the *Postural Complex* Jones (35) states that differences in leg length of ¼ in (6.35 mm) or less are considered within normal limits. In the chiropractic profession Winterstein (44) has considered 2 mm or greater as clinically significant with 5 mm being of serious concern; Herbst (45) states that "most people can adapt to a femur head deficiency of up to 6 mm." Therefore, a lower level clinical-

significance figure of 5 mm seems reasonable.

Although Rush and Steiner (42) conclude that because only 24.80% of the symptomatic group with leg deficiencies in excess of 5 mm had roentgenological evidence of pathology such pathology was not statistically correlated with the leg deficiency, the opposite conclusion can also be conjectured. In consideration of the fact that all subjects were obviously young and generally healthy soldiers, and that if even one out of the asymptomatic group with a leg deficiency in excess of 5 mm had developed spinal pathology, the possibility exists that spinal pathology is a late developmental effect of leg deficiency and that those not showing pathology at the time of the study may well show it at a later time.

### Estimation of Leg Length Equality

The most accurate method of determining leg length equality, and the procedure on which the preceding statistical data was based, is by taking an x-ray film with the central ray 90° to the film surface over the top of the femur heads. In the case of the anteroposterior full spine projection, as was discussed in the preceding chapter, the fe-

**Table 10.2.**
**Pathological conditions seen on roentgenograms[a]**

| Pathology on roentgenogram | | Equal lower extremity | Unequal lower extremities | | | Total |
|---|---|---|---|---|---|---|
| | | | Right shorter | Left shorter | Total | |
| Sacroiliac joint arthritis | | | | | | |
|   Right joint | | 1 | 4 | 3 | 7 | 8 |
|   Left joint | | 7 | 6 | 6 | 12 | 19 |
|   Bilateral | | 6 | 15 | 7 | 22 | 28 |
| Existence of an anomalous joint between the transverse process of L5 and sacrum | | | | | | |
|   No arthritis | Right side | 5 | 3 | 3 | 6 | 11 |
| | Left side | 3 | 8 | 7 | 15 | 18 |
| | Bilateral | 1 | 1 | 1 | 2 | 3 |
|   With arthritis | Right side | 0 | 2 | 2 | 4 | 4 |
| | Left side | 4 | 4 | 2 | 6 | 10 |
| | Bilateral | 0 | 1 | 0 | 1 | 1 |
| Fusion between transverse process of L5 and sacrum | | | | | | |
|   Right side | | 0 | 0 | 2 | 2 | 2 |
|   Left side | | 1 | 1 | 1 | 2 | 3 |
| Spondylolisthetic lesions | | | | | | |
|   Prespondylolisthesis | | 1 | 3 | 6 | 9 | 10 |
|   Spondylolisthesis | | 7 | 8 | 12 | 20 | 27 |
|   Reverse spondylolisthesis | | 2 | 3 | 1 | 4 | 6 |
| Flat back (loss of normal lordosis) | | 7 | 13 | 5 | 18 | 25 |
| Increased lumbosacral angle (above 50°) (elevated sacrum) | | 3 | 21 | 19 | 40 | 43 |
| Asymmetry of articular facets of L5 | | 4 | 4 | 7 | 11 | 15 |
| Structural scoliosis | | 6 | 4 | 4 | 8 | 14 |
| Narrowed intervertebral disk space | | 1 | 7 | 2 | 9 | 10 |
| Old compression fracture | | 2 | 1 | 4 | 5 | 7 |
| Biconcave disks | | 0 | 9 | 6 | 15 | 15 |
| Spina bifida (marked) | | 1 | 3 | 1 | 4 | 5 |
| Osteoarthritis of the lumbar vertebrae | | 0 | 2 | 1 | 3 | 3 |
| Schmorl's nodes | | 1 | 1 | 1 | 2 | 3 |
| Hemangioma of the lumbar vertebrae | | 0 | 0 | 2 | 2 | 2 |
| Anomalous joint between left transverse processes of L2 and L3 | | 0 | 1 | 0 | 1 | 1 |
|   Total | | 63 | 125 | 105 | 230 | 293 |
|   Complete number of cases | | 230 | 406 | 364 | 770 | 1000 |
|   Percentage with pathology | | 27.39 | 30.78 | 28.84 | 29.87 | 29.30 |

[a] From Rush and Steiner (42).

Table 10.3.
Correlation of pathology and lower extremity shortening in excess of 5 mm[a]

| Cases with lower extremity shortening in excess of 5 mm | Number | Percentage |
|---|---|---|
| With roentgenological pathology | 93 | 24.80 |
| Without roentgenological pathology | 282 | 75.20 |
| Total | 375 | 100.00 |

[a] From Rush and Steiner (42).

Table 10.4.
Measurements of lower extremity lengths (100 cases)[a]

| Lower extremity lengths | Millimeter difference | Total millimeter difference | Number of cases | Average millimeter difference |
|---|---|---|---|---|
| Equal | None | None | 29 | None |
| Right shorter than left | 0–5 | 74 | 19 | 3.89 |
| | 6–10 | 151 | 19 | 7.95 |
| | 14–20 | 35 | 3 | 11.66 |
| | 21 over | 0 | 0 | 0 |
| Subtotal | | 260 | 41 | 6.34 |
| Left shorter than right | 0–5 | 56 | 19 | 2.95 |
| | 6–10 | 74 | 10 | 7.40 |
| | 11–20 | 11 | 1 | 11.00 |
| | 21 over | 0 | 0 | 0 |
| Subtotal | | 141 | 30 | 4.70 |
| Total cases | | | 100 | |

[a] From Rush and Steiner (42).

mur heads are projected to the film via downward projecting divergent rays. Consequently, if the pelvis is rotated anterior on the femur heads on either side [left anterior pelvis/right anterior pelvis (LAP/RAP)], the femur head farthest from the film will project lower, thus simulating unequal length of the lower extremities (Fig. 10.3).

Because this simulated leg length deficiency results from bimechanical actions of the pelvis (either rotation of the pelvis as a unit or as a secondary result of bilateral innominate bone disrelationships) it is sometimes erronously referred to as a "physiological leg deficiency" as a means of distinguishing it from an actual (anatomic) leg deficiency (45). Insofar as there is no such thing as a physiological leg deficiency

(it is either actually—anatomically—short or it is not), it is best to refer to such an illusionary shortness as a "projectional" leg deficiency.

In order to arrive at an *estimate* to actual leg length inequality, various methods of line drawing analyses have been developed which attempt to mathematically deduct the projectional factor on the basis of equations derived from millimetric measurement of pelvic structures (44–46). Insofar as some of these analysis procedures are conceptually based on biomechanical and radiological projection principles which are difficult to reconcile with present-day knowledge, (47) the accuracy of their estimates of leg length deficiency are left in doubt. Although a recent study tended to support the accuracy of one of these pro-

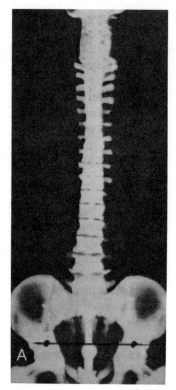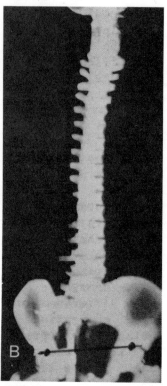

**Figure 10.3.** Projectional distortion of a model spine and pelvis taken under standard 72-in focal-film distance considerations. Note downward projection of left femur head in illustration *B* as the model was rotated anterior on the left away from the film as compared to illustration *A* which was positioned parallel to the film.

cedures on the basis of a statistical evaluation of 50 cases in which the films were taken at a nonstandard 84-in (21.3-m) focal-film distance (48), questions remain on the accuracy of that procedure in an individual case and/or at a standard 72-in (18.3-m) focal-film distance.

Therefore, this author has attempted to devise a method of pelvic measurement procedure (to determine interpelvic biomechanical deviations as well as an estimate of projected femur head deficiency) based upon the pelvic biomechanical principles previously discussed (Chapter 6: "Postural Complex of the Human Body") and a study conducted to specifically determine rates of femur head projection on a construct model which was rotated around the *pelvic center of gravity* (PCOG) at measured amounts (49). The use of the PCOG as a common point of reference for measured spino-

graphic analysis of the pelvis was considered appropriate for the following reasons:

1. It is the point of fulcrum around which all biomechanical actions of the pelvis tend to take place
2. It is a constant point of biomechanical reference within a particular patient at different times
3. It is a uniform point of biomechanical reference common to different patients
4. It is a point of minimum radiographic distortion insofar as it is generally in vertical alignment with the central ray and film
5. It allows for angular measurement of pelvic interarticular relationships in terms of degrees, as opposed to the use of more distortion-influenced millimetric measurements by which most other currently used methods attempt to ascertain interarticular disrelationships by the measurement of gross bony structures.

In order to establish the parameters of projected femur head deficiencies as they

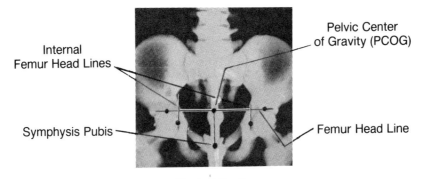

Internal
Femur Head Lines

Pelvic Center
of Gravity (PCOG)

Symphysis Pubis

Femur Head Line

Neutral Position

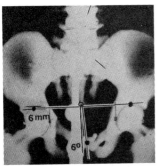

6° Left Anterior

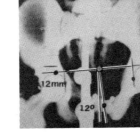

12° Left Anterior

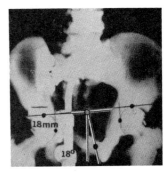

18° Left Anterior

**Figure 10.4.** Examples of the pelvis of the previous test model in which the entire spine (including pelvis) was rotated from the neutral position to 6, 12 and 18° around the pelvic center of gravity (PCOG). Note that at a standard 72-in focal-film distance, in the case of an average size adult spinal-pelvic model, the *ratio* of pelvic rotation to femur head projectional deficiency was 1:1. This is not the case where different focal-film distances may be used.

relate to rotation of the pelvis as a unit around the PCOG, a series of 72-in (18.3-m) full spine exposures were made in which the pelvis was rotated to 6, 12 and 18° as measured at the PCOG-symphysis angle (Fig. 10.4). By this method, it was determined that approximately a 1:1 ratio exists between the PCOG-symphysis angle and projected femur head deficiency; i.e. 1° of PCOG-symphysis rotation is approximately equivalent to 1° of bilateral femur head incline and 1 mm of projected femur head deficiency. Procedure and interpretation of projected femur head deficiency estimation is as follows (Fig. 10.5):

## PROCEDURE

1. Draw a horizontal line across the top of the femur heads and bisect to locate the PCOG.

2. Measure upward from the bottom edge of the film to the top of each femur head and, if a difference is shown, indicate that exact difference with a short line over the top of the lower femur head and show the measurement in millimeters.

3. Draw a vertical line from the PCOG to the center of the symphysis pubis and another line downward from the PCOG to a point below the pubic bodies. If the two lines are not superimposed, indicate amount of lateral pubic symphysis shift, as represented by the pelvic rotation angle (PRA), in degrees.

## INTERPRETATION

1. If no PRA exists (PCOG-pubic lines superimposed), the amount of femur head deficiency indicated (if any) most likely

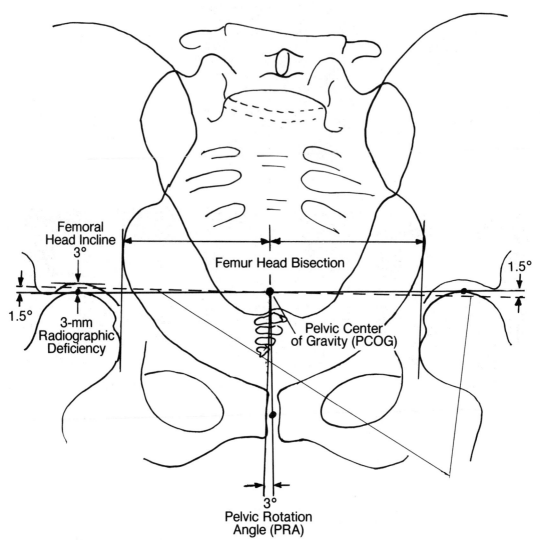

**Figure 10.5.**  Pelvic center of gravity (PCOG) method of estimating projected femur head deficiency resulting from pelvic rotation in placement. Since projectional leg deficiency is being determined on the basis of movement of the pelvis around the PCOG, half of the total deficiency is indicated from left to right of the PCOG. The total difference between the two femur heads, however, is the composite of the left anterior and right posterior rotation, or equivalent to the amount opposite the direction of pubic symphysis shift from the PCOG (– – –, dashed femur head lines indicate one-half of femur head projected deficiency around PCOG; ——, the opposite equal amount represents the total femur head deficiency, or femoral head angle).

represents actual (anatomical) leg length deficiency of approximately the amount indicated, unless qualified by pelvic pathology, trauma or abnormal development.

2. If a PRA is evident it indicates that the pelvis is in a state of RAP or LAP rotation—anterior on the side *opposite* the direction of symphysis pubis shift to the

degree indicated by the PRA measurement. To correct for projected deficiency, convert the PRA degrees to millimeters and add to the top of the femur head on the side opposite to the direction of symphysis pubis shift (the lower side if a deficiency was evident) on a 1:1 ratio basis. One of the following may be anticipated:

a. The amount of PRA will equal the millimeters of projected femur head deficiency, thus no actual femur head deficiency is indicated;

b. The amount of PRA will be less than the millimeters of projected femur head deficiency, thus the remaining deficiency is probably actual and indicates a possible anatomical shortening of that lower extremity; or

c. The amount of PRA is greater than the millimeters of projected femur head deficiency, thus an anatomical shortening of the *opposite* lower extremity may be suspected.

It should be emphasized that, in consideration of the qualifications to measurement accuracy previously discussed, the experimental nature of full spine radiographic leg length estimation and the statistical basis for application to a particular patient, this (and other similar) measurement procedure should not be taken as an absolute but only as information to assist in making a diagnostic judgement. If the estimated actual deficiency exceeds 5 mm by a significant amount, and there is a possible need for orthotic correction (heel lift, etc), further studies should be considered to determine the reason for the deficiency and its exact amount.

## Diagnosis and Measurement of Leg Length Inequality

If an actual, anatomical deficiency of a lower extremity in excess of 5 mm is indicated on the basis of full spine procedure, diagnosis and measurement of leg length inequality includes various *femur-pelvic measurements* to determine possible structural irregularities which may be implicated and certain *special radiographic procedures* to obtain exact measurement of lower extremity inequality.

## FEMUR-PELVIC MEASUREMENTS

The following femur-pelvic angle measurements and lines serve to evaluate possible developmental variations or alignments affecting the femur head and/or acetabulum which may be respnsible for lower

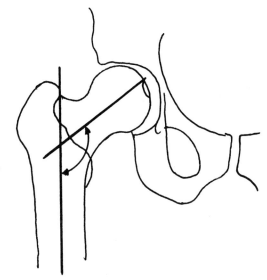

**Figure 10.6.** Method of determining normal or abnormal femoral angle in the event that an actual leg deficiency is suspect (e.g. Mikulicz's angle of declination).

extremity inequality. Other similar types of evaluations may be made on the growing hip, but are considered part of special pediatric radiology procedures and will not be included here [see *Atlas of Roentgenographic Measurement* by Lusted and Keats (50)].

Femoral Angle (Fig. 10.6)

On the posteroanterior view, bisecting lines are drawn through the long axis of the femoral shaft and neck. The angle formed by these intersecting lines are evaluated relative to the following values:

Normals*: Male 128°; Female 127°
Coxa valga: 50° or more increase
Coxa vara: 5° or less decrease

Skinner's Line (Fig. 10.7)

On the posteroanterior view, a line is drawn through the long axis of the femoral shaft and a second line is drawn across the top of the greater trochanter perpendicular to the femoral shaft line. Skinner's line

---

* Normals are based on 50 adults age 19–76 yr of age.

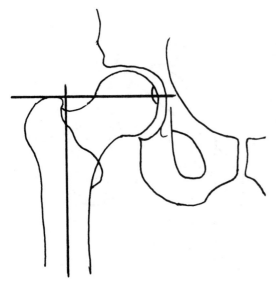

**Figure 10.7.** Skinner's line.

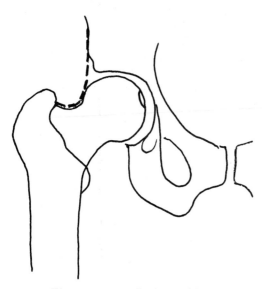

**Figure 10.8.** Iliofemoral line.

should pass through the femur head at or below the fovea centralis capitus.

Iliofemoral Line (Fig. 10.8)

On the posteroanterior view, a line drawn (or visualized) along the lateral margin of the head of the femur should pass without interruption up the lateral-inferior border of the ilium. An alteration of this line indicates possible abnormal structural alignment due to pathology, trauma or abnormal development.

Shenton's Line (Fig. 10.9)

On the posteroanterior view, a line is drawn (or visualized) along the inferior margin of the femoral neck into the superior-to-medial margin of the obturator foramen. This line is applicable to infants, juveniles and adults and is considered positive for abnormal structural alignment if line deviates.

Femoral Epiphysis Line (Fig. 10.10)

On the posteroanterior view, one line (AB) is drawn parallel to the femoral neck

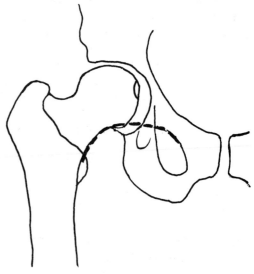

**Figure 10.9.** Shenton's line.

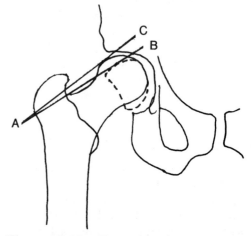

**Figure 10.10.** Femoral epiphysis line (see explanation in text).

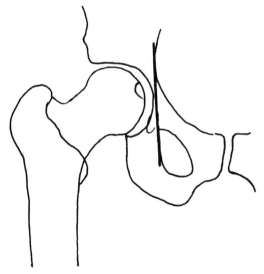

**Figure 10.11.** Kohler's protruso acetabuli line.

central ray is precisely across the top of the femur heads.

In some extreme cases where surgical correction may be considered (either to shorten the longer extremity, or staple an epiphysis to retard growth of the longer extremity in the young), a series of exposures may be taken on a 36-in film with the central ray 90° through each lower extremity articulation. This allows for a determination of which bone(s) of the lower extremity may be at fault (femur, tibia-fibula or foot), as well as provide for an exact measurement of each.

## Analysis of the Posterior Sacroinnominate Triangle

Traditionally, line drawing measurement procedures of the posterior view of the pelvis to determine innominate-sacral disrelationships incorporate linear measurements between various lines drawn on gross bony components. Some of these measurements are seemingly of questionable rationale in terms of biomechanical implications and/or of questionable accuracy in terms of radiographic distortion and structural asymmetry. With these considerations in mind, the following "posterior sacroinnominate triangle" method of analysis has been devised to collect interpretive data in accordance with the previously described interpelvic biomechanics. This procedure (Fig. 10.12) is considered more appropriate because:

1. It has its point of origin at the PCOG, the point of least radiographic distortion and point of confluence of pelvic biomechanical actions
2. It incorporates angular measurements of divergent lines which originate in close proximity to the articulations under consideration, rather than linear measurements of gross pelvic structures, both of which are more adversely influenced by radiographic distortion and developmental asymmetry
3. It only considers the primary misalignment possibilities of posteromedial/anterolateral innominate and interrelated sacral misalignments, uncomplicated by other secondary misalignments of questionable value

to intersect with the superolateral aspect of the femoral head and a second line (*AC*) is drawn tangential to the arc of the femur head. When epiphyseal slippage occurs (*dotted line*) the head descends and the neck rides upward—line *AC* disappears to overlie line *AB*, which is then a tangential line on the femoral head rather than an intersecting line.

Kohler's Protruso Acetabuli Line
(Fig. 10.11)

On the posteroanterior view, a line is drawn from the pelvic border of the ilium to the medial border of the body of the ischium. If the outline of the acetabular dome passes medial to the line, acetabular protrusion exists.

## SPECIAL RADIOGRAPHIC PROCEDURES

When the posteroanterior full spine view indicates that an actual (anatomical) leg length inequality exists for which an orthopedic correction (heel lift, etc.) is being considered, a femur head level view is mandatory insofar as the posteroanterior view provides only an *estimate* of the amount of deficiency. In taking the femoral head view, care should be exercised to ensure that the

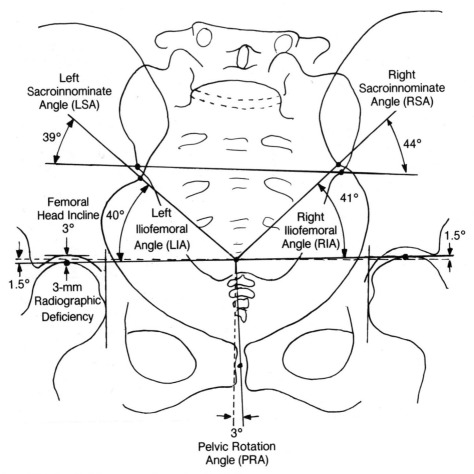

**Figure 10.12.** Pelvic center of gravity (PCOG)—triangulation method of evaluating innominate/sacral relationships (see text for procedures of measurement and advantages over other linear methods of similar procedures).

## PROCEDURE

1. Lines are drawn from the PCOG to the left and right posteroinferior iliac spines and the angles thus formed with the femur head line (left and right iliofemoral angles) are measured in degrees of divergence.

2. A line is drawn across like points on each side of the sacrum (as close as possible to the sacroiliac articulations) and the angles thus formed with the PCOG-innominate lines (left and right sacroinnominate angles) are measured in degrees of divergence.

## INTERPRETATION

1. Decreased iliofemoral angle indicates a posteromedial innominate and increased iliofemoral angle indicates an anterolateral innominate—choice of one or the other as a theoretical major for corrective purposes will be made later on the basis of lateral pelvis analysis.

2. Increased sacroinnominate angle indicates an anteroinferior sacrum relative to the ilia and decreased sacroinnominate angle indicates a posterosuperior sacrum relative to the iliac—choice of an anteroinferior or posterosuperior rotated sacrum as a

theoretical major for corrective purposes will be discussed.

## ALTERNATE PA PELVIC SPINOGRAPHIC ANALYSIS PROCEDURES

Several other PA pelvic spinographic analysis procedures have been devised to evaluate biomechanical discrepancies of the pelvis relative to the innominate bones bilaterally; the innominate bones relative to the sacrum; and/or the innominate bones and the sacrum as concerns the spine above. For the most part these alternative spinographic analysis procedures incorporate similar concepts of making linear measurements (with some modifications) of gross pelvic structures which have several deficiencies not inherent in the triangular method previously described.

### Analysis of the AP Spinal Column

Once the sacrum has been determined subluxated, or in normal position in relation to an innominate disrelation, or the sacrum is in an independent subluxation irrespective of innominate disrelation, the next step is to ascertain the position of the spinal column as a whole on a sagittal and transverse basis. These considerations primarily involve three determinations of spinal integrity: lateral or *tilted individual vertebra* relative to its supporting structure below, lateral or *tilted vertebrae* as a *unit* (scoliosis) and/or *rotated vertebrae*—usually, but not necessarily, being concomitant actions.

## LATERAL FLEXION OR LATERALLY TILTED VERTEBRAE

Initially, since the biomechanical analysis of the spinal column starts at the lowermost segment of the spinal superstructure, the evaluation begins with a determination of the state of lateral flexion and rotation of the fifth lumbar to the sacral base. Because the articulation between the sacral base and the inferior aspect of the

fifth lumbar body are not clearly visible on the anteroposterior full spine view (unless a "bow sign" of spondylolisthesis is present), it is usually necessary that a parallel line be constructed from like points at the base of the sacrum and carried upward to like points on the fifth lumbar vertebra—usually the pedicle shadows serve as appropriate landmarks for this purpose (Fig. 10.13). This procedure may be affected by a *Spinographic Parallel* device (Fig. 10.1) or more easily by the use of a *Hilmark Spinographic Protractorule* (Fig. 10.2) which eliminates the need to draw any line on the film.

After the parallel relation to the fifth lumbar with the sacrum is ascertained all space articulations are so evaluated relative to each supporting vertebra below, or only those articulations which were suspected as being subluxation on visual evaluation. For visual assesment of interarticular relationship of the spine as a whole it is sometimes helpful to mark each articular level throughout the spine in order to make a composite assessment of *primary* or *secondary* (compensatory) subluxation as is typical with the *Gonstead* "disk level" concept; e.g. "a vertebral disk wedging above a level disk is a *subluxation*, and a disk wedging below a level disk is a *compensation* (Figs. 10.14 and 10.15).

Radiographic Assessment of Scoliosis

Scoliosis, as previously discussed in this presentation is a lateral bending of the spine, usually with concomitant rotation of a severe nature. Because of its severe and often life threatening nature, it behooves the reader to review certain classic works on the subject, particularly that of the Keim (51) which will be paraphrased here in regards to radiographic assessment of what is called adolescent idiopathic scoliosis, as opposed to what is called functional scoliosis.

... "Once these initial films (full spine, lower lumbar spots, left and right lateral bending, and left hand and wrist to evaluate

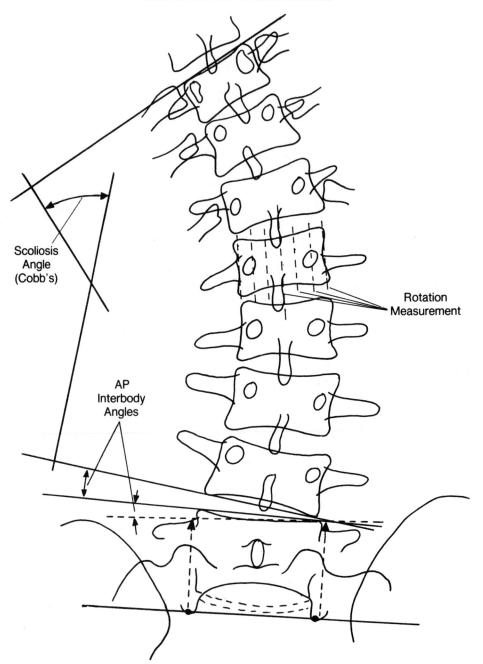

**Figure 10.13.** Basic methods for evaluating vertebral biomechanical relationships starting with the sacrum and working upward. Procedures have been held to a minimum in consideration of the many other procedures which are adequately covered in other texts.

bone growth) are taken for both diagnostic and therapeutic purposes, one can progress to actual diagnosis and measurement, which may include one of two methods—the *Risser-Ferguson* and *Cobb* methods (Figure 10.14).

"Both methods of measurement are based on determining the upper and lower 'end vertebrae.' The end vertebrae, both at the upper and lower limits of a curve, are those which have maximum tilting toward the concavity of the curve. In other words, the superior end vertebra is the last one in which the *superior* border points toward the concavity of the curve to be measured. The inferior end ver-

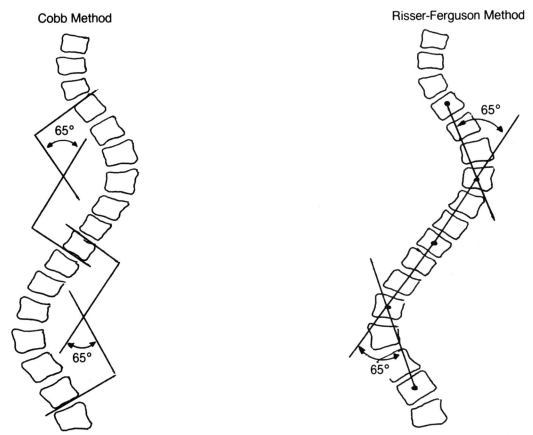

**Cobb Method**

**Risser-Ferguson Method**

**Figure 10.14.**    Comparison of Cobb and Risser-Ferguson methods of scoliosis measurement (see text for explanations).

tebra is the last one whose inferior border will point toward the concavity of the curve being measured.

"The Risser-Ferguson method of measurement is based mainly on the technique of placing a small dot in the center of the upper and lower end vertebrae. In addition, a small dot is also placed in the center of the apical vertebra. This is usually the vertebra with most wedging and deformity and is at the apex of the curve. Straight lines are drawn from the dot in each end vertebra through the dot in the apical vertebra. The intersection angle is then measured with a protractor.

"The Cobb method is more readily reproducible by multiple examiners and can be easily mastered by following these rules. A horizontal line is drawn at a superior border of the superior end vertebra. Another horizontal line is drawn at the inferior border of the inferior end vertebra. Perpendicular lines are then erected from each of the horizontal lines and the intersecting lines and the intersection angles are measured. This Cobb method gives larger angles than the Riss-Ferguson method,

and corrections can be more easily compared during treatment and following. It is this method of measurement that is advocated by the United States Scoliosis Research Society.

"Curve measurements by degrees have been standardized by the Scoliosis Research Society. The classification breaks down into seven groups.

| | |
|---|---|
| Group 1 | 0–20° |
| Group 2 | 21–30° |
| Group 3 | 31–50° |
| Group 4 | 51–75° |
| Group 5 | 76–100° |
| Group 6 | 101–125° |
| Group 7 | 126–125°"† |

## VERTEBRAL ROTATION

Since rotation is inherently a part of scoliosis, two methods have been devised to

---

† © Copyright 1978 CIBA-GEIGY Corporation. Reprinted with permission from CLINICAL SYMPOSIA by Hugo A. Keim, M.D., illustrated by Frank H. Netter, M.D.

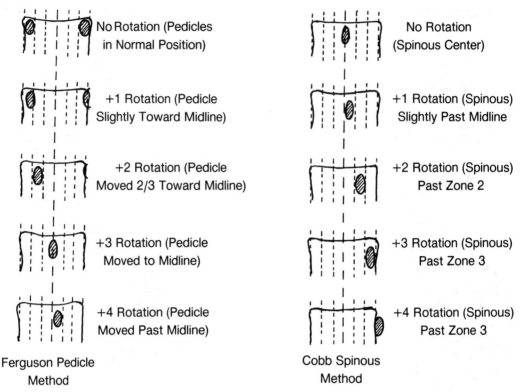

**Figure 10.15.** Comparison of Risser-Ferguson pedicle and Cobb spinous methods of vertebral rotaton measurement; bodies are divided into six equal zones (*left* or *right*); (see text for further information). [Modified from Nash et al. (52).]

standardize it. The first method, which is the most accurate, is based on the amount that the pedicles of the vertebra rotate (Fig. 10.16) as seen in the anteroposterior x-ray. If the vertebra with its pedicles rotates so that the one pedicle is in the center of the body of the vertebra, this is a 3+ rotation.

The other method is based on the spinous process. If the vertebra in question is rotated so that the spinous process is displaced one "width" from the midline of the vertebra, we call this a 1+ rotation. This method is not so accurate as measurement of the pedicles, because the spinous processes are so often deformed in severe scoliosis. By using these technics, various degrees of rotation can be standarized so that 3+ pedicle rotation means the same to different examiners.

## MATURATION

"Idiopathic scoliosis progresses rapidly during the growing years and may reach serious deformity before it is detected. Determining maturation in boys and girls is extremely important for proper treatment. Girls generally cease their growth and mature at about age 16½. Boys lag behind by 15–18 months. Knowing when maturation occurs is important because scoliosis generally ceases to progress significantly after the patient reaches maturity. Judging maturation is not easy and must be done with cumulative facts. First of all, a look at parents and siblings can sometimes be a guide as to how tall a child will probably be. Then the patient's secondary sex characteristics can also help, along with the date of menarche in female patients.

"Review of the x-rays will finally help to assess, with a reasonable degree of accuracy, how mature the patient is. The left hand and wrist can again be compared with what is called the *Gruelich and Pyle Atlas.* Also the excursion of the

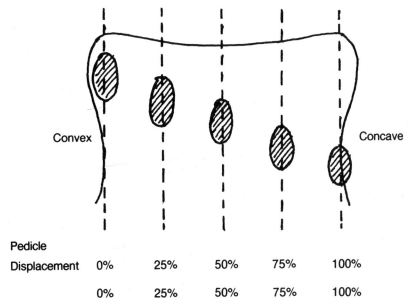

**Figure 10.16.** Nash et al.'s simplified system of describing vertebral rotation according to percentages and degrees. [Modified from Nash et al. (52).]

iliac crest, described by Risser, can be of help. The apophysis of the crests start forming their osseous centers laterally, and the development proceeds toward the sacrum. The decrease of the crest can be noted as 'incomplete.' When the apophysis joins to the sacroiliac junction and firmly seals to the ilium, maturation is nearly complete. Also, observation of the apophyseal rings of the vertebrae may be an indication of maturity" (52).

## SCOLIOSIS SCREENING

Initially, screening of adolescents for possible clinically significant scoliosis should begin with a visual observation of sitting and standing posture; noting any tilting of shoulders, leaning of the head, uneven hip levels, tendency to carry excessive weight on one leg, abnormal humping of the hips and/or shoulders on bending forward from the hips, and even any abnormal hanging of dress or slacks. Active movements should include left and right side bending ranges of motion, as well as body rotation, and ability to walk in a normally even gait. Observation with shirt or blouse open at back in front of a plumb line

and moiré contourography may be revealing. If possible these procedures should be videotaped.

Only after there is sufficient evidence that a clinically significant scoliosis is suspected should x-rays be considered, and when conducted they should be done on a full spine 14 × 36-in film so that the entire pelvis and skull can be observed for epiphyseal development. Both lateral and AP views should be taken and every possible consideration should be given in taking them to avoid excessive exposure to the radiation-sensitive organs such as the breasts, thyroid, eyes, ovaries and gonads. It is now customary to take the AP view in a PA projection to allow for tissue protective attenuation of radiation from reaching the most sensitive tissues. Where applicable, shielding should also be used.

## UPPER CERVICAL ANALYSIS

Analysis of the upper cervical area of the AP projection is basically an extension of the spine below—determinations of lateral flexion deviations and rotations, although somewhat more complex due to the architectural nature of the area. However, for

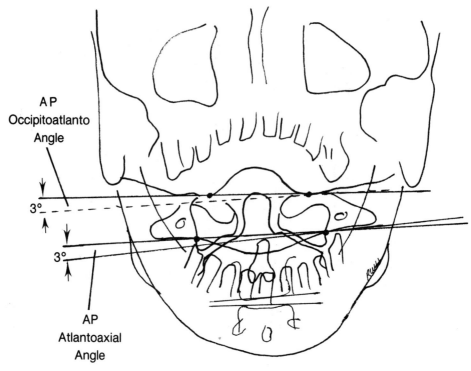

AP
Occipitoatlanto
Angle

3°

3°

AP
Atlantoaxial
Angle

**Figure 10.17.** Line drawing procedures for use on the upper cervical section of standard AP projection full spine films.

more precise analysis of this *atlanto-axial-occipital area*, the reader is referred to a number of standard upper cervical *specific* procedures which, for the most part, are taught as nonacademic entrepreneurial programs. Such procedures often encompass not only the related spinographic analysis procedures, but also include complete systems of specialized chiropractic practice, including individualized philosophies of chiropractic health care and patient management procedures (Fig. 10.17).

For these procedures, specialized spinographic equipment is required which include a positioning chair to allow for movement of the patient forward, backward and rotationally relative to a tilting 8 × 10-in or 10 × 12-in Bucky grid with specialized headclamps for precisely positioning the patient's head without distorting the body-head relationship. Unlike full spine procedure where the pelvis is the *constant* and analysis proceeds from below-upward, in upper cervical-specific procedure the head

is the positioning *constant* and analysis proceeds from below-downward; e.g. the atlas is analyzed with reference to the occiput rather than the occiput to the atlas.

At such time as there is more accepted standardized concepts of these procedures, they will be considered for more elaborate inclusion in future editions of this text.

## LATERAL FULL SPINE VIEW MEASUREMENTS

Unlike the posteroanterior view which attempts to make bilateral comparisons of like structures on each side of the body (with distortional factors in mind) lateral view interpretation is limited to a single plane of structural evaluation in accordance with what is considered a "norm" in the average patient. While certain normals may be based on studies of hundreds or thousands of normal and/or abnormal cases, others are more often based on vague empirical ideas passed on from generation to generation without question.

In the case of the posteroanterior view one deals essentially with an *ideal* normal posture in which both lower extremities are of equal length, the pelvis is level, and the spine is straight—abnormals are a matter of readily observable and measurable deviations with clinical significance being a matter of degree. Whereas in the case of the lateral view, although many analytical concepts or procedures have been proposed, few have any real basis as being representative of normal or abnormal in a particular case—it is known that the lateral spine should illustrate two anterior and posterior curves, but what is really normal to an individual is left to conjecture; the so-called L3 gravitational weight line which is supposed to fall from the center of the L3 body to the sacral promontory seldom does so even in a patient who might have relatively good posture.

Therefore, in consideraton of the philosophy that more analysis procedures are not necessarily better, but perhaps more confusing, this presentation will be limited to those basic concepts which are based on reliable statistical support or are of obvious clinical implications. Other procedures may be included at a particular instructors discretion.

## Lateral Sacral Innominate Triangle

A traditional lateral spinographic evaluation of the pelvis is *Ferguson's sacral base angle* (FSBA) which is the relationship of the sacrum to a horizontal line for reference—normally regarded as ranging from 37–42°. Ordinarily a FSBA of over 42° is equated with lumbar hyperlordosis and an FSBA of under 37° is equated with lumbar hypolordosis. This is true to a certain extent, but represents only part of the story—is the increase or decrease of the FSBA responding sympathetically to a primary involvement of the lumbar spine, or is the increase or decrease of FSBA responsible for the increase or decrease of lumbar curvature? Or is the increase or decrease in the FSBA simply a normal variation of a particular individual—apparently asymp-

tomatic individuals have been found to have FSBAs as high as 65° and others as low as 22°. Consequently, the FSBA by itself has little clinical significance, unless there are findings which indicate otherwise.

Additionally, when chiropractic diagnosis is mainly concerned with the relationship of articulations, not where a particular bone is related to a horizontal line (as with the FSBA), it is more concerned with where one bone (at its articulation) is related to an adjacent bone. Although no method of spinographic analysis can accomplish this objective to an absolute degree, the closer one attempts to evaluate the position of structures relative to the adjacent structure with which they are articulated, the more reliable will be the information relative to biomechanical values.

In the case of the *lateral sacroinnominate triangle*, effort was initiated by the author to equate the commonly used FSBA with the bones it articulates with and depends on for its support—the ilia. Thus, there was the potential of determining whether the irregularly disposed sacrum was sympathetically responding to an increase or decrease in lumbar spine curvature, or the lumbar spine irregularity was sympathetically responding to an increase or decrease of the FSBA.

The marking procedure is as follows:

1. Draw a line down the sacral base (SBL) long enough to eventually intersect with a vertical innominate line (VIL).
2. Draw a second line vertically from a point of bisection of the left and right anterosuperior iliac spine (ASISs) to a point of bisection of the left and right pubic bodies; e.g. vertical innominate line (VIL),
3. Draw a third horizontal reference line (HRL) parallel with the bottom of the film (or 90° to a true vertical gravitational line which bisects the SBL and the VIL.

These three bisecting lines, then, form the three elements of the *lateral sacroinnominate triangle*—the sacral base angle (SBA), the vertical innominate angle (VIA) and the sacroinnominate angle (SIA), which, in their entirety, integrate the biomechanical relationship of the sacrum and

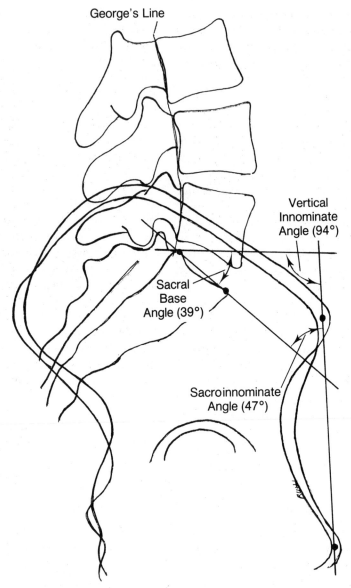

**Figure 10.18.** The lateral Sacroinnominate triangle to evaluate biomechanical relationships between the innominate bones and the sacrum (see text for further discussion).

innominate bones which provide an index of sacroiliac integrity (Fig. 10.18).

In concept the *lateral sacroinnominate triangle* was an interesting idea toward integrating the biomechanical relationship of the sacrum and ilia, but for meaningful clinical value it was necessary to establish what may be considered normal values which might be then applied to a particular case. Consequently, in 1968 the author conducted a study on 70 asymptomatic cases in order to establish, on a preliminary basis, normal parameters of the three incorporating angles comprising the triangle. The x-ray studies were taken under a then-standard 60-in FFD two-exposure lateral full spine conditions with the central ray 90° across the top of the ilia.

The findings of that study are given in Tables 10.5–10.7 which establish the fol-

**Table 10.5.**
**Vertical innominate angle (VIA) summary**[a]

| Range of measurement | Number of cases |
|---|---|
| Degrees | |
| 67–71 | 0 |
| 72–76 | 0 |
| 77–81 | 1 |
| 82–86 | 2 |
| 87–91 | 18 |
| 92–96 | 19 |
| 97–101 | 20 |
| 102–106 | 8 |
| 107–111 | 2 |
| 112–116 | 0 |
| 117–121 | 0 |
| Total Cases | 70 |

[a] Mathematical range: 74–114°; normal range: 94–99°; and median: 86.50°.

**Table 10.6.**
**Sacral base angle (SBA) summary**[a]

| Range of measurement | Number of cases |
|---|---|
| Degrees | |
| 15–19 | 0 |
| 20–24 | 1 |
| 25–29 | 5 |
| 30–35 | 6 |
| 35–39 | 16 |
| 40–44 | 21 |
| 45–49 | 13 |
| 50–54 | 8 |
| 55–59 | 0 |
| 60–64 | 0 |
| 65–69 | 0 |
| Total Cases | 70 |

[a] Mathematical range: 22–56°; normal range: 37–42°; median: 39.50°.

lowing data for each angle:

VIA (vertical innominate angle): mathematical range: 74–114°; normal range: 94–99°; median: 86.50°.

SBA (sacral base angle): mathematical range: 22–56°; normal range: 37–42°; median: 39.50°.

SIA (sacral innominate angle): mathematical range: 29–69°; normal range: 49–54°; median: 51.50°.

In applying these data to practical values,

the *mean* figures (not listed) were used. Thus, the *normal* mean for all cases was: SBA: 39°; VIA: 94°; SIA: 47° (Fig. 10.19A). Typical abnormal *mean* figures are: *B*, posterosacral rock (within the ilia); *C*, posteroinnominate rock; *D*, posteropelvic rock; *E*, anterosacral rock; *F*, anteroinnominate rock; and *G*, anteropelvic rock.

## GEORGE'S LINE

George's line is a drawn or observed line extending up the posterior aspect of all vertebral bodies from the sacrum to C2. This line should follow a smooth unbroken line up the posterior aspect of all vertebral bodies, following the normal anteroposterior spinal curves. Any deviation of this line at any one, or groups of, vertebra indicates a posterior or anterior deviation of a vertebra relative to its neighbor. Although the individual anterior or posterior normal curves of the spine may be increased or decreased, they are not in themselves too significant, as long as George's line is continuous—an increased lumbar curve may simply mean that the individual has less than good posture, possibly due to excessive weight (Fig. 10.20).

**Table 10.7.**
**Sacroinnominate angle (SIA) summary**[a]

| Range of measurement | Number of cases |
|---|---|
| Degrees | |
| 22–26 | 0 |
| 27–31 | 3 |
| 32–36 | 3 |
| 37–41 | 7 |
| 42–46 | 13 |
| 47–51 | 15 |
| 52–57 | 18 |
| 58–61 | 6 |
| 62–66 | 4 |
| 67–71 | 1 |
| 72–76 | 0 |
| Total Cases | 70 |

[a] Mathematical range: 29–69°; normal range: 49–54°; median: 51.50°.

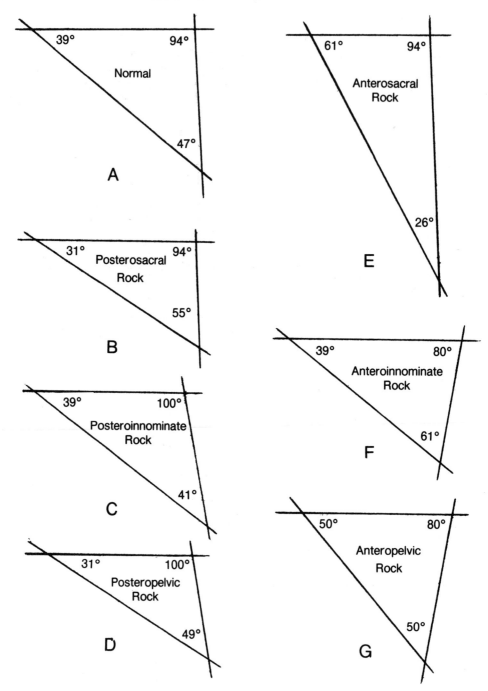

**Figure 10.19.** Various normal and abnormal configurations of the lateral sacroinnominate triangle which may be anticipated.

## VERTEBRAL INTERBODY ANGLES AND SPACES

All intervertebral body angles and spaces should be examined closely from the sacrum to the occiput, particularly at any area where there is an observable deviation in George's line, but not necessarily limited to those areas. Where desirable, lines can be drawn between the end plates of each of the vertebral bodies and measured for comparison and/or recordings of findings. Spe-

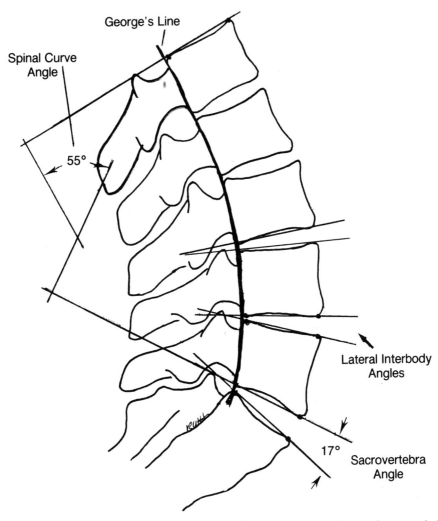

**Figure 10.20.**   Analysis procedures for the lateral lumbar spine which may be extended up to and including the cervical spine.

cific observation should be made for any abrupt deviations indicating possible flexion or extension subluxations which may or may not be consistent with a break in George's line.

Particular attention should be given to general signs of osseous or soft tissue pathology, trauma and/or abnormality, in particular; recent or healed fractures, osteophytosis, paraspinal or intervertebral disk (IVD) calcific infiltrate, erosive conditions of the vertebral bodies and appendages, etc. In such concerns, it is important to discuss any unusual findings with an instructor and refer to a well recommended text on general radiology—in a book of this nature it is not possible to cover all considerations of importance.

## LATERAL CERVICAL SPINE

For the most part, the evaluation of the lateral cervical spine is an extension of the lumbar and thoracic spine sections, the first effort being to evaluate George's line—regardless of the extent of the cervical spine curve, George's line should scribe a smooth, unbroken line from C7 to C2. Any break in George's line, particularly in the presence of an abnormal intervertebral appearance, should be suspect as a stressed vertebral motor unit (Fig. 10.21).

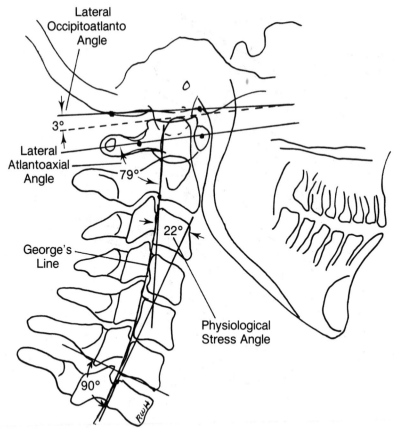

**Figure 10.21.**   Special analytical considerations which may apply to the cervical spine, particularly the atlas-axis-occiput.

Because the cervical spine as a whole is the most flexible spinal unit, special attention should be given to the normal lordotic curve as represented by the *physiological stress angle* which is normally about 22°. Also because they do not ascribe to the alignment of George's line, the atlantoaxial and axiooccipital units bear special attention. Normally, a line drawn up the posterior aspect of the axis body (the superior cervical physiological stress line), should intersect with a horizontal atlas line at about 79°, and the atlas itself should converge anteriorly with the base of the occiput at about a 3° angle. Even slight variations in these measurements bear further study.

## References

1. Anderson M, Green WT, Messner MB: Growth and predictions of growth in lower extremities. *Clin Orthop* 136:7, 1978.
2. Bailey HW, Beckwith CG: Short leg and spinal abnormalities and effects on spinal biomechanics. *J Am Osteopath Assoc* 36:319–327, 1937.
3. Bailey HW: Theoretical significance of postural imbalance, especially the short leg. *J Am Osteopath Assoc* 77:452–55, 1978.
4. Beal MC: A review of the short leg problem. *J Am Osteopath Assoc* 50:109, 1950.
5. Beal M: The short leg problem. *J Am Osteopath Assoc* 73:745–751, 1972.
6. Cathie AG: The influence of the lower extremities upon the structural integrity of the body. *J Am Osteopath Assoc* 150:49:443–446, 1950.
7. Cox W: On the want of asymmetry in the length of opposite side of persons who have never been subject of disease or injury to their lower extremities. *Am J Med Sci*
8. Day JW, Schmidt GL, Lehmann T: Effect of pelvic tilt on standing positions. *Phys Ther* 64:510–516, 1984.
9. Delacerda FG, et al: Effect of lower extremity asymmetry on the kinimatics of gait. *JOSP* 105:7, 1982.
10. Giles LGF: Leg length inequality associated with low back pain. *J Can Chirop Assoc* 20:25–37, 1976.
11. Giles LGF: Low back pain associated with leg

length inequality. *Spine* 6:510–521, 1981.
12. Giles LF: Lumbosacral facetal joint angles associated with leg length inequality. *Rheumatol Rehabil* 20:233–238, 1981.
13. Giles LGF, Taylor JR: Lumbar spine: structural changes with associated leg length inequality. *Spine* 7:159–182, 1982.
14. Gofteon, JP, et al: Studies in osteoarthritis of the hip and leg length disparity. *Can Med Assoc J* May:791–991, 1971.
15. Grice A: Posture and posture mechanics. *J Can Chirop Assoc* July, 1970.
16. Ladermann JP: About irregularities of the lower extremities. *Ann Swiss Chirop Assoc* 6:37–58, 1976.
17. Lawrence D: Lateralization of weight in the presence of structural short leg: a preliminary report, *J Manipulative Physiol Ther* 7:105–106, 1984.
18. Mazwell TD: The piriformis muscle and its relation to the long legged sciatic syndrome. *J Can Chirop Assoc* 22:51–55, 1978.
19. Mersden R: Etiology and pathophysiology of leg length discrepancies. In *Progress in Orthopaedic Surgery*, vol 1, *Equal Length Discrepancy—the Injured Knee.* New York, Springer-Verlag 1977, pp 9–19.
20. Murphy JP: Letter: short leg and sciatica. *JAMA* 242:1257–1258, 1979.
21. Nichols PJR: Short leg syndrome. *Br J Med* 1:1863–1868, 1960.
22. Pauwels PA: A correlation between disk degeneration and short leg. *J Clin Chiropractic* 2:3–13, 1978.
23. Vernon H, et al: A radiographic study of the incidence of low sacral base and lumbar lateral curvature related to the presence of apparent short leg. *J Clin Chiropractic* 27:1145, 1983.
24. Seeman DC: C1 subluxations, short leg and pelvic distresses. *Int Rev Chiropractic* April/June: 37–41, 1979.
25. Redler I: Clinical significance of minor inequalities in leg length. *New Orleans Med Surg J* 104:308, 1952.
26. Sharpe CR: Leg length inequality. *Can Fam Physician* 29:333–336, 1983.
27. Sicuranza BJ, Richards J, Tischl LH: The short leg syndrome in obstetrics and gynecology, *Am J Obstet Gynecol* 107:217–219, 1970.
28. Simon S, Whiffen J, Shapiro F: Leg length discrepancies in monarticular and pariarticular juvenile rheumatoid arthritis. *J Bone Joint Surg* 63A:209–215, 1981.
29. Stoddard A: The short leg and low back syndrome: *Proceedings of the International Congress of Physical Medicine*, 1952, City and State.
30. Clarke GR: Unequal leg length: an accurate method of detection and some clinical results. *Rheum Phys Med J* 2:385–390, 1972.
31. Denslow JS, et al: Methods in taking and interpreting weight bearing x-ray films. *J Am Osteo-path Assoc* 54:663–670, 1955.
32. Fisk JW, Baigent ML: Clinical and radiological assessment of leg length. *NZ Med J* vol 81, 1975.
33. Green WT, Wyatt GM, Anderson M: Orthoroentgenography as a method of measuring the bones of the lower extremities. *J Bone Joint Surg* 28:60–65, 1946.
34. Hirsberg GG, Robertson, KB: Device for determining difference in leg length. *Arch Phys Med Rehabil* 53:45–46, 1972.
35. Jones LB: Radiologic measurement of pelvic positions. In *The Postural Complex.* Springfield, Ill, Charles C Thomas, 1977, pp 33–42.
36. Kraus ER: A postural roentgenography study. *J Am Osteopath Assoc* 49:231–235, 1949.
37. Mann M, Glashheen Wray, M, Nyberg R: Therapist agreement for manipulation and observation of iliac crest heights. *Phys Ther* 64:334–338, 1984.
38. Moseley CF: A straight line graph for leg discrepancies. *Clin Orthop* 136:33, 1978.
39. Nichols PJR, Bailey NTS: The accuracy of measuring leg length differences: an observer error experiment. *Arch Med J* 2:124–178, 1955.
40. Smith DJ, Zindrick MR, Lambert RW, Miller EA: Assessment of three techniques to predict leg length discrepancy. *Clin Orthopedics* 5:737–738, 1982.
41. Van EK, et al: A comparative study of leg length defects. *Eur J Chiriropractic* 31:68–80, 1983.
42. Rush WA, Steiner HA: A study of lower extremity length inequality. *AJR* 56:621–623, 1946.
43. Rush WA: Roentgenographic spinal fixation and stabilizing device. *Am J Roentgenol Rad Ther Nucl Med* 11:87–149, 1946.
44. Winterstein JF: Chiropractic spinographology. Lombard, Ill, National College of Chiropractic, 1970, pp 20–30.
45. Herbst RW: *Gonstead Chiropractic Science and Art: Femur Head Height Changes with Ilium Misalignment.* Mt. Horeb, Wisc, Sc-Chi Publication, 1974, pp 25–36.
46. Macrae J: *Roentgenometrics in Chiropractic.* Toronto, Canadian Chiropractic College, 1974.
47. Schramm SB, Hosek RS, Silverman HL: Spinographic positioning errors in Gonstead pelvic x-ray analysis. *J Manipulative Physiol Ther* 4:179–181, 1981.
48. Phillips RB: An evaluation of the graphic analysis of the pelvis on three AP full spine radiographic analyses. *ACA J Chiropractic*, 9:S139–S148, 1975.
49. Hildebrandt RW: *Chiropractic Spinography: A Manual of Technology and Interpretation.* Des Plaines, Ill, Hilmark, 1977.
50. Lustead LB, Keats, TE: *Atlas of Roentgenographic Measurement*, ed 3. Chicago, Medical Year Book, 1972.
51. Keim HS: Scoliosis. *Ciba Clin Symp* 30:22–24, 1978.
52. Nash CL, Moe JH: A study of vertebral rotation. *J Bone Joint Surg* 51A:222–229, 1969.

# Appendix A:
# International System of Units (SI)

## HISTORY OF MEASUREMENT SYSTEMS

The measurement system commonly used in the United States today is nearly the same as that brought from England by the colonists. These measures had their origin in a variety of cultures—Babylonian, Egyptian, Roman, Anglo-Saxon, and Norman French. The ancient "digit," "palm," "span," and "cubit" units evolved into the "inch," "foot," and "yard" through a complicated transformation not yet completely understood (1).

Roman contributions include the use of the number 12 as a base for the 12-inch foot, and words from which we derive many of the names for our weights and measures. For example, the 12 divisions of the Roman "pes" or foot were called "unciae," Our words "inch" and "ounce" were both derived from that Latin word.

The "yard" as a measure of length can be traced back to the early Saxon kings. They wore a sash or girdle around the waist that could be removed and used as a convenient measuring device; thus the word "yard" comes from the Saxon word "gird," or the circumference of a person's waist.

Standardization of the various units and their combinations into a loosely related system of weights and measures sometimes happened in fascinating ways. Tradition holds that King Henry I decreed that the yard should be the distance from the tip of his nose to the end of his thumb. The length of the furlong (furrow long) was established by early Tudor rulers as 220 yards. This led Queen Elizabeth I to declare in the 16th century that, henceforth, the traditional Roman mile of 5000 feet would be changed to 5280 feet. This made the mile exactly 8 furlongs and provided a convenient relationship between two previously ill-related measurements.

Consequently, through such royal edicts, England by the 18th century had achieved a greater degree of standardization than the continental countries. The English units were well suited to commerce and trade because they had been developed and refined to meet specific commercial needs.

Through colonization and dominance of world commerce during the 17th and 18th centuries, the English system of weights and measures was spread to many parts of the world, including the American colonies. However, standards still differed to some extent and the need for greater uniformity for commerce among the 13 colonies led to clauses in the Articles of the Confederation and the Constitution, ratified, respectively, in 1781 and 1790. This gave Congress the power to fix uniform standards which today are regulated by the National Bureau of Standards.

However, although various countries of the world have given similar effort to standardization of weights and measures within their respective domains, the need for a single worldwide coordinated measurement system has been well recognized for over 300 years. In 1670 Gabriel Mouton, Vicar of St. Paul in Lyons first proposed a comprehensive decimal measurement system based on the length of 1 minute of arc of a great circle of the earth. This was essentially the beginning of the "metric" system of weights and measures.

The metric system as such can be traced back to 1791, in which year a committee of the Academie des Sciences in Paris adopted as the unit of length, the metre (meter). The metre was defined by the committee as "one forty-millionth part of the earths meridian passing through Paris," and was redefined by the first "international governmental Conference generale des Poids et Mesures (CGPM) in 1889 as "the distance between two marks engraved on a special bar of platinum-iridium alloy kept in the Bureau International des Poids et Mesures" (BIPM).

The search for a "universally acceptable" system of measurement began in 1862 with the convening of an international committee under the sponsorship of the British Association for the Advancement of Science. In 1863 this committee recommended a system based on the metre (meter), the gram and the second. In 1873 a similar comittee, also sponsored by the British Association, recommended a system based on the centimetre (centimeter), the gram and the second, which became widely used and was known as the CGS system.

The CGS system, however, did not satisfactorily meet the need for a universal system of units, and the international studies and conferences continued. In 1901 Italian physicist G. Giorgi proposed a system based on the metre (meter), the kilogram, the second, and an electrical unit. Following its endorsement by a number of international organizations, this system also came into widespread use under the official names MKS system or "Giorgi system." The fourth base unit of the system, the ampere, was not finally selected until 1950, after which date the name MKSA system was also used. The Conference generale des Poids et Mesures adopted this system (adding other units to it) in 1954, and renamed it Systeme international d'Unites (SI) in 1960.

# INTERNATIONAL SYSTEM OF UNITS—SI

The SI is essentially an expanded version of the MKS/MKSA/Giorgi systems that have been used to some extent since 1901. The SI is comprised of seven "base" units, an indefinite number of "derived" units, and two "supplementary" units. (2)

## Base Units

The base units of the SI are the *meter* for length, *kilogram* for mass, *second* for time, *ampere* for electrical current, *kelvin* for thermodynamic temperature, *candela* for luminous intensity, and *mole* for amount of substance. These units, along with their symbols, are listed in Table A.1.

The base units are defined very precisely, and the constant progress of science makes it necessary to redefine them even more precisely from time to time. Currently, these base units are defined as follows:

***Meter.*** The length equal to 1 650 763.73 wavelengths in vacuum of the radiation corresponding to the transition between the levels $2p_{10}$ and $5d_5$ of the krypton-86 atom (11th CGPM, 1960).

**Table A.1.**
**SI base units**[a]

| Quantity | Name of unit | Symbol for unit |
|---|---|---|
| Length | meter | m |
| Mass | kilogram | kg |
| Time | second | s |
| Electric current | ampere | A |
| Thermodynamic temperature[b] | kelvin | K |
| Luminous intensity | candela | cd |
| Amount of substance | mole | mol |

[a] From *Brief History of Measurement Systems.* Washington DC, US Department of Commerce, National Bureau of Standards, Special Publication 304-A.

[b] The thermodynamic temperature scale is based on the relationship between heat and mechanical work, and is independent of the properties of any particular working substance, such as alcohol or mercury. It should be noted that the unit of measurement is "kelvin," not "degree kelvin," and that its symbol is K, not °K.

**Table A.2.**
**Some SI derived units**[a]

| Quantity | Name of derived unit | Symbol for unit |
|---|---|---|
| Area | square meter | $m^2$ |
| Volume | cubic meter | $m^2$ |
| Speed | meter per second | m/s (or $m\text{-}s^{-1}$) |
| Acceleration | meter per second squared | m/s (or $m\text{-}s^{-2}$) |
| Substance Concentration | mole per cubic meter | $mol/m^3$ (or $mol\text{-}m^{-2}$) |

[a] From *Brief History of Measurement Systems.* Washington DC, US Department of Commerce, National Bureau of Standards, Special Publication 304-A.

*Kilogram.* The mass of the international prototype of the kilogram; a cylinder of platinum alloy kept by the International Bureau of Weights and Measures in Paris, with a duplicate in the United States Bureau of Standards (1st CGPM, 1889; 3rd CGPM, 1901).

*Second.* The duration of 9 192 631 770 periods of the radiation corresponding to the transition between the two hyperfine levels of the ground state of cesium—133 atom (13th CGPM, 1967).

*Ampere.* That constant electric current which, if maintained in two straight parallel conductors of infinite length, of negligible cross-section, and placed 1 meter apart in vacuum, would produce between these conductors a force equal to $2 \times 10^{-7}$ newton per meter of length (9th CGPM, 1948).

*Kelvin.* The fraction 1/273.16 of the thermodynamic temperature of the triple point of water (13th CGPM, 1967).

*Candela.* The luminous intensity, in the perpendicular direction of a surface of 1/600 000 square meter of a blackbody at the temperature of freezing platinum under a pressure of 101 325 newtons per square meter (13th CGPM, 1967).

*Mole.* The amount of substance of a system which contains as many elementary entities as there are atoms in 0.012 kg of carbon-12. When the mole is used, the elementary entities must be specified and may be atoms, molecules, ions, electrons, or other particles or groups (14th CGPM, 1971).

## Derived Units

By multiplying a base unit by itself, or by combining two or more base units by simple multiplication or division, it is possible to form a large group of "SI-derived units." Taking two examples, the derived unit of speed is meter divided by seconds, or meter per second; the derived unit of meter cubed, or cubic meter.

Derived units may be divided into "sample derived units" as in the foregoing examples and in Table A.2, or into "derived units with special names" as in Table A.3.

The combination of base units to form derived units exemplifies one of the main advantages of the SI system. Within this system, there is not a single conversion factor to be memorized—the formation of derived units does not involve any mathematical factor other than 1 (unity), and such a system is said to be "coherent."

There are a number of rules for writing symbols for SI units and if one is unfamiliar with these rules, reference to the booklet *The SI for the Health Professions* (2) published by the World Health Organization is suggested.

## Supplementary Units

In addition to the base units and derived units, two "supplementary units" have been designated—the unit of plane angle, the radian (symbol: rad), and the unit of solid angle, the steradian (symbol: sr). However, at the present time, these supplementary units are considered somewhat anomalous

**Table A.3.**
**SI derived units with special names**[a]

| Quantity | Name of unit | Symbol for unit | Derivation of unit[b] |
|---|---|---|---|
| Frequency | hertz | Hz | $s^{-1}$ |
| Force | newton | N | $m \cdot kg \cdot s^{-2}$ |
| Pressure | pascal | Pa | $N/m^2$ |
| Work; energy; quality of heat | joule | J | $N \cdot m$ |
| Power; radiant flux | watt | W | $J/s$ |
| Electric charge; quantity of electricity | coulomb | C | $A \cdot s$ |
| Electric potential; potential difference | volt | V | $W/A$ |
| Capacitance | farad | F | $C/V$ |
| (Electric) resistance | ohm | Ω | $V/A$ |
| Conductance | siemens | S | $A/V$ |
| Magnetic flux | weber | Wb | $V \cdot s$ |
| Magnetic flux density | tesla | T | $Wb/m^2$ |
| Inductance | henry | H | $Wb/A$ |
| Luminous flux | lumen | lm | $cd \cdot sr$ |
| Illuminance | lux | lx | $m^{-2} \cdot cd \cdot sr$ |
| Celsius temperature | degree Celsius | °C | K |
| Absorbed dose; absorbed dose index; kerma; specific energy imparted (radiation) | gray | Gy | $J/kg$ |
| Activity (of a radionuclide) | becquerel | Bq | $s^{-1}$ |

[a] From *Brief History of Measurement Systems.* Washington DC, US Department of Commerce, National Bureau of Standards, Special Publication 304-A.

[b] With the exception of those units that can be expressed only in terms of base units, the derived units are expressed in this column, in terms of other derived units. (These units can, of course, be expressed in terms of base units; thus, the expression for the newton can be substituted for N in the expression N·m for the joule, giving $m2 \cdot kg \cdot s^{-2}$ as the expression of the joule base units, and so on down the list.) It will be noticed that two units in this table—the lumen and the lux—are expressed in terms of a unit (steradian) whose symbol is sr (not a base unit).

in that the CGPM has not as yet concluded whether they are to be regarded as base units or derived units.

In any case, the supplementary units can be used to form derived units in the same manner as the base units.

## SI Prefixes

In order to form decimal multiples and submultiples of SI units, 16 prefixes have been designated to allow for convenient application to exceedingly large or small factors. For example, it would not be convenient to use kilometer (factor $10^3$) for measurement of the size of a bone lesion, but rather one would use the centimeter (factor $10^{-2}$) or millimeter (factor $10^{-3}$) (Table A.4).

When the 16 prefixes, listed in Table A.4, are used they are joined directly to the unit name with punctuation; i.e. millimeter, not milli-meter. The same is true for the prefix symbols, i.e. mm not m.m.

When the SI prefix is joined to a particular unit, it multiples that unit by the factor used; i.e. the millimeter is $10^{-3}$ or 0.001 meter.

The units that are formed by the use of the prefixes should not be called SI units. The SI units are confined to the base, derived and supplementary units which form a "coherent set." The result of using a pre-

**Table A.4.**
**Multiples and prefixes; these prefixes may be applied to all SI units E[a]**

| Amount | Name | Symbols |
|---|---|---|
| 1 000 000 000 000 000 000 = $10^{18}$ | exa (ĕx′ a) | E[b] |
| 1 000 000 000 000 000 = $10^{15}$ | peta (pĕt′ a) | P |
| 1 000 000 000 000 = $10^{12}$ | tera (tĕr′ a) | T |
| 1 000 000 000 = $10^{9}$ | giga (jĭ′ ga) | G |
| 1 000 000 = $10^{6}$ | mega (mĕg′ a) | M |
| 1 000 = $10^{3}$ | kilo (kĭl′ ŏ) | k |
| 100 = $10^{2}$ | hecto (hĕk′ tŏ) | h |
| 10 = 10· | deka (dĕk′ a) | da |
| Base unit 1 = 10 | | |
| 0.1 = $10^{-1}$ | deci (dĕš′ ĭ) | d |
| 0.01 = $10^{-2}$ | centi (sĕn′ tĭ) | c |
| 0.001 = $10^{-3}$ | milli (mĭl′ ĭ) | m |
| 0.000 001 = $10^{-6}$ | micro (mī′ krŏ) | $\mu$ |
| 0.000 000 001 = $10^{-9}$ | nano (năn′ ŏ) | n |
| 0.000 000 000 001 = $10^{-12}$ | pico (pē′ kŏ) | p |
| 0.000 000 000 000 001 = $10^{-15}$ | femto (fĕm′ tŏ) | f |
| 0.000 000 000 000 000 001 = $10^{-18}$ | atto (ăt′ tŏ) | a |

[a] From *Brief History of Measurement Systems*. Washington DC, US Department of Commerce, National Bureau of Standards, Special Publication 304-A.
[b] E applies to gram in case of mass.

**Table A.5.**
**Non-SI units retained for general use with the SI[a]**

| Quantity | Name of unit | Symbol for unit | Value in SI units |
|---|---|---|---|
| Time | minute | min | 60 s |
| | hour | h | 3 600 s |
| | day | d | 86 400 s |
| Plane angle | degree | ° | $\pi/180$ rad |
| | minute | ′ | $\pi/10\ 800$ rad |
| | second | ″ | $\pi/648\ 000$ rad |
| Volume | liter | l | 1 dm$^3$ = $10^{-3}$ m$^2$ |
| Mass | ton | t | 1 000 kg |

[a] From *Brief History of Measurement Systems*. Washington DC, US Department of Commerce, National Bureau of Standards, Special Publication 304-A.

fix is considered a multiple or submultiple of an SI unit.

## Writing Symbols and Numbers

Symbols for units are always written in Roman (up-right) type, even if they appear in text that is set in italics. Symbols for units are the same for both singular and plural (5 mm, not 5 mms), and are never followed by a period unless appearing at the end of a sentence (5 mm not 5 mm.).

In writing numbers, either a comma or a period may be used as the decimal marker; most international bodies have indicated a preference for the use of the comma because the period may be confused with an elevated dot which is the indicator for multiplication.

Digits should be separated into groups of three, to the left or right of the decimal marker, and separated by spaces rather than commas or periods. Examples:

*Correct:* 1 000,350 1 (one thousand, comma or period, three five zero one)

*Incorrect:* 1,000.350,1

## Non-SI Units

Some non-SI units are so widely used that they are difficult to discontinue. Consequently, in adopting the SI, eight such units were retained. These non-SI units are given in Table A.5.

Some of these units, particularly the liter and units of time, are of great importance to health professions. It should be explained, however, that the *liter* is a "special name" given to the submultiple "cubic decimeter" of the SI unit of volume, and

**Table A.6.**
**Non-SI units accepted for use for a limited time that are of concern in the healing professions[a,b]**

| Unit name | Unit symbol | Value in SI units |
|---|---|---|
| Ångström | A | $10^{-10}$ m (0, 1 nm) |
| barn | b | $10^{-28}$ m$^2$ (100 fm) |
| bar | bar | 100 000 Pa (0, 1 MPa) |
| normal atmosphere | atm | 101 325 Pa |
| curie | Ci | $3.7 \times 10^{10}$ Bq (or $3.7 \times 10^{10}$ s$^{-1}$) |
| roentgen | R | $2.58 \times 10^{-4}$ C/kg |
| rad | rad or rd[c] | $10^{-2}$ Gy (or $10^{-2}$ J/kg) |

[a] From *Brief History of Measurement Systems*. Washington DC, US Department of Commerce, National Bureau of Standards, Special Publication 304-A.

[b] It has often been asserted in the medical literature that the liter is "the fundamental SI unit of volume." This is untrue; the misunderstanding arises from the fact that the liter has been widely adopted by the health professions as the unit of volume to be used with the SI in those professions. (It should also be reiterated that there are no "fundamental" units in the SI.) Also, the commonly used term "metric ton" is a misnomer.

[c] Symbol rd if there is any danger of confusion with the symbol rad for radian.


**Table A.7.**
**Radiation quantities and units[a]**

| Quantity | SI unit | Old unit | Example |
|---|---|---|---|
| Absorbed dose; absorbed dose index; kerma; specific energy imparted | gray | rad | 15 $\mu$Gy (1, 5 mrad) |
| Absorbed dose rate | gray per second | rad per second | 15 $\mu$Gy/s (1, 5 mrad/s) |
| Dose equivalent | joule per kilogram | rem | 10 mJ/kg (1 rem) |
| Activity | becquerel | curie | 37 MBq (1 mCi) |
| Exposure | coulomb per kilogram | roentgen | 0, 258 $\mu$C/kg (1 mR) |
| Exposure rate | coulomb per kilogram second (or ampere per kilogram) | roentgen per second | 0, 258 $\mu$C(Kg·s) (1 mR/s) |

[a] From *Brief History of Measurement Systems*. Washington DC, US Department of Commerce, National Bureau of Standards, Special Publication 304-A.


that the *ton* is a special name given to a multiple of the SI unit of mass.

An additional group of 12 non-SI units have been retained for use with the SI for a limited period of time; the length of that time to depend upon circumstances of phasing-out processes. Some have already been largely superseded, and for others a time limit has been set by international organizations. The units of this group that may have particular interest to the health professions are given in Table A.6.

The remaining five units of this group are the *nautical mile* (no symbol), 1 852 m; the *knot* (no symbol), approximately 1,514 m/s; the *arc* (symbol: a), 100 m$^2$; the *hectare* (symbol: ha), 10 000 m$^2$; and the *gal* (symbol: Gal), $10^{-2}$ m/s$^2$.

Table A.8.
Miscellaneous "old" units that should no longer be used[a]

| "Old" unit (symbol) | Amount | "New" unit (symbol) |
|---|---|---|
| Ångström (Å) | 0.1 | nanometer (nm) |
| atomic weight unit (awul); dalton | 0, 992 1 | unified at omic mass unit ($\mu$) |
| micron ($\mu$) | 1 | nicrometer ($\mu$m) |
| millimicron (m$\mu$) | 1 | nanometer (nm) |
| svedberg, Svedberg unit (S, Sv) | 10–12 | second (s) |
| | 0, 1 | picosecond (ps) |
| | 100 | femtosecond (fs) |
| torr (Torr) | 0, 133 3 | kilopascal (kPa) |
| $\gamma$ (gamma) | 1 | microgram ($\mu$g) |
| $\lambda$ (lambda) | 1 | microliter ($\mu$l) |

[a] From *Brief History of Measurement Systems*. Washington DC, US Department of Commerce, National Bureau of Standards, Special Publication 304-A.

## Radiation Units

In radiology and allied fields, the joule per kilogram replaces the rad and the rem; the reciprocal second replaced the curie; and the *coulomb per kilogram* replaces the roentgen. However, in 1975 the CGPM adopted, at the request of the International Commission on Radiation Units and Measurements (ICRU), the *gray* (symbol: Gy) as a special name for the joule per kilogram for the measurement of absorbed dose. It added a note to the effect that the gray could also be used for other physical quantities in the field of ionizing radiation that are expressed in joule per kilogram. This means that absorbed dose index, kerma and specific energy imparted are also expressed in terms of the gray (as listed in Table A.7). Also in 1975, the CGPM adopted the *becquerel* (symbol: Bq) as a special name for the reciprocal second for the measurement of activity. No special name was adopted for the coulomb per kilogram. Following these CGPM decisions, ICRU recommended that the units curie, rad, and roentgen be abandoned and replaced by the SI units over a period of no less than 10 years (i.e. the old units should not be completely abandoned before 1985). At the same time, it requested all international and national organizations to assist in implementing the change (3).

The present situation is summarized in Table A.7. It is recommended that, as an

Table A.9.
Year of introduction or anticipated introduction (after 1975) of SI units[a,b]

| Year | Country |
|---|---|
| 1970 | Netherlands |
| 1971 | Denmark, Finland |
| 1974 | Australia |
| 1975 | United Kingdom |
| 1976 | New Zealand, South Africa, Sweden |
| 1977 | Norway |
| 1978 | Federal Republic of Germany |
| 1979 | Czechoslovakia, Democratic Republic of Germany |
| 1980 | Hungary, Italy |
| 1981 | Japan, Switzerland, Yugoslavia |
| 1982 | Ecuador |

[a] From *Brief History of Measurement Systems.* Washington DC, US Department of Commerce, National Bureau of Standards, Special Publication 304-A.
[b] SI indicates International Systems of Units

interim measure, numerical values should, for most purposes, be quoted in the literature as in the examples in the right-hand column of this table. Attention is drawn to the recommendation that, in order to avoid confusion, dose equivalent (for which the old unit was the rem) should be expressed in joule per kilogram, and not gray.

## Miscellaneous Old Units That Should No Longer Be Used

As the SI is adopted for use, a number of old units would be dropped completely,

**Table A.10.**
**Common conversions: accurate to six significant figures**[a]

| Symbol[b] | When you know number of | Multiply by | To find number of | Symbol[b] |
|---|---|---|---|---|
| in | inches | 25.4[c] | millimeters[d] | mm |
| ft | feet | 0.3048[c] | meters | m |
| yd | yards | 0.9144[c] | meters | m |
| | | | | |
| mi | miles | 1.609 34 | kilometers | km |
| $yd^2$ | square yards | 0.836 127 | square meters | $m^2$ |
| | acres | 0.404 686 | hectares[e] | ha |
| $yd^3$ | cubic yards | 0.764 555 | cubic meters | $m^3$ |
| qu | quarts (1q) | 0.946 353 | liters[f] | l |
| oz | ounces (avdp) | 28.349 5 | grams | g |
| 1b | pounds (avdp) | 0.453 592 | kilograms | kg |
| F | degrees Farenheit | 5/9[c] (after subtracting 32) | degrees Celsius | C |
| | | | | |
| mm | millimeters | 0.039 370 1 | inches | in |
| m | meters | 3.280 84 | feet | ft |
| m | meters | 1.093 61 | yards | yd |
| km | kilometers | 0.621 371 | miles | mi |
| $m^2$ | square meters | 1.195 99 | square yards | $yd^2$ |
| ha | hectares[e] | 2.471 05 | acres | |
| $m^3$ | cubic meters | 1.307 95 | cubic yards | $yd^3$ |
| l | liters[f] | 1.056 69 | quarts (lq) | qt |
| g | grams | 0.035 274 0 | ounces (avdp) | oz |
| kg | kilograms | 2.204 62 | pounds (avdp) | lb |
| C | degrees Celsius | 9/5[c] (then add 32) | degrees Farenheit | F |

[a] From *Brief History of Measurement Systems.* Washington DC, US Department of Commerce, National Bureau of Standards, Special Publication 304-A.

[b] Note: Most symbols are written with lower case letters; exceptions are units named after persons for which the symbols are capitalized. Periods are not used with any symbols.

[c] Exact

[d] For example, 1 in = 25.4 mm, so 3 in would be 3 in × 25.4 mm = 76.2 mm.

[e] Hectare is a common name for 10 000 square meters

[f] Liter is most common name for fluid volume of 0.001 cubic meter

being replaced by new designations as given in Table A.8.

## DISCUSSION

Most countries have already made, or are in the process of making, the International System of Units (SI) the legal system of measurement in their jurisdictions. The years of introduction, or scheduled introduction, in those countries where it has been officially adopted are given in Table A.9.

Although the United States has committed itself to eventual changeover to SI on the basis of the Metric Conversion Act of 1975, no specific target date has been set. Instead, because of the reluctance of the populace in general to accept the change in toto, the present effort is to "encourage" rather than "require." It is in this spirit of "encouragement" that the health professions are transitioning into the SI, primarily through educational efforts of scientific and clinical journals. This is being done by first publishing editorials and/or instructional matter on the SI and then requiring all submitted papers to express units in the "new system" with the old factors following in parentheses. (See Table A.10 for conversion factors for some common, current measurements.)

In the health profession sector in general, it is anticipated that dual reporting of the new and old measurements will continue for an indefinite period of time until the majority of individuals are well oriented to SI, after which the old measurements (in parentheses) will be dropped.

### References

1. *Brief History of Measurement Systems*. Washington DC, US Department of Commerce, National Bureau of Standards, Special Publication 304-A.
2. *The SI For the Health Professions*. Geneva, World Health Organization, 1975.
3. Wychoff, HO: The international system of units (SI). *Radiology* 128:833–835, 1978.

# Appendix B:
# Glossary

**achalasia:** Failure to relax, said of muscles such as sphincters, the normal function of which is a persistent contraction with periods of relaxation of visceral openings.

**adenopathy:** Enlargement or disease of lymphatic glands.

**adhesion:** Sticking together of two surfaces in an inflammatory process, as for example, the adhesions of the pleura from pleurisy, or of peritonitis.

**adynamic:** Lacking in movement, such as in ileus when the bowel distends with gas which is not expelled.

**adynamic ileus:** (*see* ileus)

**agenesis:** Complete absence of a part resulting from failure of development during the early blastemic stage. Weakness resulting from agenesis of a part is frequently compensated for by anomalous or overdevelopment of an adjacent structure.

**aluminum filter:** Various thicknesses of aluminum used as filtration in the x-ray beam to absorb the longer, ineffective rays. Minimum of 5 mm recommended in spinography.

**aluminum step wedge:** Graduated steps of the same thickness of added aluminum which may be used to measure penetration of a given beam of x-rays and the tonal scale, on film, of various qualities of x-ray beams.

**amorphous:** Aplastic state of matter having no regular form; shapeless.

**amphiarthrosis:** A joint in which the opposing ends of the bones, tipped with articular cartilage, are united together with fibrous or fibrocartilaginous tissue; movement is limited.

**anatomical vertical axis:** A hypothetical line perpendicular to the horizontal plane about which the body would rotate in theoretical ideal posture. It is defined by the vertical intersection of the midsagittal and midcoronal body planes.

**aneurysm:** An abnormal sacculation or outpouching of a blood vessel.

**angiography:** Roentgenographic demonstration of blood vessels utilizing radiopaque contrast medium.

**angle:** Area or point of junction of two intersecting borders or surfaces; the degree of divergence of two intersecting lines or planes.

**basal:** An angle measured between the glabella and the midpoint of the pituitary fossa joined with a line extending to the basion (anterior margin of the foramen magnum). The mean of this angle is 137°, minimum 123°, and maximum 152°.

**Cobb's:** Angle of lateral curvature of the spine in scoliosis; also used to measure kyphotic and lordotic spinal curves.

**costovertebral:** That formed on either side of the vertebral column between the last rib and the lumbar vertebrae.

**critical:** Incidence at which a ray of

light passing from one medium to another of different density changes from refraction to total reflection.

**Ferguson's:** An angle formed between bisecting lines across the sacral base and a horizontal line. Normal range is 35–43°. Mean average 39.5°. Variation denotes instability of the low back.

**iliofemoral:** Angle between a line across both femor heads and a line from the pelvic center of gravity to the left or right posteroinferior iliac spine as viewed on a PA pelvic roentgenograph—indicates possible opposed disrelation of the innominate bone on a symphysis pubis pivot.

**kyphotic:** The superior angle formed by intersection of two lines drawn on the lateral chest roentgenogram, tangential to the anterior borders of the second and eleventh intervertebral spaces, an index of the degree of deformity in thoracic kyphosis.

**lumbosacral:** The angle of the fifth lumbar vertebra relative to the sacral base, as viewed from the side.

**Martin's basilar:** The angle formed between bisecting lines drawn from the root of the nose to the midportion of the sella turcica, and from the sella to the anterior margin of the foramen magnum. Normal angulation averages 135° (115–150°): flattening of the angle in excess of 150° is consistent with platybasia.

**Mikalicz's:** Angle formed by two planes, one passing through the long axis of the epiphysis of the femur and the other through the long axis of the diaphysis, normally 130°—also called angle of declination.

**of incidence, light:** The angle made with the perpendicular line by a ray of light which strikes a denser, or rarer, medium.

**of incidence, spinographic:** That angle of a divergent primary x-ray beam relative to the central ray which projects anatomic structures to a point of implantation on the film.

**of inclination:** Angle at pelvic saggital plane attitude relative to a horizontal line.

**pelvic rotation:** Angle formed by lines drawn from the pelvic center of gravity to the symphysis pubis and a vertical line—indicates pelvic rotation on a PA pelvis radiographic view.

**sacral base:** Angle between sacral base and a horizontal line as viewed from the side; normal range or 39–42°.

**sacral rotation:** Angle formed by a line across like bilateral sacral points on an AP full spine radiograph and the iliofemoral lines—decreased angle on one side relative to the other side indicates anteroinferior rotation at the sacrum within the ilia.

**sacroinnominate:** Angle formed by intersection of a vertical innominate line and Ferguson's sacral base line—indicates position of the sacrum relative to the innominate bones.

**sacrovertebral:** (*see* Angle, lumbosacral)

**vertical innominate:** Angle formed by a line drawn from the anterior superior iliac spines to the symphysis pubis and a vertical line as viewed on a lateral pelvic radiographic view—indicates AP rocking of the pelvis on the femur heads.

**ankylosis:** Stiffness or fixation of a joint usually complicating trauma or infection.

**annular:** A circular or ring-like structure, such as the anulus fibrosis of the intervertebral disk.

**anomaly:** An unusual anatomical variation in the development of a structure or organ.

**antero-:** A combining form meaning in front.

**anteroposterior:** From front to back direction with reference to the x-ray tube, abbreviated AP, and frequently used to designate the path of x-rays through a part being examined. Opposite of PA projection.

**aortic knob:** That portion of the aortic arch which curves posterolaterally as seen in the PA or AP projections, presenting a knob or knuckle as it joins the descending portion of the thoracic aorta.

**aortic window:** A radiolucent area seen below the curving arch of the thoracic aorta in the lateral view, through which may be seen the right and left main bronchi and vascular roots of the lung.

**AP:** (*see* anteroposterior)

**AP film:** Roentgenogram made in the AP projection with reference to the x-ray tube, i.e. where the front of the part is directed toward the x-ray tube.

**apex:** The point of a pyramidal structure, the upper portion of the lung; the end of a root of a tooth.

**aplasia:** Signifies defective or incomplete development of tissues.

**apophyseal:** Pertaining to apophysis or secondary center of ossification; also the lateral articulating joints of the spine.

**architecture:** Normal arrangement of the component parts of a structure. There may be pathologic alterations of normal architecture.

**arteriosclerosis:** Calcium deposits in the walls of the arteries; "hardening" of the arteries. Pathologic aging process of the arterial vessels.

**arthrodesis:** The surgical fixation of a joint; artificial ankylosis.

**arthrography:** Injection of air or radiopaque contrast material into joint spaces for purposes of x-ray examination of them.

**arthropathy:** Disease of a joint.

**articular:** Pertaining to a joint.

**articular cortex:** (*see* cortex)

**articular facets:** (*see* facet)

**articular process:** (*see* process)

**artifact:** A mark foreign to the image of which is imposed on film by the action of x-rays.

**asthenic:** The habitus of an individual who lacks normal tone.

**asymmetry:** Lack or absence of symmetry of position or motion. Dissimilarity in corresponding parts or organs on opposite sides of the body which are normally alike. Of particular use when describing position or motion alteration resulting from somatic dysfunction.

**asymptomatic:** Lacking in symptoms; having no symptoms or complaints.

**atlantooccipital fusion:** Ankylotic union of the atlas to the base of the skull, frequently accompanied by asymmetrical development.

**atonic:** Without tension or evidence of normal muscle contraction.

**atresia:** Narrowing of an opening of a passage or tube, or congenital absence of such an opening.

**atrophy:** Wasting away of a tissue or part.

   **Sudeck's:** Acute bone atrophy after an injury related to trophic disturbance through reflex phenomenon.

**atypical:** Not typical; of unusual type.

**avulsion:** The tearing away, as in avulsion fracture of a bone.

**bamboo deformity.** Spoken of the bamboo appearance of the spine in advanced rheumatoid arthritis of the Marie-Strümpell variety.

**basal angle:** (*see* angle)

**basilar invagination:** An upward depression of the base of the occiput and foramen magnum with invagination of the upper cervical vertebra due to congenital malformation or disease processes resulting in a softening of the bone.

**benign:** Innocent; not malignant.

**biconcave:** Concave on each side, as a lens.

**bifid:** Cleft or split into two parts or forked, as a rib, or cervical vertebrae spinous process.

**biomechanics:** The application of mechanical laws to living structures. The study and knowledge of biological function from an application of mechanical principles. Distinguished from somatology.

**biopsy:** A surgical procedure involving removal of a small particle of tissue from a living subject for microscopic examination.

**bipedism:** The erect posture characteristic of Man which is representative of a highly developed musculoskeletal and proprioceptive nervous system.

**bizarre:** Of odd or irregular shape, as the duodenal bulb in chronic ulcer.

**bleb:** A small air cyst or blister.

**block vertebra:** (*see* vertebra)

**bone:**

   **absorption:** Evidence of demineralization of bone manifested by increased radiolucency.

   **age:** The degree of maturation of growth of bones as shown by comparison of epiphyses with tabulated standard.

   **cancellated:** The soft, spongy portion, usually ends of long bones, having a lattice-like structure.

   **chalky:** This is a rare condition of unknown cause characterized by excessive calcium deposit and can be diagnosed by x-ray examination.

   **demineralization of:** Loss of calcium and phosphorus salts by excessive excretion and absorption.

   **erosion:** Evidence of beginning destruction, as of the surface of a bone.

   **innominate:** The large, irregular pelvic bones comprised of the ilium, ischium and pubis.

   **limbus:** An ununited vertebral ring epiphysis. It is visualized as a separate triangular ossicle most commonly at the anterosuperior aspect of the vertebral body on a lateral roentgen view.

   **supernumerary:** Greater number of bones than normal; extra bones.

   **sutural:** These are supernumerary or wormian bones found principally in the lambdoid suture and occasionally in the coronal and sagittal sutures.

**bow sign:** A "bow-like" line appearing below the base of the sacrum on the anteroposterior projection which is indicative of spondylolisthesis of the fifth lumbar vertebra. The bow-line is actually the anteroinferior aspect of the body of L5 which has moved anteriorly down the base of the sacrum.

**Bucky diaphragm:** Invented in 1909 by Dr. Gustav Bucky. It is an ingenious piece of roentgenographic apparatus consisting of a grid of parallel strips of lead arranged on the radius of curvature of a cylinder whose center is at the focal spot of the x-ray tube. The purpose of this is to reduce the effects of scattered radiation.

**butterfly vertebra:** (*see* vertebra)

**calcarea:** Lime or calcium, usually as a deposit (as in peritendinitis calcarea)

**calcareous:** Of the nature of lime; chalky.

**calcific:** Lime or made of lime:

**calcification:** The laying down of calcium salts in a tissue.

**calcinosis:** Deposit of calcium salts in soft tissues in locations where they are not normally found.

**calcium salts:** Chiefly calcium phosphate and calcium carbonate which are deposited in bony structures.

**calculus:** Commonly called "stones." Any abnormal concretion within the animal body, and usually composed of mineral salts.

**callus formation:** Development of new bone with calcium depositions, uniting fragments of a fracture.

**cancellated bone:** (*see* bone)

**cardiothoracic ratio:** Refers to the relation of the measurement of the greatest transverse diameter of the heart to the intrathoracic measurement. This is also described as Groedel's index.

**caudad:** Toward the tail or away from the head.

**cephalad:** Toward the head.

**cephalic indices:** These are percentage relationships of the breadth of the skull to the length of the skull, and determine whether a skull is brachycephalic, dolichocephalic or mesocephalic.

**cervical rib:** Riblike formation extending from the seventh cervical transverse processes, occasionally the sixth cervical transverse processes, which develop from independent ossification centers. Differentiated from abnormally long transverse processes by the appearance of an articulation.

**chalky:** The quality of a radiograph which presents an extreme degree of contrast between the highlights and shadows.

**chalky bone:** (*see* bone)

**Chamberlain's line:** (*see* line)

**Chamberlain's technique:** A roentgenologic procedure to ascertain mobility of the symphysis pubis by making exposures first in the neutral standing position and then with a block placed alternately under each foot. Normal movement is 0–0.5 mm in the male and 0–1.5 mm in the female.

**chemical fog:** A blurred appearance of the radiograph produced by contaminated developer or other chemicals, not by light or x-rays.

**chip fracture:** (*see* fracture)

**cineradiography:** Recording serial cineflurographic studies as a record on moving picture film, either 16- or 35-mm size.

**cleft vertebra:** (*see* vertebra)

**closed fracture:** (*see* fracture)

**Cobb's scoliosis measurement:** (*see* scoliosis)

**Codman's triangle:** A subperiosteal point of reactive bone formation caused by pressure of a tumor within bone elevating the periosteum and forming an angle with the normal periosteum of the shaft of the bone.

**collimation:** Restriction of a beam, as in x-rays, by square or rectangular diaphragming or by use of cone or cylinder.

**comparison film:** One made of the opposite side of the body of the part in question, especially where epiphyses of bones are involved, so that a comparison with the affected side may be made.

**compensating filter:** A filter of aluminum or plastic x-ray opaque material which is interposed between the x-ray tube and patient so as to shield less dense areas, and thereby produce a more uniform quality in the radiography.

**compression band:** A broad band of heavy cloth or similar material used to immobilize, and/or decrease thickness of, a part during x-ray examination.

**condensation:** This refers to an abnormal deposit of bony elements, as at the site of inflammation.

**cone:** A metallic tubular extension placed between the x-ray beam and the patient to the limit the field of examination to that of the structures desired and to aid in the proper centering of the rays; an antiquated x-ray beam collimation device.

**contralateral:** On the opposite side, as distinguished from ipsilateral, on the same side.

**contrast:** The difference in density between the highlights and shadows seen in a roentgenogram. The ratio of light intensity between the brightest and darkest portions of an image.

**contrast medium:** Various forms of radiopaque substances used to delineate anatomical structures roentgenographically. Barium sulfate is commonly used to opacify the GI tract. Telepaque or Chologrfin is given by mouth to opacify the gall bladder and ducts; Conray or Renografin I.V. to delineate the kidneys, ureters, and bladder or directly into blood vessels for angiography.

**coronal plane:** (*see* plane)

**cortex, articular:** The end of a long bone over which the articular cartilage extends.

**cortical atrophy:** Thinning of the boney cortex due to systemic or local disease.

**coxa valga:** Curvature of the neck of the femur causing abduction of the femora and bowlegs.

**coxa vara:** A deformity produced by decrease in angle made by the head and neck of the femur with the shaft. Normally it should be 120° but in coxa vara it may be 80–90°. It occurs in rickets or may be due to bone injury.

**craniosacral mechanism:** A term used by W. G. Sutherland, D.O., to describe the synchronous movement of the sacral base with the cranial base. This synchrony is accomplished by the attachment of the dural tube to the foramen magnum and sacral canal, and is probably aided by cerebrospinal fluid fluctuation. It is thought that the foramen magnum moves forward and upward during flexion of the splenobasilar articulation, which, through the dural tube, pulls the sacral base superior and posterior around a transverse axis at this articular process posterior to the canal through the second sacral segment.

**decubitis:** This term means that the patient is lying horizontally, either face up or face down. Roentgenograms made with the patient lying in this position will be, therefore, either AP or PA with respect to the x-ray tube. A position in roentgenography in which the patient is recumbent. The words ventral, dorsal or lateral are employed in conjunction to describe the particular recumbent position and the x-ray beam is directed "cross-table". Example: left lateral decubitus implies the patient is positioned left side down.

**degenerative:** Pertaining to the change of tissue to a lower or less functionally active form.

**degenerative spondylosis deformans:** (*see* spondylosis deformans)

**demarcated:** Sharply defined or well and distinctly separated from associated structures; marked by bounds.

**demineralization of bone:** (*see* bone)

**densities:** Referring to multiple radiopaque shadows within a structure, such as lung, brain or other organs.

**density:** Compactness of the structure of a substance, or darkness or lightness of film image.

**decreased:** A roentgenographic term used to denote a part relatively more permeable to x-rays.

**increased:** A roentgenographic term used to denote less permeability to x-rays, hence producing a white shadow on the x-ray film or one of less brightness on the fluoroscopic screen.

**deossification:** This refers to loss of mineral substance of a bone, also spoken of as demineralization.

**depressed fracture:** (*see* fracture)

**derangement:** Disordered function of structure.

**developmental:** Something which occurs during development of an individual.

**diaphysis:** The shaft of a long bone, as distinguished from the ends of epiphysis.

**diarthrodial:** A synovial line articulation which characteristically has relatively free movement.

**differential diagnosis:** Consideration of a number of possible diagnoses to explain presenting signs and symptoms. Such diagnoses are usually listed by the examiner in the order of those most likely to be present to those considered least likely to be present.

**discogenic disease:** Progressive degenerative intervertebral disk thinning.

**discography:** Injection of air or aqueous contrast medium into an intervertebral disk in order to show the presence of herniation of the nucleus pulposus.

**discopathy:** Degenerative or infectious disk thinning with reactive changes of the vertebral body articular surfaces and margins.

**discrete:** Well defined and clear-cut in appearance. Lesions which are not blended together.

**disk deficiency:** A congenital lack of disk material representing a manifestation of spinal transitionalization.

**disk protrusion:** Bulging of the annulus and protrusion of the nucleus pulposus through the endplates into the vertebral bodies. Also called disk pulsion.

**disseminated:** Scattered areas or points of involvement.

**distortion:** Variation from normal contour; misshapen appearance of the radiographic image, as from motion.

**divergence:** Radiating outward from any point source of radiation.

**dorsal:** Back or posterior, as opposed to ventral or anterior.

**dose:** The word "dose" in metric (SI) measurement connotes the disposition of energy per unit mass of absorber and replaces the term "absorbed dose." The unit is the rad, defined as 100 ergs/g or 0.01 J/kg.

**air:** X-ray or $\gamma$-ray dose expressed in roentgens delivered at a point in free air. In radiologic practice it consists of the radiation of the useful beam and that scattered from surrounding air.

**cumulative:** The total dose resulting from repeated exposures to radiation of the same region or of the whole body.

**erythema:** Amount of x-rays applied to the skin which will cause reddening in 7–10 days. This dose varies with quality of the radiation.

**permissible:** The amount of radiation which may be received by an individual within a specific period with expectation of no significantly harmful result to himself. That amount of radiation which may be received by an individual in a certain period of time without harmful results ensuing. Latest recommendation (1956) by the International Commission on Radiation Units, was recommended as no more than 0.1 R (100 mR) measured in air, per week.

**skin:** Dose of radiation measured on the skin, either in diagnosis or therapy, and representing the sum of the air dose and backscatter, measured at the center of the radiation field.

**double-focus tube:** A tube having two focal spots; one, small for greater detail; the other, broad to permit greater energy to be applied to the tube.

**dysarthria:** Term used to describe a speech disorder; sometimes misused to denote biomechanical irregularity of a vertebral motor unit.

**eburnation:** A dense sclerotic change of bone commonly noted at joint interfaces and margins as a result of increased or abnormal weight-bearing stresses associated with loss of articular cartilage.

**encroachment:** The invasion of tissue into the confines of another tissue; as "encroachment" of the body of a vertebra into the confines of the intervertebral foraminal contents.

**endosteum:** The fibrous lining of the medullary cavity of the bones.

**endplate:** The bony cortex on the superior and inferior surfaces of each vertebral centra body.

**enostosis:** A bony tumor within a bone resembling a dense bone island.

**epiphyseal:** Pertaining to or of the nature of an epiphysis. Also, epiphyseal ring or line.

**epiphyseal separation:** Abnormal separation of the epiphysis from the shaft, usually from injury (trauma).

**epiphyseolysis:** Disruption or absorption of an epiphysis of bone. Slipping or loosening of an epiphysis from the shaft of a bone.

**epiphysis:** The portion of a long bone developed from a separate center of ossification distinct from that of the diaphysis from which it is separated by a layer of cartilage.

**erosion:** The destruction or wearing away of bone or other tissues due to localized action of infectious, malignant or degenerative processes.

**exostosis:** An outgrowth of bone.

**extension:** Straightening of a curve or angle; bending movement that increases a curve or internal angle.

**craniosacral:** Anterior movement of the sacral base around a transverse axis in relation to the ilia, occurring during sphenobasilar extension.

**sacral:** Posterior movement of the base of the sacrum in relation to the ilia.

**facet:** A small, smooth area, or face, on a bone or other hard surface.

**articular:** Small rounded articulation surfaces of vertebrae.

**facet asymmetry:** Vertebral structure in which the orientation of the facets is not anatomically bilaterally comparable.

**facet symmetry:** Describes the structure of a vertebra in which the facets are anatomically bilaterally comparable.

**Ferguson's angle:** (*see* Angle)

**Fergusons' line:** (*see* line)

**FFD:** (*see* focal-film distance)

**flattening:** Spoken of as flattening of an intervertebral disk or the body of a vertebra. This may also describe change in contour of a surface.

**fleck formation (fleck sign):** This refers to a collection of barium or other opaque substance within the crater of an ulcer which may remain after the main portion of the opaque medium has passed from stomach or duodenum. Same as "barium fleck."

**Focal-film distance (FFD):** Focus of x-ray tube or target to the film.

**fog:** Hazy appearance of a radiograph due to exposure to light or x-rays, or subjection to unusual chemical action.

**fracture:**

**chip:** A small fracture where only a fragment or piece of cortex has been separated from the main body of the bone.

**closed:** A fracture in which the bone fragments are not protruding through the soft tissue structures. Same as a "simple fracture." This is the opposite of a compound fracture.

**complete:** A fracture which extends completely through the bone.

**compound:** A fracture of bone which penetrates the skin or communicates with the outside air.

**compression:** Usually seen in the mid-thoracic vertebrae following extreme or sudden flexion or involving the outer or inner table (or both) of the skull from external violence.

**depressed:** The fracture of a flat bone in which one edge of the bone fragment is depressed below the other as in skull fracture.

**diastatic:** Separation of bones as at a suture.

**greenstick:** An incomplete fracture with one side broken and other side of the bone intact.

**incomplete:** A fracture which does not extend completely through a bone.

**insufficiency:** A stress or march fracture.

**pseudo-:** An apparent, but not actual, fracture; a false fracture.

**Shoveler's:** (Clay Shoveler's fracture): Fracture of the C7 spinous by a lifting action, as in shoveling heavy clay, resulting in an avulsion fracture by muscle action.

**simple:** Having no complicating features; a fracture not connected with the outside air. Same as "closed fracture."

**spontaneous:** One occurring with little or no evidence of trauma and usually secondary to pathological fracture.

**stress:** This fracture occurs at site of maximal strain in bone, usually in connection with unaccustomed activity.

**union of:** Growing together of two ends of a fractured bone with callus formation.

**fusion:** Union of two parts, by development, disease process or operative intervention.

**gibbus:** A sharp dorsal kyphotic angulation commonly associated with infective spondylitis, especially Pott's disease.

**deformity:** This is a posterior angulation of the vertebral column similar to a kyphos but without definite disturbance in the line of weight bearing.

**gravitational line:** Viewing the patient from the side, an imaginary line in a coronal plane which, in the theoretical ideal posture, starts at the external auditory canal, passes through the lateral head of the humerus at the tip of the shoulder, across the greater trochanter, the lateral condyle of the knee, and slightly anterior to the lateral malleolus. If this were a plane through the body, it would intersect the middle of the third lumbar vertebra and the anterior one-third of the sacrum. It is used to evaluate the AP curves of the spine.

**greenstick fracture:** (*see* fracture)

**gynecoid pelvis:** Female-type pelvis.

**half-valve layer:** Used in radiation physics and therapy as an indication of the average penetrability of the beam of x-rays coming from an x-ray tube; its value is determined by finding the thickness of a given filter, such as aluminum or copper, which will reduce the ionizing effect of the primary x-ray beam to one-half of its value. The HVL is a measure of the "hardness" or penetrating ability of radiation; the thickness of any given absorber that will reduce the intensity of a beam of radiation to one-half its initial value.

**"hard" radiation:** (*see* radiation)

**hemivertebra:** A half-vertebra resulting from inadequate genetic control or other developmental aberration. Commonly, the hemivertebra is noted to be united with the segment next caudad.

**homeostasis:** (*a*) Maintenance of static or constant conditions in the internal environment. (*b*) The level of well being of an individual maintained by internal physiologic harmony. It is the result of a relatively stable state or equilibrium among the interdependent body functions.

**hyperimbrication:** Excessive overlapping.

**hyperlucency:** Darker appearance of parts more easily penetrated by x-rays on x-ray film as compared with other denser structures.

**hypermotility:** Increased movement of a part.

**hyperostosis:** Excessive production of bone.

**hyperplastic:** Associated with an overgrowth of tissue.

**hypersthenia:** High position of an organ such as the stomach.

**hypertonic:** Having more than normal muscular tone; also an increase of osmotic pressure.

**hypertonicity:** Excessive contraction or tonus, as of the stomach or bowel.

**hypertrabeculation:** Excessive number of, or increased density in, the appearance of the tiny partitions of bone usually seen near the metaphyses, in response to chronic inflammatory disease and/or tumor.

**hypertrophic:** Inflammation of a joint associated with overgrowth of bone at the joint margin.

**hypocondylar arch:** A characteristic manifestation of occipital vertebrae. When present, it is located anterior to the foramen magnum and may be partially or completely fused. Frequently it may bear a "third condyle" for articulation with the odontoid.

**hypoplasia:** Incomplete or inadequate development of a tissue as a result of a failure during the early blastemal stage of development. Such a deformity is usually reflected in weakness or instability of the part. Adjacent tissues may be overdeveloped in compensation.

**hyposthenic:** Having less than normal tone or strength or referring to low position of an organ, as of the stomach.

**ileus, adynamic:** Ballooning of the small and large intestine by gas, usually in response to painful somatic stimuli, to be distinguished from dynamic or mechanical ileus in which there is an actual obstructive lesion producing distention of the bowel.

**iliosacral motion:** Motion of the ilia on a transverse axis of the sacrum, as occurs in walking. Considered to be primarily influenced by the attachments and movements of the pelvis, hips and lower extremities.

**imbrication:** Over-riding or over lapping of one structure or another. Often used to describe the characteristic mechanical changes of a telescoping nature at the posterior facets after disk thinning has occurred.

**incomplete fracture:** (*see* fracture)

**infiltrating:** Invasion of the tissue or organ as by a neoplastic or infectious process.

**infraction:** An incomplete fracture of a bone without displacement of the fragments.

**inherent filtration:** The glass envelope of an x-ray tube through which x-rays must pass is described as the inherent filter to be distinguished from the added primary and secondary filters.

**inion:** A prominence on the external surface of the occipital bone; the external occipital protuberance.

**innominate bones:** (*see* bone)

**insufficiency fracture:** (*see* fracture)

**interarticular:** Between joints.

**interarticular ossicle:** (*see* ossicle)

**interarticularis pars:** The portion of the neural arch, or isthmus, that connects the superior and the inferior articular processes of a vertebra. Translated as the part between.

**intercalary:** Inserted between two others.

**intercalary ossicle:** (*see* ossicle)

**interchondral:** Between cartilages.

**interface:** A boundary separating two substances. The plane or surface forming the boundary of two adjacent media of different impedances.

**interosseous:** Space between two bones as the interosseous membrane between the radius and ulna.

**interpedicular distance:** This is a gradually varying distance in millimeters between the inner margins of the pedicles as shown on AP radiographs of the thoracic and lumbar vertebrae.

**intersegmental motion:** Designates relative motion taking place between two adjacent vertebral segments or within a vertebral unit (q.v.). Described as the upper vertebral segment moving on the lower.

**interspace:** Interval between two parts, such as between ribs.

**interstitial:** Relating to the spaces or interstices in any structure.

**intertrochanteric:** A fracture extending between the trochanters of the upper end of the femur.

**intervertebral:** Situated between two adjacent vertebrae as the cartilaginous disk.

**intra-articular:** Within a joint.

**intracapsular:** Refers to a process, usually inflammatory, within the soft tissue borders of a joint.

**intramedullary:** Within the central portion or medullar cavity of a bone.

**intramural:** Pertaining to a location within the wall of a structure.

**intraspinal:** Within the spinal canal.

**involucrum:** A covering or sheath, such as contains the sequestrum of a necrotic bone.

**ipsolateral:** On the same side. As distinguished from contralateral, on the opposite side.

**isthmus:** The pars interarticularis connecting the superior and inferior articular processes of a vertebra; a narrow passage or band connecting cavities or parts. The part between.

**joint:**

   **Luschka's:** Synovially lined joint cavities in the region of the posterolateral borders of the lower five segments.

   **uncovertebral, of Luschka:** These are amphiarthrodial joints beginning between C2 and C3 and extending to the level of C6–C7, formed between the uncus of the lower vertebrae and the lateral inferior surfaces of the vertebrae above, forming posterolateral articulations between the cervical vertebrae referred to as Luschka's joints, or sometimes the intervertebral joints of Luschka.

**juxta-articular:**   Near a joint.

**kinesthesia:**   The sense by which muscular motion, weight, position, etc., are perceived.

**kinetics:**   The body of knowledge that deals with the effects of forces that produce or modify body motion.

**kissing impingement:**   Weight-bearing interspinous pseudoarthrosis (Baastrup's disease). Such impaction and degenerative deformity is principally the result of a hyperlordotic attitude.

**Klippel-Feil deformity:**   A congenital abnormality of the cervical spine characterized by irregularities of the lamina and spinous process, fusion of the vertebra, shortening of the neck, cervical ribs, etc.

**krinkl mark:**   A crescentic mark on an x-ray film produced by the film being wrinkled before exposure.

**KUB film:**   An abbreviation indicating a plain radiograph of the abdomen to the kidneys, ureters and urinary bladder (KUB).

**Kümmell's disease:**   A delayed, compressive type of vertebral deformity subsequent to trauma. The initial radiograph reveals no change in the bony architecture. Later, hyperemia causes osteoporosis and demineralization. Collapse and compression result; callus formation ensues. Disk changes may occur later.

**kypholordosis:**   Double curve with a kyphosis and lordosis appearing where only a lordosis should be present. Most commonly found in the neck associated with a sway back.

**kyphoscoliosis:**   Combined angular and lateral spinal curvature, commonly seen in conjunction with the Klippel-Feil deformity and the Sprengel deformity.

**kyphosis:**   A spinal curvature with a dorsally directed convexity; the usual connotation is that of an abnormal or excessive curve.

**kyphotic:**   Pertaining to, or characterized by, hyphosis.

**lacuna:**   A depression in a bone as a defect or gap.

**lamina:**   The flattened part of either side of the arch of a vertebra; bony covering on a neural arch.

**laminagram:**   A radiograph made with only one plane or lamina of a part in clear focus. (cf. planigram, tomogram, stratigram, ordogram, and body section radiography).

**LAO:**   Left anterior oblique, referring to a position of the part either with reference to the x-ray tube or the film, at discretion of the radiologist. Usually implies that the left shoulder is touching the cassette. With reference to the fluoroscopic screen, taken to mean the left shoulder turned forward.

**latent image:**   The invisible image produced on photographic or x-ray film by the action of light or x-rays, before development.

**lateral decubitus:**   A position in which the patient lies on either side and the x-ray beam is directed in a posteroanterior or an anteroposterior direction across the table, especially for the purpose of demonstrating change in fluid level.

**lateral flexed:**   A term used to describe a position of a vertebral body. Defined as the movement of a point on the anterosuperior aspect of the vertebral body about an anteroposterior axis in a coronal plane.

**lateral oblique:**   A projection in which a part is turned from a true lateral position a varying number of degrees in order to more clearly outline a particular structure or organ.

**lateral recumbent:** A position in which the patient is supine or prone and the x-ray beam is directed horizontally across the table at right angles to the x-ray film. This position is utilized in myelography and in cases of intestinal obstruction.

**latitude:** The range of exposure of an x-ray film permissible for a good diagnostic result.

**lead apron:** A lead-impregnated rubber apron to protect personnel working in x-ray exposure room.

**lead equivalent:** The thickness of lead required to affect the same reduction in radiation dose rate under specified conditions as the material in question.

**lead glass:** Lead-impregnated glass used in windows of control booths and in protective shields on fluoroscopic screens to protect radiologists and their technical assistants from scattered radiation.

**lead gloves:** Leather protective gloves made by special process for impregnating the material with lead equivalent to at least 0.3 mm, used during fluoroscopy for handling patient.

**leg deficiency:**

 **anatomical;** acutal deficiency due to lack of development, trauma or pathology.

 **physiological:** a biomechanical "retraction" of the leg in the reclining position due to innominate disrelationship or muscle contraction.

 **projectional:** a radiographic impression on the AP full spine view which simulates a leg deficiency due to the pelvis being torsioned relative to the film.

**lesion:** A diseased structure, morbid change, injury, or wound.

**ligamentum nuchae ossification:** This may occasionally be posterior to the fifth and sixth cervical spinous processes.

**limbus:** The border or edge of a part.

**limbus bone:** (*see* bone, limbus)

**line:**

 **Chamberlain's:** A line drawn from the hard palate to the posterior aspect of the foramen magnum on the lateral cervical projection should normally pass above the odontoid process of axis. Passage of the line through the odontoid process indicates possible basilar invagination.

**Ferguson's:** A vertical line from the center of the body of L3 on the lateral lumbar roentgenograph should fall approximately at the anterior third of the sacral base.

**McGregor's:** A line drawn on true lateral skull roentgenograms from the hard palate to the external aspect of the squamous occipital cortex. The dens should be situated 1.32–2.62 mm below this line. Should the dens reside above such a line, suspicion is directed towards the possibility of basilar invagination.

**midheel:** A vertical line used as a reference in standing AP x-rays, passing equidistant between the heels.

**midmalliolar:** A vertical line passing through the lateral malleolus, used as a point of reference in standing lateral x-rays.

**Shenton's:** The curved line representing the relationship between the undersurface of the neck of the femur and the upper margin of the obturator foramen.

**Skinner's:** A horizontal line is drawn from the top of the greater trochanter of the femur, as seen in the AP view, to the top of the obturator foramen of the pelvis in a question of fracture through the neck of the femur. A perpendicular line is dropped through the axis of the shaft of the femur to the horizontal line. In fractures with shortening of the femur, the greater trochanter will be displaced above this line.

**linear:** Like a line, such as a linear fracture. Also a linear shadow.

**lipping:** This term refers to small bony excrescences or osteophytes on the margins of the articular surfaces of bone in degenerative arthritis. Lipping is the earliest manifestation of this degenerative change.

**lith-:**  A combining form meaning stones or calculi, as broncholiths.

**lithiasis:**  A combining form meaning the presence of calculi or stones, as in methrolithiasis or cholelithiasis.

**longitudinal:**  A term used to describe a fracture extending along the long axis of a bone. In the long axis of the body or an organ.

**lordosis:**  The exaggerated (or pathologic) posterior concavity in the anteroposterior curvature of the lumbar and cervical spine.

**lordosis posture:**  Frequently called the swayback posture, this attitude may compensate for a dorsal kyphosis or postural fatigue. It may help to balance an enlarged abdomen. Shearing stresses, facet imbrication, joint capsule tension, and spinous impingement are common subsequent changes.

**lordotic:**  Pertaining to, or characterized by, lordosis.

**lordotic curvature:**  Having a convex curvature anterior to a vertical line.

**lordotic position:**  Usually an AP view of the chest of apices of lungs, made with the patient leaning backward.

**lumbarization:**  A congenital attempt at forming an additional lumbar-like segment from the superosacral segment. Such a transitionalization permits a greater anteroposterior movement and tends to reduce the tension on the posterior aspect of the intervertebral disks.

**lumbar ribs:**  Ribs arising from lumbar vertebrae.

**lumbosacral instability:**  Predisposition to low back disorders due to biomechanical deviations or maldevelopment.

**Luschka's joint:**  (*see* joint)

**luxation:**  Abnormal slipping of one structure on another at a joint or place of natural division.

**lysis:**  A combining form meaning breaking down or dissolution.

**malformation:**  Imperfect development of a part, usually congenital.

**malposition:**  This term usually refers to the fragments of a fracture if they are in defective or abnormal position.

**malunion:**  Healing of a fracture in an undesirable position.

**manipulation:**  Therapeutic application of manual force.

**Martin's basilar angle:**  (*see* angle)

**McGregor's line:**  (*see* line)

**metaphysis:**  The part of a long bone between the epiphyseal plate and the diaphysis.

**midheel line:**  (*see* line)

**midmalliolar line:**  (*see* line)

**motion:**  An act or process of changing position. An act of moving the body or its parts.

  **active:**  Movement produced voluntarily by the patient.

  **inherent:**  That spontaneous motion of every cell, organ, system, and their component units within the body.

  **passive:**  Motion induced by the operator while the patient remains passive or relaxed.

  **physiologic:**  Normal changes in the position of articulating surfaces taking place within a joint or region.

  **translatory:**  Uniform motion in one direction (in a straight line) without rotation. Used in describing the physiologic straight line motion of vertebrae in a horizontal plane or of other structures along a plane passing between two opposing structural surfaces.

**mottling:**  Irregular; of uneven density.

**MPD:**  Maximum dose of radiation which may be permitted for persons working with ionizing radiations.

**neoplastic:**  Of, or pertaining to, a new growth, tumor.

**neutral:**  The point of balance of an articular surface from which all the motions physiologic to that articulation may take place. Substitute term for easy normal in relation to physiologic motion of the spine.

**niche:** A crater or hole as seen in an ulcer eroding a surface. In a roentgenographic study where a hollow viscus is filled with opaque medium, the niche projected beyond the normal lumen of the organ thus indicating excavation as by a crater.

**nidus:** A cluster, nestlike in structure; a focus of infection; a nucleus or origin of a nerve. Also the radiopaque center of an osteoid osteoma.

**nonsegmentation:** A growth deficiency and synostosis of vertebral segments resulting from a failure of proper segmentation of the mesodermal tissues. Commonly used synonyms are congenital or developmental block vertebra.

**opaque:** Impenetrable by light or x-rays of diagnostic quality range.

**orthodysarthria:** Functional inadequacy of an articulation characterized by fixation, hypomobility, hypermobility or aberrant movement. The biomechanical aspect of a chiropractic subluxation syndrome.

**os odontoideum:** Congenital nonunion of the odontoid process with the body of the axis. The upper surface of the axis usually presents a cone-shaped formation which serves as a pivot for rotation. The separate odontoid may lie within the foramen magnum or be attached to the anterior arch of the atlas.

**ossicle:**

**interarticular:** a separate bony formation within the confines of a diarthrodial joint. In contradistinction to a joint mouse, the interarticular ossicle is more specifically an ununited secondary ossification center, which has become avulsed and malpositioned.

**intercalary:** Irregularly shaped, isolated osseous formations in the anterior peripheral portion of the intervertebral disk, between two apposing vertebrae. They are closely associated with degenerative changes in the annular tissue. Most probably they are related to penetrating vascular granulation tissue and bone-forming elements.

**ossiculum terminali:** An anomalous structure occurring as a separate ossicle, originated from an notochordal remnant in the terminal ligament of the odontoid process. Normally, this unites with the dens by 6 yr of age. When fusion fails, it persists as a separate triangular bony segment associated with shortening and blunting of the dens. It must be differentiated from a third condyle.

**ossification:** The formation of bone or of a bony substance.

**secondary, center:** small epiphyseal growth centers located at the tips of the spinous, transverse, articular, and mammillary processes, as well as the vertebral surfaces, are seen early in the second decade. They become united between the ages of 16–21 yr. Their primary importance lies in their differentiation from avulsion type fractures. They commonly fail to unite, remaining as separate ossicles; rarely, they may form interarticular ossicles.

**osteoblastic:** Bone forming. Formation of new bone, as by osteoblasts.

**osteoclastic:** Bone destroying.

**osteogenic:** Bone forming.

**osteolysis:** Softening and destruction of bone.

**osteolytic:** Of, or pertaining to, bone softening or destruction, e.g. by a metastasis from breast or thyroid carcinoma.

**osteophyte:** A bony excrescence or outgrowth, usually branched in shape; a bony spur on the articular margins.

**osteophytosis:** An abnormal marginal bony protuberance as a result of excessive and abnormal ligamentous stresses at periosteal attachments.

**osteoporosis:** Diminished bone tissue ascribed to a disorder of metabolism characterized by failure of osteoblasts to lay down adequate bone matrix (osteoid). Thus, the bones appear more radiolucent and are frail and fragile. There is a secondary diffuse and generalized demineralization with an increased density at the bony periphery. Normal contour is maintained in the early stages but later, deformity may be expected. Serum calcium and phosphorus levels, as well as alkaline phosphatase, usually remain within the limit of normal.

**circumscripta:** A form of early osteitis deformans (Paget's disease) of the skull and where there is a confluent maplike resorption of bone.

**of disuse:** Increased radiability of bone secondary to disuse and/or immobilization.

**osteosclerosis:** Increased bone density of radiopacity. This may be due to increased calcium deposition within the bone, as in osteopetrosis, or may be due to increased bone formation in the periosteum on the external portion of the bony cortex, or endosteal, causing narrowing of the marrow cavity or thickening of the compact bone itself.

**overpenetration:** Too great penetration (kilovoltage) used in radiography, thus producing a radiograph that is too dense and lacking contrast.

**PA:** (*see* posteroanterior)

**palpation:** The application of variable manual pressure through the surface of the body for the purpose of determining the shape, size, consistency, position, inherent mobility, and health of the tissues beneath.

**palpatory diagnosis:** a term used by osteopathic physicians to denote the process of palpating the patient to evaluate the neuromusculoskeletal and visceral systems.

**palpatory skills:** The sensory skills used in performing palpatory diagnosis and osteopathic manipulative therapy.

**paraoccipital process:** (*see* process)

**paraspinal:** Usually a swelling or tumor mass along the side of the vertebral column, commonly seen in tuberculous disease of the vertebrae.

**paravertebral:** Situated adjacent to a vertebra or the vertebral column such

as a soft tissue mass, tumor or calcification.

**pars interarticularis:** An osseous region located immediately below the superior articular facets of lumbar vertebrae at the superolateral corner of the laminae. A defect or interruption in the normal bony continuity of this region of the neural arch is the usual cause of true spondylolisthesis.

**part thickness:** A measurement usually made with a metal caliper for determining kilovoltage settings relative to centimeter thickness of a part being examined.

**pathogenic:** Capable of producing disease.

**pathognomonic:** Indicative of a disease, especially of one or more of its characteristic symptoms.

**pedicle erosion:** A thinning, demineralization or disappearance of a pedicle from pressure of a tumor, frequently a neurogenic tumor of the spinal canal, and visible on plain AP roentgenograms of the thoracic or lumbar vertebrae.

**pelvic rotation:** Movement of the entire pelvis in a relatively horizontal plane on the base of the sacrum.

**pelvic sideshift:** Deviation of the pelvis to the right or left of the central vertical axis, usually observed in the standing position.

**pelvic tilt:** Pelvic rotation about a transverse (horizontal) axis (forward or backward tilt) or about an anteroposterior axis (right or left side tilt).

**penetration:** The ability of radiation to extend down into, and go through, substances; as the penetration of x-rays. The voltage factor in radiography.

**penumbra:** Partial shadow about the umbra or true shadow of an object whether produced by light or x-rays. In radiography, it is determined by the size of the focal spot, the focus-film distance and the object-film distance.

**periarticular:** Surrounding a joint.

**periosteal proliferation:** Bone formation in the periosteum or beneath it which may be caused by trauma, toxic agents like phosphorus, chronic pulmonary and cardiac ailments, chronic inflammatory changes as in syphilis, subperiosteal hemorrhage, or tumor. When sharply localized, bone spicules are formed which are termed osteophytes, or larger ones, exostosis.

**periostitis:** Inflammation of the covering of a bone.

**peritendinitis calcarea:** Calcification in or around a tendon sheath. (Frequently, and incorrectly, often referred to as "bursitis").

**permissible dose:** *see* dose

**photographic effect:** The effect of light or x-rays on a photographic emulsion, as in radiography.

**plane:** A flat surface determined by the position of three points in space. Any of a number of imaginary surfaces passing through the body and dividing it into segments.

  **coronal:** Frontal plane.

  **frontal:** A plane passing longitudinally through the body from one side to the other, and dividing the body into anterior and posterior portions.

  **saggital:** A plane passing longitudinally through the body from front to back and dividing it into right and left portions. The median, or midsagittal, plane divides the body into approximately equal right and left portions.

  **transverse:** A plane passing horizontally through the body perpendicular to the sagittal and frontal planes, dividing the body into upper and lower portions.

**platybasia:** Flattening and widening of the base of the skull with an exaggeration of Martin's basilar angle. It is not to be confused with, or used synonymously with, basilar invagination.

**poker spine:** Straight like a poker in rheumatoid arthritis of the vertebral column.

**polyarthritis:** Arthritis of many joints.

**polyarticular:** Involving many joints.

**polyostotic:** Multiple bony involvement as in fibrous dysplasia.

**poor visualization:** Term used in cholecystography when the gall bladder is not clearly seen on the roentgenogram following ingestion of opaque medium.

**ponticulus lateralis:** An abnormal bony arch extending from the superior articular surface of the atlas to its transverse process; based on a congenital ligamentous ossification.

**ponticulus posticus:** A similar but more commonly bony arch from the posterior margin of the superior articular surface of the atlas to the upper margin of the posterior arch of the atlas. It represents an ossification of the posterior portion of the atlantooccipital ligament.

**postero-:** A combining form meaning behind.

**posteroanterior:**

  **films:** Roentgenograms made in the PA projection with reference to the x-ray tube; i.e. where the back of the part is directed toward the x-ray tube.

  **projection of the x-rays:** That is, from back to front of the part with respect to the x-ray tube. Opposite of AP projection.

**postural balance:** A condition of optimal distribution of body mass in relation to gravity.

**posture:** Position of the body. The distribution of body mass in relation to gravity.

**prespondylolisthesis:** This condition exists when the patient demonstrates the defects in the isthmi which could lead to a frank spondylolisthesis, but which has not yet developed.

**pressure atrophy:** Atrophy of bony structure from pressure of an abnormal soft structure such as a tumor.

**prevertebral:** In front of, or anterior to, the vertebra.

**principal ray:** The central ray coming from the target of an x-ray tube perpendicular to its long axis; these rays show the least divergence and, therefore, produce the least distortion in roentgenography.

**process:**

    **articular:** Processes of bone (as of the vertebrae) bearing articular surfaces or facets.

    **paraoccipital:** An abnormal congenital ligamentous ossification with observable bony connection between the occiput and the first transverse process.

    **pronation:** In relation to the anatomical position, as applied to the hand, the act of turning the hand palmar surface backward (medial rotation). Applied to the foot, a combination of eversion and abduction movements taking place in the tarsal and metatarsal joints, resulting in lowering of the medial margin of the foot.

**prone:** Lying with the ventral surface downward.

**proprioception:** The sensing of motion and position of the body.

**proprioceptor:** Sensory nerve terminals that give information concerning movements and position of the body. They occur chiefly in the muscles, tendons, joints, and labyrinth.

**prosthesis:** An artificial device used as a substitute for a part of the body.

**protrusio acetabuli:** Protrusion of the femoral head through the floor of the acetabulum.

**proximal:** Near to the central portion, or trunk, of the body, as the proximal fragment of a fracture; the fragment nearest the body.

**pseudoarthrosis:** A false joint developing after a fracture that has not united; also a congenital false joint as between a transverse vertebral process and the sacrum.

**pseudofracture:** (*see* fracture)

**pseudospondylolisthesis:** An anterior gravitational displacement of a vertebral segment on its caudad fellow on the basis of changes other than isthmus separation. There may be a deficiency in the size (hypoplasia), or an imperfection in the shape or disposition of the lumbosacral facets. A traumatic event is usually necessary to initiate the anterior deviation.

**quality:** In electricity, pressure represented by the voltage. Also, the degree of "hardness" of an x-ray beam specified by its half-value layer.

**R:** The unit of quantity of roentgen rays; the unit for measuring x-ray exposure.

**R unit of roentgen rays:** The unit of x-ray exposure; see roentgen or R.

**rachischisis:** A posterior vertebral deviation peculiar to the fifth lumbar segment and dependent upon the normal coronal or frontal facet disposition. Any lumbosacral disk thinning allows the fifth lumbar vertebra to settle upon the sacrum and be guided posteriorly by the backward slope of the superior sacral facets.

**rad (radiation absorbed dose):** The radiation energy absorbed by a small volume of tissue, divided by this volume. Its unit is 100 ergs/g, or 0.01 J/kg.

**rad-equivalent man (rem):** (*see* rem)

**radiation:** The projection through space of any form of electromagnetic waves. This may be primary, as that emanating directly from the focal spot of an x-ray tube; or scattered, which is produced by anything in the path of x-rays. The emission and propagation of energy through space or through a material medium in the form of waves; for instance, the emission and propagation of electromagnetic waves, or of sound and elastic waves. The term radiation or radiant energy, when unqualified, usually refers to frequency, as hertzian, infrared, visible (light), ultraviolet x-ray and $\gamma$-ray. By extension, corpuscular emissions, such as $\alpha$- and $\beta$-radiation or rays of mixed or unknown type, as cosmic radiation.

    **burn:** Reaction of skin or mucous membranes to cancericidal doses of radiation. These reactions will vary with the quality and amounts of radiation used, and will usually heal completely within weeks of completion of treatment.

    **"hard":** A term applied to x-radiation of short wave length, having high energy and ability to penetrate deeply. Opposite of "soft" x-rays.

**scattered:** A term used in radiology which refers to secondary radiation produced as radiation is deviated in direction, causing a modification resulting in an increase in wave length.

**"soft":** Long wave length x-rays of low penetrability found as components of relatively low kV (40–80) x-ray beams.

**radiolucent:** Easily penetrable by x-radiation, not radiopaque.

**radiopaque:** Impenetrable to the x-ray or other forms of radiation.

**RAO:** (*see* right anterior oblique)

**rarefaction:** An area of decreased density, hence more radiable.

**reciprocating grid:** A Bucky grid which moves throughout an x-ray exposure and which does not require presetting.

**rectify:** To change from an alternating to an unidirectional current, either by mechanical rectifying apparatus or by valve tubes.

**reflex:** An involuntary nervous system response to a sensory input. The sum total of any particular involuntary activity.

**conditioned:** one that does not occur naturally in the organism or system but that may be developed by regular association of some physiological function with an unrelated outside event. Soon, the physiological function starts whenever the outside event occurs.

**red:** the erythematous reaction of the skin in an area that had been mildly stimulated mechanically (e.g. by palpatory examination). The reflex is greater in duration in an area of acute somatic dysfunction.

**somatosomatic:** localized somatic stimulation producing patterns of reflex response in segmentally related visceral structures.

**viscerosomatic:** localized visceral stimuli producing patterns of reflex response in segmentally related somatic structures.

**viscerovisceral:** localized visceral stimuli producing patterns of reflex response in segmentally related visceral structures. Also called viscerosomatovisceral reflex.

**rem (RAD-equivalent man):** The rad, multiplied by the biological effectiveness of a particular quality of radiation, relative to that of conventional radiation.

**resorption:** Absorption of mineral elements, such as calcium from bone in osteoporosis. The act of soaking up; the removal of an exudate, a blood clot, pus, etc., by absorption.

**retropulsion:** Backward displacement of a part such as intervertebral disk herniation.

**rib, bifid:** A congenital anomaly usually of the third, fourth, or fifth ribs seen in frontal projections of the chest and rib cage, sometimes resembling a cavity because of margination of the lung parenchyma produced by the rib anomaly.

**right anterior oblique:** The RAO position with the right side closest to the film or screen, at a 45° angle.

**right lateral:** A position for x-ray examination with the right side closest to the film or screen, at a 90° angle.

**right lateral decubitus:** A roentgenogram exposed with the patient lying on the right side with the film in front of him and the x-rays directed from back to front producing a PA view.

**right posterior oblique:** A roentgenographic position with right side of the part posterior and nearest to the film at a 45° angle.

**ring epiphysis:** Two secondary centers of ossification at each vertebral body, located at the upper and lower surfaces, are noted by the 16th yr. They allow for the insertion of strong ligamentous structures without interfering with the underlying growth processes. The ring may be absent posteriorly. The rings eventually fuse between years 18–25 and form an elevated rim at the periphery of the vertebral endplates.

**Roentgen, Wilhelm Konrad:** Born

March 27, 1845; Died February 10, 1923. The physicist who discovered x-rays on November 8, 1895, in the Physical Institute of the University of Wurzburg, Germany.

**roentgen:** The roentgen is a special unit of exposure, not of dose; i.e. 1 e.s.u./ 0.001293 g of air or $2.58 \times 10^{-4}$ C/kg. The recommended abbreviation of the roentgen is R, in place of r. This change, adopted with considerable reluctance, brings the ICRU into line with a number of other international bodies concerned with nomenclature, which have agreed that abbreviations for units named after individuals should be capitalized.

  **diagnosis:** That part of the science of roentgenology which uses roentgen rays (x-rays) to make a diagnosis.

**roentgenogram:** A film transparency recording in its emulsion varying densities of a body traversed by x-rays.

**roentgenography:** Use of x-rays in making x-ray films of a part.

**roentgenologist:** A physician who limits his work to the use of x-rays in the diagnosis and treatment of a disease after following a prescribed course of instruction in the specialty.

**roentgenology:** The science which deals with the use of x-rays in examination and treatment of disease.

**rotary:** Having a circular movement around a central axis. Turning or rotation about a central axis as a rotatory scoliosis.

**rotating anode tube:** An x-ray tube in which the target area constantly rotates during exposures, thus preventing overheating and permitting use of higher energy.

**rotoscoliosis:** Lateral deviation of the vertebral column, usually the lumbar vertebrae with, in addition, rotation of several degrees from the central axis. Rotatory twisting of the lumbar vertebrae.

**routine:** An examination done without special indication as, for example, a routine film of the chest in a survey.

**rudimentary:** A part arrested in its development, i.e. rudimentary rib.

**sacralization:** A congenital non-segmentation of the first presacral vertebra. The malformation may be unilateral or bilateral; with total fusion or pseudoarthrosis formation. Articulation may take place at the sacral alae or ilium.

**scattered radiation:** (*see* radiation)

**Scheuermann's disease:** A dystrophy of the early teens wherein the enchondral bone growth of the midthoracic area is restricted. Radiographically, there is characteristically noted some degree of kyphotic deformity, flattening or wedging of the vertebral bodies, undulation of the vertebral endplates, and increased anteroposterior vertebral body diameter and Schmorl's nodes.

**Schmorl's nodes:** An intraspongy herniation of nuclear matrix; usually central in location. It is commonly associated with Scheuermann's disease and traumatic episodes. Some authorities believe there may exist weakened areas in the cartilaginous endplate as the result of vascular channel remnants.

**sclerotic:** Pertaining to, or affected with, sclerosis. Hard.

**scoliosis:** A lateral curvature of the spine. The scolioses are commonly divided into postural, congenital, acquired, and idiopathic varieties.

  **Cobb's measurement of:** Calculation of magnitude of a scoliosis as determined by lines drawn at right angles to the top and bottom vertebrae involved in the lateral curvature.

**segmentation:** The normal process of separation into individual segments during the blastemal stage.

**sesamoid bone:** A bone formed in a tendon; small, flat bone developed in a tendon which moves over a body surface.

**sharply marginated:** A structure or lesion having a definite, clearly outlined border with no tendency to merge with its surroundings.

**shear:** An action or force causing, or tending to cause, two contiguous parts of an articulation, such as the pubic symphysis, to slide relative to each other in a direction parallel to their plane of contact (e.g. symphyseal shear).

**Shenton's line:**   (*see* line)

**Shoveler's fracture:**   (*see* fracture)

**simple fracture:**   (*see* fracture)

**skin dose:**   (*see* dose)

**Skinner's line:**   (*see* line)

**"soft" radiation:**   (*see* radiation)

**soft tissue shadows:**   The record of density of soft tissue as compared with bone shown on the roentgenogram. Breast shadows are shown contrasted against the air in the lungs around them.

**somatology:**   The study of the naturally organized self-sustaining human body.

**spicule:**   A small fragment, as a small spicule of bone.

**spina bifida:**   A congenital defect consisting of failure of fusion of the laminae over the lower vertebral column with herniation of the meninges.

**spina bifida occulta:**   Hidden or obscure spina bifida without herniation of meninges.

**spinogram:**   A myelogram or injection of an opaque medium into the subarachnoid space of the spinal cord.

**spondylitis:**   Inflammation of the spine; arthritis of the spine. In tuberculous, it is known as Pott's disease. Pathologic changes begin in the vertebrae and intervertebral joints.

**spondylizema:**   Downward settlement of a vertebral segment caused by the disintegration of the segment next caudad.

**spondylolisthesis:**   (*also see* pseudospondylolisthesis) Anterior displacement of one vertebral segment on its caudad fellow, usually as the result of a defect in the neutral arch at the pars interarticularis.

**spondylosis:**   Detection of an observable isthmus separation, but without anterior gravitation of the vertebral segment.

**spondylosis deformans:**   Degenerative arthritis of the vertebral column as compared with spondylitis deformans caused by rheumatoid arthritis of the Marie-Strümpell type.

**degenerative:**   Degenerative disorder of the spine characterized by narrowing of the disk spaces, lipping or spurring at the margins of the vertebral bodies and secondary involvements of the posterior facet structures. A common finding in the aged.

**spondylolysis interarticularis:**   A congenital defect or break in the neural arch at the isthmus or pars.

**spontaneous fracture:**   (*see* fracture)

**Sprengel's deformity:**   A developmental deformity due to the failure of the scapula to descend from its embryonic position in the neck to the upper part of the thorax. As a rule, it is rotated so that the inferior angle is nearer to the spine than the superior angle; but the rotation may occur in the opposite direction. Sprengel's deformity is often associated with the Klippel-Feil deformity.

**spur:**   An osteophyte, or lip, or beak, on the articular margin of a projecting bone; a horny outgrowth from the skin.

**stationary anode:**   An x-ray tube in which the target is fixed, compared with a rotating anode tube in which the target constantly turns on a rotor.

**stationary grid:**   A thin wafer grid placed between the cassette and the part to be examined in order to absorb secondary radiation.

**sthenic:**   Strong, active, normal. Eutonic or orthotonic.

**stippled calcification:**   Small flecks or dots of calcium seen without a breast tumor and usually indicating carcinoma. Also refers to flecks or irregular opacities within hilar glands, lung or brain tumors.

**stress fracture:** (*see* fracture)

**subluxation:** (*a*) a partial or incomplete dislocation. (*b*) a restriction of motion of a joint in a position exceeding normal physiologic motion although the anatomic limits have not been limited.

**subperiosteal:** Beneath the periosteum.

**Sudeck's atrophy:** (*see* atrophy)

**superior position:** Higher or above.

**supernumerary bones:** (*see* bone)

**supernumerary vertebra:** (*see* vertebra)

**supine:** Lying with the ventral surface upward.

**sutural bones:** (*see* bone)

**symmetry:** Similarity in corresponding parts or organs on opposite sides of the body.

**symphyseal shear:** Any mechanical action causing or tending to cause the pubic symphysis to slide in a direction parallel to its plane of contact. This is usually in an inferior or superior direction.

**synarthrosis:** The union of two bones without a joint and without the possibility of movement.

**synostosis:** Union or articulation of formerly separate bones by osseous tissue.

**tangential projections:** These are produced by directing the central x-ray beam to the margin or edge of an area under study as, for example, the skull or the rib cage to demonstrate the presence of fracture or fluid.

**target-film distance (TFD):** Distance between anode of an x-ray tube and the x-ray film.

**teleroentgenogram:** A film, usually of the chest, made at a distance of 6 ft.

**tendinitis:** Inflammation of a tendon sheath or tendon. Also used interchangeably, but incorrectly, with bursitis.

**TFD:** (*see* target-film distance)

**thinning:** Spoken of diminished thickness of a part, such as cartilage space or intervertebral disk.

**thoracolumbar:** Comprising the thorax and the lumbar vertebrae, a segment of the vertebral column.

**tomography:** An x-ray apparatus used for making x-ray examinations of layers of tissue in depth, without interference of tissues above or below that level.

**tonus:** The slight continuous contraction of muscle which, in skeletal muscles, aids in the maintenance of posture and in the return of blood of the heart.

**torsion:** (*a*) a motion or state where one end of a part is turned about a longitudinal axis while the opposite end is held fast or turned in the opposite direction. (b) a specific sacral motion.

**trabeculation:** A pattern marked by trabeculae or interlacing cross-bars.

**traction:** A force acting on a longitudinal axis to draw structures apart.

**transitional vertebra:** (*see* vertebra)

**tubercle (or tuberosity):** small, rounded projections on a bone, as the tubercle of the anterosuperior surface of the tibia.

**ultra fine focus tube:** One having a 0.3-mm, or smaller, focal spot which can be used for direct radiographic enlargements because of absence of penumbra effect.

**uncovertebral joints of Luschka:** (*see* joint)

**unilateral:** On one side only.

**union of epiphysis:** The joining of the epiphysis with the shaft, then it ceases to function as a bone-forming structure.

**union of fracture:** (*see* fracture)

**ununited:** Not grown or placed together, as in an ununited fracture.

**useful beam:** A term used in radiology to indicate that part of the primary radiation which passes through a collimating cone or diaphragm.

**ventral:** Of, or pertaining to, the anterior or frontal surface of any structure or part.

**vertebra:** (*also see* prevertebral)

**block:** An abnormally developed vertebral motor unit, characteristically due to developmental anomaly, as opposed to acquired fusion of traumatic arthritis, tuberculosis, etc. Also referred to as congenital nonsegmentation, developmental block vertebra and congenital block vertebra.

**butterfly:** 1. developmental defect in which the vertebral body develops bilaterally in two separate triangular components. The adjacent segments and disks may assume a compensatory configuration. 2. the appearance of a vertebra with two biconcave deformities of the endplates as seen in the AP view. This appearance is due to persistence of a remnant of the fetal notochord.

**cleft:** This is a hemivertebra due to lack of fusion or partial fusion of the right and left halves during embryonic development.

**supernumerary:** An extra vertebral segment.

**transitional:** The first or last vertebra of a spinal region may take on the characteristics of the adjacent region and is then said to be in a state of transitionalization; e.g. sacralization, lumbarization.

**wedge-shaped:** One having a short anterior vertical height as compared with its posterior measurement, and usually representing a compression fracture.

**wedging, traumatic:** Compression fracture of a vertebra with marked shortening of the anterior vertical height.

**vertebra plana:** A very flat vertebra.

**vertebral notching:** Notches, both superiorly and inferiorly, seen in the preadolescent vertebral body to receive the epiphyseal ring. This is of no pathological significance.

**vertebral motor unit:** Two vertebral segments, along with their associated musculature, which are activated to purposeful function by an interplay of their sensory and motor nerve supply.

**wedging, traumatic:** (*see* vertebra)

**whole body irradiation:** Uniform exposure of the whole body to ionizing radiation, contrasted to local irradiation as in x-ray therapy.

**window:** The transparent opening in an x-ray tube transmitting the beam of x-rays with little (inherent) filtration, and generally made of beryllium.

**x-radiation:** The broad spectrum of x-rays from the longest (grenz rays) to the shortest (supervoltage).

**x-ray:** (roentgen rays) Electromagnetic radiations discovered by W. K. Roentgen of Wurzburg, November 8, 1895, are generated at the point of impact of a stream of high speed cathode rays or electrons on the focal spot or target of the annode of an x-ray tube. These invisible rays carry no charge, are not refracted as are light rays, and have the ability to penetrate opaque materials and affect photographic film emulsion, recording shadows of varying densities, depending upon absorption by the specific components of the substances. Although not explicitly stated, the usage for x-rays seems to be "x-rays" as a noun, and "x-ray" as an adjective—thus "a beam of x-rays" but "an x-ray beam" and "x-ray therapy". Similarly, "$\gamma$-ray" should be hyphenated when used adjectivally.

**beam:** Primary beam of x-rays composed of heterogenous qualities.

**image intensifier system:** The x-rays are allowed to fall on a fluorescent screen which is mounted in contact with the window in the end of a cathode ray tube (CRT). On the inner surface of this window is a photoelectric layer of the transparent type, i.e. light entering the surface from one side ejects electrons from the opposite side. These electrons are accelerated by a high potential placed across the highly evacuated tube, and are focused by a constant magnetic field applied axially. The electrons impinge on a phosphor layer on the opposite end, where they form an image identical to the original pattern. If the efficiencies of the fluorescent screen, the photoelectric surface, and the phosphor are high enough and sufficient accelerating energy is supplied, a gain in brightness will result.

**tube:** A vacuum or cathode ray tube used for the production of x-rays. It may be a gas tube relying on gas in the tube for its source of electrons, or a hot cathode tube which develops its electrons from a heated filament.

# Index

10